ADVANCES IN CHEMICAL ENGINEERING

Volume 19

ADVANCES IN
CHEMICAL ENGINEERING

Editor-in-Chief

JAMES WEI

School of Engineering and Applied Science
Princeton University
Princeton, New Jersey

Editors

JOHN L. ANDERSON
Department of Chemical Engineering
Carnegie Mellon University
Pittsburgh, Pennsylvania

KENNETH B. BISCHOFF
Department of Chemical Engineering
University of Delaware
Newark, Delaware

MORTON M. DENN
College of Chemistry
University of California at Berkeley
Berkeley, California

JOHN H. SEINFELD
Department of Chemical Engineering
California Institute of Technology
Pasadena, California

GEORGE STEPHANOPOULOS
Department of Chemical Engineering
Massachusetts Institute of Technology
Cambridge, Massachusetts

Volume 19

ACADEMIC PRESS
San Diego New York Boston
London Sydney Tokyo Toronto

This book is printed on acid-free paper. ∞

Academic Press, Inc.
A Division of Harcourt Brace & Company
525 B Street, Suite 1900, San Diego, California 92101-4495

United Kingdom Edition published by
Academic Press Limited
24-28 Oval Road, London NW1 7DX

International Standard Serial Number: 0065-2377

International Standard Book Number: 0-12-008519-4

PRINTED IN THE UNITED STATES OF AMERICA
94 95 96 97 98 99 BB 9 8 7 6 5 4 3 2 1

CONTENTS

A Systems Approach to Multiphase Reactor Selection

R. Krishna

Pollution Prevention: Engineering Design at Macro-, Meso-, and Microscales

David T. Allen

Tropospheric Chemistry

John H. Seinfeld, Jean M. Andino, Frank M. Bowman, Hali J. L. Forstner, and Spyros Pandis

CONTRIBUTORS

Numbers in parentheses indicate the pages on which the authors' contributions begin.

DAVID T. ALLEN, *Department of Chemical Engineering, University of California at Los Angeles, Los Angeles, California 90024* (251)

JEAN M. ANDINO, *Department of Chemical Engineering, California Institute of Technology, Pasadena, California 91125* (325)

FRANK M. BOWMAN, *Department of Chemical Engineering, California Institute of Technology, Pasadena, California 91125* (325)

K. E. FORSTEN, *Department of Chemical Engineering, Virginia Polytechnic Institute and State University, Blacksburg, Virginia 24061* (51)

HALI J. L. FORSTNER, *Department of Chemical Engineering, California Institute of Technology, Pasadena, California 91125* (325)

RAKESH K. JAIN, *Department of Radiation Oncology, Harvard Medical School and Massachusetts General Hospital, Boston, Massachusetts 02114* (129)

R. KRISHNA, *Department of Chemical Engineering, University of Amsterdam, 1018 WV Amsterdam, The Netherlands* (201)

ROBERT LANGER, *Department of Chemical Engineering, Massachusetts Institute of Technology, Cambridge, Massachusetts 02139* (1)

D. A. LAUFFENBURGER, *Department of Chemical Engineering, University of Illinois at Urbana-Champaign, Urbana, Illinois 61801* (51)

J. J. LINDERMAN, *Department of Chemical Engineering, University of Michigan, Ann Arbor, Michigan 48109* (51)

P. A. MAHAMA, *Department of Chemical Engineering, University of Toledo, Toledo, Ohio 43606* (51)

SPYROS PANDIS, *Departments of Chemical Engineering and Engineering and Public Policy, Carnegie Mellon University, Pittsburgh, Pennsylvania 15213* (325)

JOHN H. SEINFELD, *Department of Chemical Engineering, California Institute of Technology, Pasadena, California 91125* (325)

PREFACE

Volume 19 of *Advances in Chemical Engineering* features a variety of articles on chemical engineering, with a special theme on biomedical engineering. Chemical engineers have worked to apply their science to biomedicine since World War II. In the past decade, their impact on the practice of medicine has been unprecedented and useful. Langer writes about pioneering work on using polymer systems for the controlled release of macromolecules, for immobilized enzymes, for medical bioreactors, and for tissue engineering. Linderman *et al.* address receptor binding and signaling. Jain writes about transport phenomena in tumors, a topic that has been recognized as the key to effective treatment with drugs. These three chapters prove that chemical engineering in medicine has advanced from an academic exercise to widespread clinical practice.

Krishna has worked for the Shell Oil Company for many years; his chapter on the selection of multiphase reactors carries the knowledge of a skilled practitioner, which complements his theoretical teachings as a professor at the University of Amsterdam. Allen is one of the early pioneers in the application of engineering design to pollution prevention, and his chapter deals with macro-, meso-, and microscales. Seinfeld *et al.* write on tropospheric chemistry, the arena where a great many of our air pollution problems reside.

Together, these six chapters provide an expanding horizon for the intellectual scope of chemical engineers, in topics from oil refining to biomedicine, in scale from transport in tumors to the troposphere, and in approach from scientific analysis to practical design selections.

James Wei

POLYMER SYSTEMS FOR CONTROLLED RELEASE OF MACROMOLECULES, IMMOBILIZED ENZYME MEDICAL BIOREACTORS, AND TISSUE ENGINEERING

Robert Langer

Department of Chemical Engineering
Massachusetts Institute of Technology
Cambridge, Massachusetts 02139

Recent advances in biology and medicine have created new challenges and opportunities for engineers. With these advances occurring more and more at a cellular and molecular level, the chemical engineer, in particular, has a unique training to address these challenges in a creative fashion. Research in chemical aspects of biomedical engineering is growing rapidly. Numerous biotechnology and bioengineering companies are being formed; this creates and should continue to create an increasing demand for scientists with interdisciplinary training in biology and engineering. There are numerous efforts involving research in this area. Our research at M.I.T. provides one of many such examples. In this chapter we discuss the following areas of our research: controlled release systems; immobilized enzyme medical bioreactors; and tissue engineering using degradable polymers.

I. Controlled Release Systems

Over the past decade there has been increasing attention devoted to the development of controlled release systems for drugs, pesticides, nutrients, agricultural products, and fragrances. However, nearly all of the systems that have been developed have not been capable of slowly releasing drugs of large molecular weight (MW > 600). In fact, up until 1976 it was a fairly common conception in the field of controlled release that effective systems could not be developed for macromolecules (1). However, after several years of effort an approach was discovered that permitted the continuous release of biologically active macromolecules as large as 2,000,000 daltons from normally impermeable, yet biocompatible, polymers for more than 100 days (2). Three areas of our drug delivery research are reviewed here: systems that release large molecules through porous polymer matrices, novel biodegradable polymeric delivery systems; and pulsatile controlled release polymer systems.

A. Porous Delivery Systems for the Release of Proteins and Macromolecules

Our interest in creating controlled release systems for polypeptides and other macromolecules began in 1974 and stemmed from studies on the growth of solid tumors. Most solid tumors require ingrowth of new blood vessels from the host for further tumor development, and we were attempting to isolate a drug that prevents the growth of new blood vessels. This substance is derived from cartilage, a tissue that contains no blood vessels. The bioassay used for this substance involved placing a tumor in the cornea of a rabbit and monitoring the growth of new vessels toward the tumor. It was desired to deliver the drug to the tumor to see if it decreased the rate of blood vessel growth. The assay takes 30 days.

Purified fractions of the cartilage material were highly soluble, so that they disappeared quickly after they were added. Therefore, a small sustained-release system was needed to provide steady diffusion into the tumor. Such a system had to be inert and noninflammatory. In early work (3), polyacrylamide pellets had been tried for this purpose. The test protein was mixed with acrylamide before polymerization. After polymerization, however, the small pellets were often highly inflammatory. The inflammation could be reduced by extensive washing, but it could never be completely eliminated. Furthermore, washing leached out most of the test protein.

At that time, the only polymer systems reported for administering large molecules were those described by Davis (4), polyacrylamide or polyvinylpyrrolidone. However, these systems damaged the cornea and permitted only brief periods of sustained release (2, 5). Therefore, other polymers and new ways of placing drugs in these polymers were examined. However, one problem was that large molecules would only diffuse through highly porous and permeable membranes (e.g., Millipore filters). In these cases diffusion was too rapid to be of value. A new approach was developed that permitted sustained release of large molecules from biocompatible polymers (2). The polymer was dissolved in an appropriate solvent, and the macromolecule was added in powder form. The resulting mixture can be cast in a mold and dried. When the pellets are placed in water, they release the molecules trapped within the polymer matrix.

A number of polymer systems were tested for tissue biocompatibility and release kinetics. The best long-term release results were obtained with hydrophobic polymers. Examples included non-degradable ethylene–vinyl acetate or biodegradable polylactic acid. Certain hydrogels such as polyhydroxyethylmethacrylate or polyvinylalcohol also worked effectively, but released proteins for shorter time periods. With the hydrophobic polymers, biologically active protein was released for more than 100 days (2). In other tests, larger molecules (2 million MW), such as polysaccharides and polynucleotides, were also successfully released for long time periods (2).

While these initial studies demonstrated the feasibility of releasing macromolecules from biocompatible polymers, the kinetics were often not reproducible; controlled release was not achieved. The irreproducibility results from drug settling and redistribution during casting and drying, caused by the insolubility of the incorporated macromolecule powder in the polymer solvent. At room temperature, the drug migrated vertically, and visible lateral motion was caused by currents (possibly thermal) in the mixture. A low-temperature casting and drying procedure was developed to minimize this drug movement during matrix formation. When the dissolved polymer–solid drug powder mixture was cast in a mold at −80°C, the entire matrix froze before any settling could occur. These matrices were then dried at −20°C for 2 days until almost all the solvent was gone. Final drying was conducted under vacuum at room temperature (6).

1. Factors Affecting Release Kinetics

With this reproducible method, factors that regulated release kinetics could now be accurately assessed. Such factors were found to be drug powder particle size and drug loading (drug : polymer ratio) (6). Coating drug-containing polymeric matrices by dropping them into polymer solutions of differing concentrations and drying them, also affected release kinetics. By combining these simple fabrication parameters—drug particle size, loading, and coating—release rates for any drug could be changed several thousandfold (6).

To understand the release mechanism, cryomicrotomy was used to slice 10 μm-thick sections throughout the matrices. Viewed under an optical microscope, polymer films cast without proteins appeared as nonporous sheets. Matrices cast with proteins and sectioned prior to release displayed areas of either polymer or protein. Matrices initially cast with proteins and released to exhaustion (e.g., greater than 5 months) appeared as porous films. Pores with diameters as large as 100 μm, the size of the protein particles, were observed. The structures visualized were also confirmed by Nomarski (differential interference contrast microscopy). It appeared that although pure polymer films were impermeable to macromolecules (2), molecules incorporated in the matrix dissolved once water penetrated the matrix and were then able to diffuse to the surface through pores created as the particles of molecules dissolved. Scanning electron microscopy showed that the pores were interconnected (7).

Next investigated were changes in pore structure over time. Sections were prepared from matrices in the process of release. It was observed that (i) the pore structure changes minimally as a function of time; (ii) after 16–40 h there is no evidence of a receding interface between dissolved and dispersed drug; and (iii) none of the drug remains undissolved at 40 h (30% release). Observations (ii) and (iii) differ from those reported for less soluble low molecular-weight drugs such as certain steroids, and are probably due to the high solubilities of many proteins such as bovine serum albumin (BSA) (solubility > 500 mg/mL). Thus, the widely used moving zone models developed by Higuchi may not be applicable to the situation of macromolecules because of observations (ii) and (iii).

A number of assumptions were made and then verified to develop a model: (i) The rate-limiting step for transport is drug diffusion through pores (other steps such as water penetration into the matrix and drug dissolution occur in less than 40 hours). (ii) The effect of concentration dependence on the drug diffusion coefficient is not significant. This was verified by an analysis of diffusion effects at the concentrations in the matrix. (iii) No drug diffusion occurs through the polymer backbone (2). (iv) The pores are interconnected, the porosity is uniform, and pore size changes minimally with time. (v) The initial drug distribution is uniform. This was also verified by cryomicrotomy. (vi) No boundary layer effects exist. This was verified by stirring, which would have disrupted boundary layers had they been present. Release rates of matrices stirred in containers at 2000 rpm were identical to unstirred release rates, indicating the lack of boundary layer effect. (vii) Infinite sink conditions exist. The volume of the release medium is approximately 100 times the volume of the polymer/protein matrix. Increasing the volume of the release medium does not alter measured release kinetics. (viii) Minimal effects exist as a result of osmosis due to solutes in the surrounding environment or charge interaction of the drug with the polymer. Consonant with this assumption, no effect on release rate was found to result from increasing the ionic strength of the medium from 0 to 1 M NaCl.

For these assumptions, permitting release from only one side of the slab, the boundary conditions are those of zero flux at the coated edges, and $C = 0$ at the releasing face.

If diffusion through pores occurs, the Fick diffusion equation can be solved:

$$\frac{\partial c}{\partial t} = D_{\mathrm{e}} \frac{\partial^2 c}{\partial x^2}, \qquad 0 < x < L; \tag{1}$$

$$\frac{M_{\mathrm{t}}}{M_{\infty}} = 1 - \frac{8}{\pi^2} \sum_{n=0}^{\infty} \frac{1}{(2n+1)^2} \exp\left[-(2n+1)^2 \pi^2 D_{\mathrm{e}} t / 4L^2\right], \tag{2}$$

where M_t is the cumulative drug mass released, M_∞ is the drug mass originally incorporated in the matrix, t is time (hours), and L is the thickness of the slab (centimeters). In addition, D_{e}, the effective diffusion coefficient (cm^2/hour) of the drug in the matrix is set equal to $D_0 F$, where D_0 is the bulk diffusion coefficient of the same drug in the release media that has filled the pores, and F is a factor accounting for the geometric effects of the pore structure of the matrix (i.e., tortuosity, dead-end pores, and constrictions between pores). F was determined via a regression analysis for several cases of BSA released from polymer slabs at several porosities (Fig. 1). A log–log plot of F versus porosity was well fitted by the function

$$\log_{10} F = 0.463 + 5.64 \log_{10} \varepsilon, \tag{3}$$

where ε is the porosity. Knowing this equation for F, it can then be

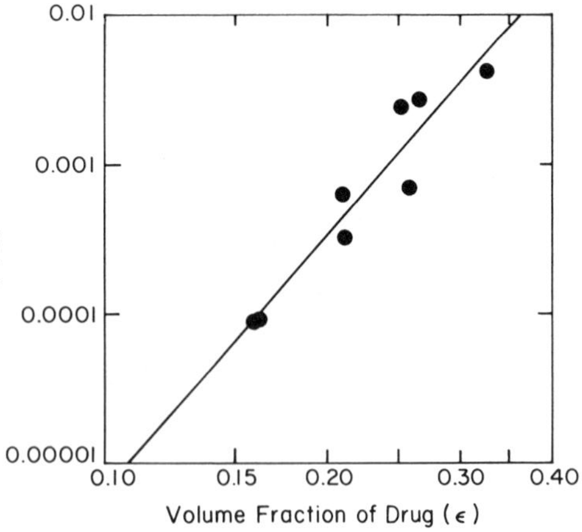

FIG. 1. Log–log plot of factor $F = D_e/D_0$ as a function of porosity for BSA matrices [from Bawa *et al.* (7), with permission of Elsevier Science Publishers BV].

written

$$D_e = D_0(2.904\varepsilon^{5.64}), \tag{4}$$

and this value of D_e can be substituted into Eq. (2).

Both the slab thickness L and the porosity ε were measured. For a given macromolecule, the bulk diffusivity, D_0, is measurable or obtainable from the literature. Thus, a test of the model is to cast slabs using other proteins, measure the parameters L, ε, and D_0, and see whether the release kinetics follow Eq. (2). This has been done for β-lactoglobulin and lysozyme (Fig. 2). The solid lines are predictions based on Eq. (2) which show general agreement with the data (7).

An additional check of the model is to determine if it can predict not only the time-dependent release of the drug, but also the time-dependent position of the drug within the matrix. If Eq. (2) is valid, then the drug distribution within the matrix can be described by

$$c(x,t) = \frac{4C_0}{\pi}\sum_{n=0}^{\infty}\frac{(-1)^n}{2n+1}\exp\left[-(2n+1)^2\pi^2 D_e t/4L^2\right]\cos\frac{(2n+1)\pi x}{2L}, \tag{5}$$

where C_0 is the initial concentration of drug in the matrix (mg/cm^3 matrix), and $C(x,t)$ is the concentration (the concentrations C and C_0 are expressed in terms of the volume of the whole matrix, including both pore and polymer volumes) at time t and distance x (centimeters) into the matrix from the exposed face. To test Eq. (5), cryomicrotomy was used to

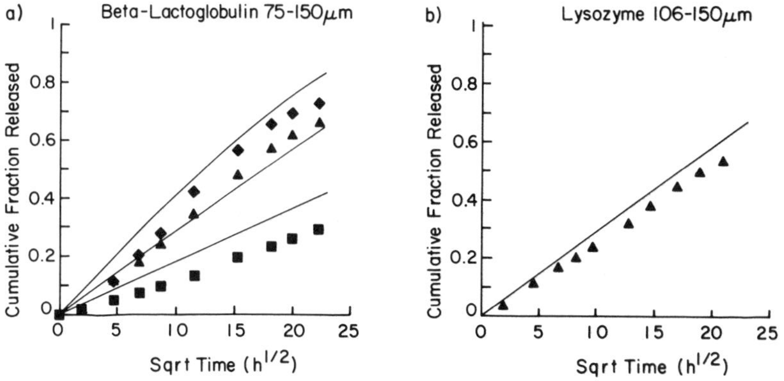

FIG. 2. Release kinetics of β-lactoglobulin and lysozyme [from Bawa *et al.* (7), with permission of Elsevier Science Publishers BV].

determine the drug concentration profiles within the polymer matrix for several cases of loading and release time. Partially released matrices were sectioned at 10 μm intervals, and the remaining protein in each section was assayed and plotted against its normalized (x/L) position within the matrix to yield internal concentration profiles. The data and the predictions from Eq. (5) are within experimental error (7).

The diffusion equations just used are simplifications of more complex processes. The F factor was empirically derived and must take into account those matrix pore geometric factors contributing to decreases in diffusion rates. Such factors may include pore "tortuosity," dead-end pores, and pore constrictions. Initial modeling studies suggest that constrictions, in particular, have large effects in retarding release (8, 9).

2. *In Vivo and in Vitro Release Kinetics and Biocompatibility*

In vitro and *in vivo* release kinetics were compared using two different approaches. In the first approach (the recovery approach) polymer implants containing a radioactively labeled substrate—^{14}C-labeled bovine serum albumin, β-[^{14}C]-lactoglobulin, or [^{3}H]-inulin—were implanted subcutaneously into rates (*in vivo*) or released in phosphate-buffered saline, pH 7.4, at 37°C (*in vitro*). At various time points, the polymer implants were removed from the rats or the saline. They were then lyophilized to remove residual water and dissolved in xylene. When the polymer dissolved, the unreleased macromolecules precipitated to the bottom of the vial. Water was then added to dissolve the macromolecules; scintillation fluid was next added, resulting in a homogeneous translucent emulsion which was counted via liquid scintillation.

Release rates determined in this manner were essentially identical in the *in vivo* and *in vitro* implants. In addition, for the *in vitro* experiments, release was also measured directly by analyzing the radioactivity in the release media. The release rates determined in this way correlated precisely with the *in vitro* and *in vivo* release rates determined by the recovery experiments (last paragraph). Furthermore, they demonstrated that the material balance was completed, showing no material was lost (10).

One limitation of the foregoing approach, however, was that the amount of macromolecules "directly" released *in vivo* could not be assayed. This

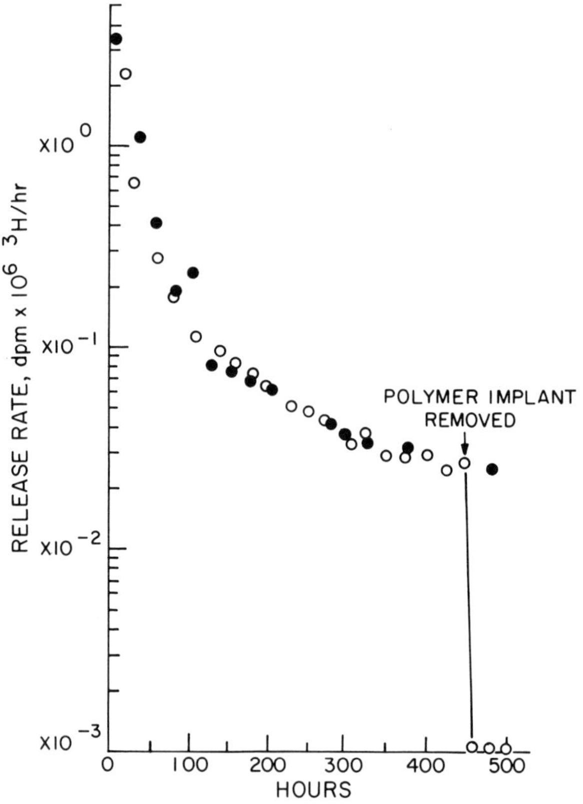

FIG. 3. *In vivo* and *in vitro* comparison of release rates from 44% loaded (w/w) [^{3}H]inulin. Each *in vivo* point (○) represents the average release rate obtained by the collection of urine from five rats. Each *in vitro* point (●) represents the average release rate from four polymer squares in phosphate-buffered saline. The polymer squares were removed from the rats after 450 h [from Brown *et al.* (10), reproduced with permission of the copyright owner, the American Pharmaceutical Association].

is because macromolecules such as proteins are metabolized, making direct *in vivo* release measurements difficult. To solve this problem, [^{3}H]-inulin was used as a model.

Inulin is a polysaccharide of molecular weight 5200. It is one of the very few molecules that is neither metabolized *in vivo* nor reabsorbed or secreted by kidney tubules. Thus, all inulin released from the polymer should be recovered in the urine. An *in vivo–in vitro* comparison was made by making nine identical inulin–polymer pellets. Five pellets were implanted in rats housed in metabolic cages. Four pellets were released into a physiological solution of phosphate-buffered saline (PBS) at pH 7.4 at 37°C. Both urine and PBS were collected daily. The [^{3}H]-inulin was measured by scintillation counting. The experiment was carried out for 500 hours. (Additional experiments have been carried out for 1500 hours with similar results.) Over this period, *in vivo* and *in vitro* release rates agreed to within 1% (10) (Fig. 3).

Furthermore, as an internal control, inulin pellets were removed from several animals at 450 h and the urine analyzed 4.5 h later. Within that time, the inulin recovery rate had dropped by a factor of over 50 (Fig. 3).

The polymer slabs were examined histologically in two different *in vivo* sites at times as long as 7 months after implantation. Nearly no inflammation or fibrous encapsulation was observed (10).

Thus, these experiments show that *in vitro* and *in vivo* release kinetics of macromolecules from ethylene–vinyl acetater copolymer matrices are essentially identical, and they establish a methodology which can be applied to other *in vitro–in vivo* release comparisons.

3. *Approaches for Achieving Zero-Order Release*

One important goal is the development of a zero-order release device. The difficulty is that the preceding systems contain drug evenly distributed through polymer slabs, and thus, release rates will decrease with time because the drug diffusion distance from the matrix surface increases with time. In order to obtain zero-order release, one could either compensate for the distance-dependent diffusion in a matrix device, or employ a different kind of release system such as a reservoir device (a system in which all drug is centered inside a membrane). Variations of the latter approach have been reported for low molecular-weight drugs in which matrices have been laminated with rate-controlling outer barriers. However, such an approach might prove difficult for macromolecules because the barriers would decrease, if not eliminate, the permeability of these high molecular-weight drugs. Therefore, ways of compensating for the distance-dependent diffusion were developed. The approaches considered

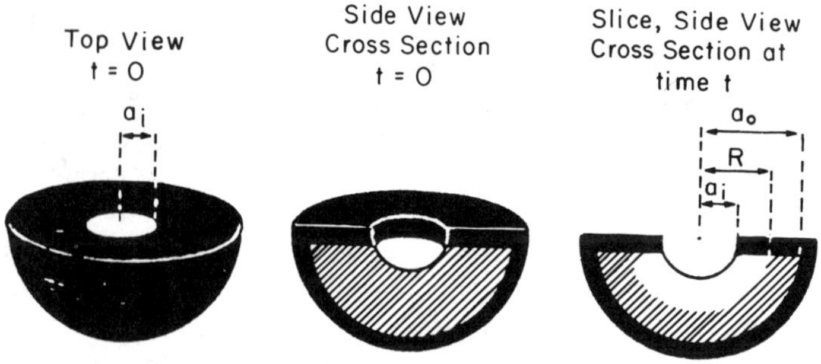

FIG. 4. Diagram of an inwardly-releasing hemisphere; a_i is the inner radius, a_o is the outer radius, and R is the distance to the interface between the dissolved region (white area) and the dispersed zone (diagonal lines). Black represents laminated regions through which release cannot occur [from Hsieh *et al.* (11), reproduced with permission of the copyright owner, the American Pharmaceutical Association].

were altering the drug distribution pattern or the matrix geometry. The idea of altering matrix geometry is experimentally more attractive, particularly if it were possible to design a shape in which an increased area of drug would be available as the drug diffusion distance increased.

Models were therefore developed for predicting release from systems of various shapes, and a special hemisphere system [coated everywhere with an impermeable coating except for an aperture in the center face (Fig. 4)] worked best. An experimental method for making the special hemisphere device was then developed to test the predictions. In this procedure the bottoms of test tubes were cut off and used as molds. A low-temperature casting and drying procedure was used. Using this approach, a constant release rate of 0.5 mg/day for 2 months (the duration of the experiment) for test macromolecules (11) was obtained.

4. *Additional Formulation Procedures*

A number of additional formulation procedures have been developed. One of these does not require solvents. The method consists of mixing drug and polymer powders below the glass transition temperature of the polymer, and compressing the mixture at a temperature above the glass transition point. The macromolecule is not exposed to any organic solvent during the fabrication process.

The advantages of this sintering method, when compared to solvent casting methods used in previous studies, include (i) elimination of shrinkage, (ii) elimination of the need for potentially expensive scale-up steps such as vacuum drying, (iii) reduction of processing time (slabs have been produced in 2 h, compared to 4 days required for solvent casting), and (iv) lack of the necessity to expose the macromolecule to a solvent. The kinetics, microstructure, bioactivity, and effects of polymer and drug particle size have all been studied (12).

A simple technique has also been devised for preparing ethylene–vinyl acetate copolymer microspheres containing macromolecular drugs. Beads with good sphericity were formed by a simple extrusion process that can easily be repeated without special equipment. Drug release kinetics and polymer microstructure were also investigated with this technique. The kinetic trends were as would be predicted from earlier studies (13). Degradable polymers such as lactic–glycolic acid copolymers can also be formed into microspheres which can release proteins (14). Such microspheres may be more desirable than slabs or hemispheres in many situations because they can be injected through a small needle.

A technique for insuring the controlled release of small amounts of macromolecules such as polypeptides from polymeric delivery systems was also developed. Incorporating albumin in milligram quantities into these delivery systems can facilitate the sustained release of nanogram or microgram quantities of model macromolecules such as epidermal growth factor (EGF) (15). The albumin can be used to create the pore structure in the polymer matrix through which the EGF can subsequently migrate. Such a technique may be valuable for highly potent precious macromolecules for which little drug needs to be released.

5. *Applications*

Studies have also been conducted to explore numerous applications of these systems. These include release of insulin (16), anticalification agents (17), interferons (18), growth factors (19) and inhibitors (20), and neurologically active agents (21). Several polymer-based systems for releasing luteinizing-hormone–releasing hormone analogues for treating prostate cancer and endometriosis are now available clinically.

B. New Biodegradable Polymers

Biodegradable controlled release systems have an advantage over other systems in obviating the need to surgically remove the drug-depleted device. In many cases, however, the release is augmented by diffusion through the matrix, rendering the process difficult to control—particularly if the matrix is hydrophilic and thereby absorbs water, promoting degradation in the matrix interior. To maximize control over the release process, it is desirable to have a polymeric system which degrades only from the surface and deters the permeation of the drug molecules. Achieving such a heterogeneous degradation requires the rate of hydrolytic degradation on the surface to be much faster than the rate of water penetration into the bulk. With this in mind, an ideal polymer should have a hydrophobic backbone, but with water-labile linkages connecting monomers. Many classes of polymers, including polyesters, polyamides, polyurethanes, polyorthoesters, and polyacrylonitriles, had been studied for controlled-delivery applications, but only polyorthoesters eroded from the surface and then only if additives were included in the matrix. Other than polyesters, none of these polymers have yet received FDA approval for human implantation. In designing a biodegradable system that would erode in a controlled heterogeneous manner without requiring any additives, polyanhydrides were suggested as a promising candidate because of the high lability of the anhydride linkage.

1. Polyanhydrides

Several approaches were examined for synthesizing polyanhydrides: melt polycondensation, dehydrochlorination, and dehydrative coupling. A report of polyanhydride synthesis techniques and polymerization conditions for polyanhydrides appears in Leong *et al.* (22).

One major drawback in previous work on polyanhydrides was their low molecular weight (MW < 40,000), which made them impractical for many applications. A systematic study was therefore conducted to determine the mechanism of polymerization and factors affecting polymer molecular weight. The highest molecular-weight polymers were obtained by using extremely pure prepolymers and by operating under conditions which optimize the polymerization process while at the same time minimizing the depolymerization process. With careful understanding of the factors affecting both these mechanisms, much higher molecular weights of polyanhydrides—as determined by gel permeation chromatography, GPC, and viscosity measurements—were obtained. For example, by reacting pure individually prepared prepolymers to produce P(CPP:SA) (a copolymer of carboxyphenoxypropane and sebacic acid) (1:4), a molecular weight of 116,800 was achieved, in comparison to 12,030 when an unisolated prepolymer mixture was used. The use of catalysts in polyanhydride synthesis was also studied. Since the reaction is an anhydride interchange which involves a nucleophilic attack on a carbonyl carbon, a catalyst which will increase the electron deficiency under the carbonyl carbon will affect the polymerization. More than 20 coordination catalysts were examined in the synthesis of the 1:4 (CPP-SA) copolymer. Significantly higher molecular weights in shorter times were achieved by utilizing cadium acetate, earth metal oxides, and $ZnEt_2$-H_2O. The molecular weights ranged from 140,935 to 245,010 with catalysts, in comparison to 116,800 without catalysts. When acidic *p*-toluene sulphonic acid (*p*-TSA) or basic 4-dimethyl amino pyridine(4-DMAP) catalysts were tested, the acid catalyst *p*-TSA did not show any effect, while the basic catalyst (4-DMAP) caused a decrease in molecular weight. Since the polymerization and depolymerization reactions involve anhydride interchange, which leads to a high molecular weight polymer with the removal of acetic anhydride as the condensation product (polymerization) and internal ring formation (depolymerization), catalysts affect both reactions, and optimizing the reaction time in the presence of catalysts is critical (23).

Two approaches for one-step solution polymerization of polyanhydrides at ambient temperature were also developed. In the first approach, highly pure polymers (> 99.7%) were obtained by the use of sebacoyl chloride, phosgene, or diphosgene as coupling agents and poly(4-vinyl-pyridine) or K_2CO_3 as insoluble acid acceptors. The second approach for one-step synthesis of pure polyanhydrides was the use of an appropriate solvent where the polymer is exclusively soluble, but the corresponding polymerization by-product (e.g., $Et_3N \cdot HCl$) is insoluble (24).

2. *Degradation Characteristics*

More hydrophobic polymers, PCPP and PCPP-SA 85:15, displayed constant erosion kinetics over eight months. By extrapolation, 1 mm thick disks of PCPP will completely degrade in more than three years. The degradation rates were enhanced by copolymerization with sebacic acid. An increase of 800 times was observed when the sebacic acid concentration reached 80%. By altering the CPP/SA ratio, nearly any degradation rate between 1 day and 3 years could be achieved (25) (Fig. 5).

The effect of different backbones on erosion rates was demonstrated in a study of the homologous poly[*p*-(carboxyphenoxy)alkane] series. As the number of methylene groups in the backbone increased from 1 to 6, thus decreasing the reactivity of the anhydride linkage and rendering the polymer more hydrophobic, the erosion rates underwent a decrease of three orders of magnitude (25).

3. *Release Characteristics*

The release behavior depended on the formulation procedure. The best results were obtained with injection-molded samples. The drug release pattern followed closely that of the polymer degradation over a period of

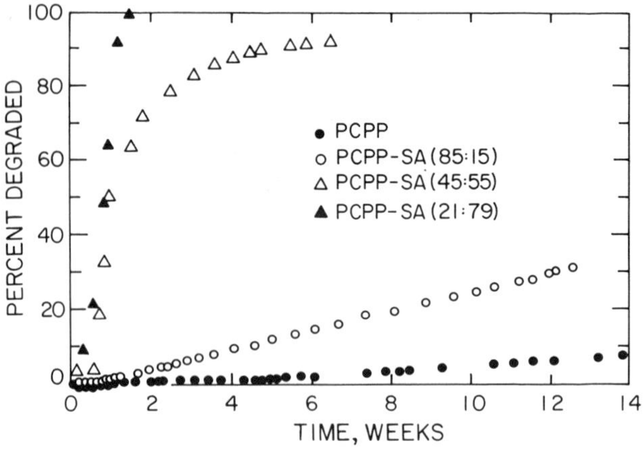

FIG. 5. Degradation profiles of compression molded poly[bis(*p*-carboxyphenoxy)propane anhydride] and its copolymer with sebacic acid in 0.1 *M* pH phosphate buffer at 37°C [from Leong, K. W., Brott, B. C., and Langer, R., *J. Biomed. Mater. Res.* (25). Copyright © 1985 John Wiley & Sons, Inc. Reprinted by permission of John Wiley & Sons].

8 months for PCPP. The correlation between release and degradation was still maintained in the more hydrophilic PCPP-SA 21:79, where both processes were completed in two weeks. Compression molding can also be used, but the correlation between drug release and polymer degradation is not as good (25).

4. *Microspheres*

Several approaches for producing polyanhydride microspheres were developed. One was a hot-melt technique. This process yielded spherical microspheres, and the capsule yield was almost quantitative. The release of acid orange and insulin from PCPP-SA was studied. This approach is most useful for molecules that are exposed to the polymer melting temperature (76°C) without inactivation (26).

A second method to prepare polyanhydride microspheres—via solvent removal—has also been developed. Polyanhydrides composed of the following diacids were used: sebacic acid (SA), bis(*p*-carboxyphenoxy)propane (CPP), and dodecanedioic acid (DD). Drug release was affected by polymer composition, physical properties of the microspheres, and type of drug. The potential for injectable microspheres (size range 1–300 μm) made of CPP-SA (50:50) for the controlled release of insulin was assessed. Both 5% and 10% w/w insulin loaded microspheres were prepared. The best clinical response was produced by 10% loaded microspheres, which demonstrated five days of urine glucose control and four days of serum glucose control in diabetic rats (27).

5. *Stability*

The stability of poly(anhydrides) (PA) composed of the diacids: sebacic acid (SA), bis(*p*-carboxyphenoxy)methane (CPM), 1,3-bis(*p*-carboxyphenoxy)propane (CPP), 1,6-bis(*p*-carboxyphenoxy)hexane (CPH), and phenylenedipropionic acid (PDP), in solid state and in organic solutions, was studied for more than a one-year period. Aromatic PA [poly(CPH) and Poly(CPM)] maintained their original molecular weight in both solid state and solution, while aliphatic PA [poly(SA) and poly(PDP)] decreased in molecular weight over time. The decrease in molecular weight shows first-order kinetics, with activation energies of 7.5 kcal/mol K. The decrease in molecular weight was explained by an internal anhydride interchange mechanism as revealed from elemental and spectral analysis (IR and ^{13}C, ^{1}H-NMR). The depolymerization in solution can be catalyzed by metals. Among several metals tested, copper and zinc were the most effective. Studies on the stability of aliphatic poly(esters) in chloroform showed that poly(orthoesters) depolymerized over time, whereas poly(α-esters) and poly(ethylenesuccinate) remained intact. Interestingly, the solid-state stability of the polymers did not correlate with their hydrolytic stability (28).

6. *Toxicity and Clinical Studies*

Initial biocompatibility studies were conducted on polyanhydrides. As evaluated by mutation assays (29), the degradation products of the polymer were non-mutagenic and non-cytotoxic. Teratogenicity tests were also negative. Growth of mammalian cells in tissue culture was also not affected by these polymers (29).

The possibility of implanting polyanhydride disks containing the nitrosoureas, BCNU an CCNU, for brain cancer following surgery was considered as one potential clinical application of these polymers. Surface erosion would be critical for such drugs because if bulk erosion occurred, uncontrolled amounts of this potentially toxic drug could be released during breakup of the matrix. Following additional safety studies, Institutional Review Board (IRB) approval was given to conduct human clinical trials with polyanhydrides at five American hospitals. In 1987, the FDA approved polyanhydrides for human clinical trials. Clinical studies showed that this approach was safe in humans and that it increased lifespan in the first 21 patients tested (29). Based on these initial promising results, 56 hospitals are now testing this system in hundreds of patients in several different clinical trials.

7. Pseudopolyaminoacids and Other Biopolymers

Several other novel biodegradable polymer systems were also developed. One of these stems from the observation that many polymers used in medicine today were not initially designed for that purpose. It may be particularly useful to have available biodegradable polymers that are composed of, and will break down into, naturally occurring substances. One example is the synthesis of structurally new poly(amino acids) in which L-amino acids or dipeptides are polymerized by nonamide bonds (e.g., ester, iminocarbonate) involving the functional groups located on the amino acid side chains, rather than the extensively used approach involving the amino acid termini.

This approach was considered because it would permit the synthesis of biomaterials (for drug delivery systems, sutures, artificial organs, etc.) which are derived from nontoxic metabolites (amino acids and dipeptides) while also having other desirable properties; for example, the incorporation of an anhydride linkage into the polymer backbone could result in rapid biodegradability, an iminocarbonate bond may provide mechanical strength, and an ester bond may result in better film and fiber formation.

Several polymers were synthesized to initiate the development of this concept (30). In one case (single amino acid), poly(palmitoyl-hydroxyproline [(Pal-Hpr)-ester] was obtained by melt transesterification of *N*-Pal-Hpr-Me in the presence of aluminum isopropoxide as catalyst. In a second case (dipeptide), the tyrosine (Tyr) dipeptide carbobenzyoxy-Tyr-Tyr-Hex was cyanylated at the tyrosine side chain hydroxyl groups, to yield carbobenzoxy-Tyr-Tyr-Hex-dicyanate. By solution polymerization of equimolar quantities of carbobenzoxy-Tyr-Tyr-Hex and carbobenzoxy-Tyr-Tyr-Hex-dicyanate in tetrahydrofuran, poly(carbobenzoxy-Tyr-Tyr-Hex-iminocarbonate) (polyCTTH) was obtained with M_n = 11,500 and M_w = 19,500.

One interesting example of this class of polymer system stems from a study using controlled release systems for immune adjuvants (31). Many adjuvants such as aluminum oxide, surfactants, and incomplete Freund's adjuvant rely on a simple "depot" effect, releasing adsorbed antigen over a short period of time, ranging from several hours to a few weeks at most. It had previously been shown in mice (31) and rabbits (32) that the prolonged release of small amounts of antigen from a polymeric antigen delivery device [made of ethylene-vinyl acetate copolymer (EVAc)] resulted in sustained production of antibodies over a period of 6 months.

Since EVAc is a non-biodegradable polymer, the implanted device has to be surgically removed from the host after completion of the immunization process. Hence, it would be advantageous to use biodegradable devices for the controlled release of antigen.

This concept is particularly attractive considering that the polymer degradation products could be intentionally designed to have adjuvant properties. This would make it possible to design a device capable of stimulating the immune response while simultaneously releasing antigen over prolonged periods of time. Considering the known adjuvanticity of L-tyrosine and its derivatives, it occurred to us that a polymeric antigen delivery system which would degrade into tyrosine or a tyrosine derivative could provide sustained adjuvanticity while simultaneously serving as a repository for antigen. In order to test this hypothesis, poly(CTTH–iminocarbonate) was selected as a candidate material for a polymeric antigen delivery system. Poly-(CTTH–iminocarbonate) is a structurally new, biodegradable polymer in which tyrosine dipeptide units are linked together by hydrolytically labile bonds via the tyrosine side-chain hydroxyl groups (33). The release of antigen from poly(CTTH–iminocarbonate) gave rise, in mice, to higher antibody titers than release of the same dose of antigen from a comparable control polyiminocarbonate or complete Freund's adjuvant over a one-year period even though a single injection was used (33).

In addition to these studies, polyiminocarbonates (34) and polyphosphazenes (35) were evaluated as new biomaterials and drug delivery systems.

C. Pulsatile Release Systems

Several polymeric systems capable of delivering drugs at increased rates on demand were studied and developed.

1. Magnetic Systems

One system consists of drug powder dispersed within a polymeric matrix (generally ethylene–vinyl acetate copolymer, EVAc), together with magnetic beads (Fig. 6). Release rates were controlled by an oscillating external magnetic field, which is generated by a device that rotates permanent magnets beneath the vials. By placing small plastic cages containing animals on the top of the device, it can also be used for *in vivo* studies. Polymer matrices containing drug and magnets can release up to

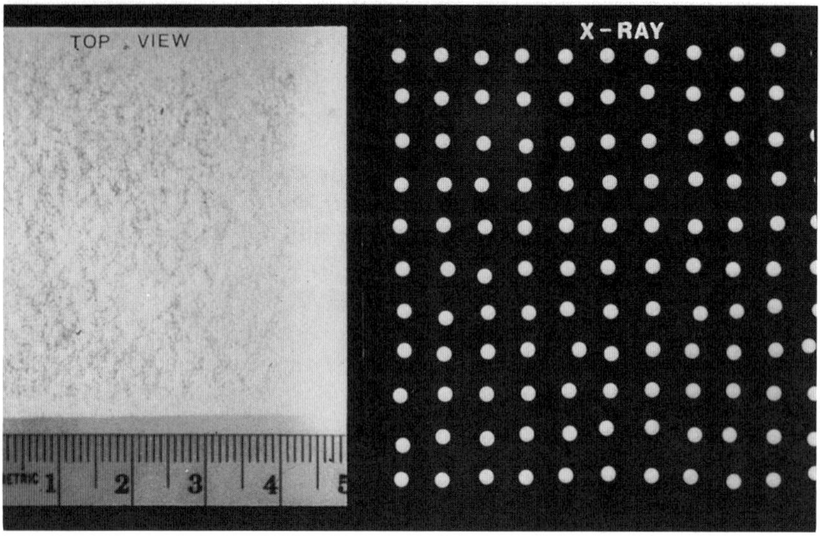

FIG. 6. Top view and x-ray of a controlled release polymer matrix containing magnetic beads and a drug.

30 times more drug when exposed to the magnetic field, and release rates return to normal when the magnetic field is discontinued. The magnetically controlled implant does not cause inflammation *in vivo*. This was confirmed by the lack of edema, cellular infiltrate, and neovascularization as judged by gross and histologic examination in animals (36).

a. Magnetic Field Characteristics. The amplitude of the magnetic field was varied by increasing the distance between the external and embedded magnets or by changing the embedded magnets' strength. The extent of release enhancement increased as the field amplitude rose. For example, at a field frequency of 11 Hz, a release rate enhancement of 12.4 times was obtained for matrices containing 1100 G magnets, as opposed to 1.5 times for matrices containing less than 100 G magnets (37).

When the frequency of the applied field was increased from 5.0 to 11.0 Hz, the rate of release rose linearly (37).

To study magnet orientation, samples containing a single 1100 G magnet were used. In half the cases, the magnet was placed perpendicular to the applied field, and in the other half it was oriented parallel to the field. The mean release rate enhancement (also termed "modulation") was 2.1 times in the parallel cases, and 12.4 times in the perpendicular cases. The difference between the two is presumably due to rotational torque. When placed in parallel the magnet rotates in an attempt to align its pole vector with the field; therefore, the displacement is smaller (37).

b. Polymer Properties. The mechanical properties of the polymeric matrix also affect the extent of magnetic enhancement. For example, the modulus of elasticity of the polymeric matrix can be altered by changing the vinyl acetate content of the polymer. The release rate enhancement induced by the magnetic field increases as the modulus of elasticity of the EVAc decreases (38).

c. Mechanism. The release of macromolecules from EVAc systems not containing magnetic beads has been studied extensively. It was found that although molecules with molecular weights greater than 300 cannot permeate through the polymer, the direct incorporation of macromolecules in the polymer–macromolecule casting procedure caused a tortuous and complex series of pores to form within the matrix. Factors affecting permeation of water into the polymer and drug out of these pores determine the release rates.

Video recordings of the polymer matrix surface show that the beads actually move within the matrix in response to the external magnetic field and move adjacent material containing polymer and drug with them, "squeezing" the dissolved drug out through the pores (37).

McCarthy *et al.* (39) proposed a model for the enhanced release and suggested that the major effect stems from the alternate compression and expansion deformation of the pores, causing the fluid within to undergo a pulsatile flow which alone (no net convection) is able to greatly improve diffusive mass transfer. A mathematical model was developed based on ideal axial diffusion in a cylinder with pulsed flow, which describes the observed trend of increasing release rate with increasing frequency. This provides a preliminary estimate of drug release rate enhancement as a function of frequency of the oscillating magnetic field (39).

d. Release Dynamics. A flow-through spectrophotometer provided a continuous recording reflecting BSA release. Release rates were very stable at baseline. When a matrix was exposed to a 390-G magnetic field for 20 min, the absorbance of BSA rose after the magnetic field was applied, plateaued at this elevated level, and then returned to baseline after the field was withdrawn. Within the time constants of the system, the rise and fall were instantaneous, and the increased release remained at a constant elevated level for the duration of field exposure (40).

e. Field Amplitude. When the strength of the magnetic field was altered by adjusting the input voltage to an electromagnet, modulation changed accordingly. The relationship between modulation and the strength of the applied magnetic fields ranging from 200 to 700 G, is linear (40).

f. Controls. Heat had little effect on the rate of BSA release. The rate of BSA release was nearly constant from polymer matrices transferred every 2 h from 25 to 37°C. The heat generated by the electromagnet did not alter release rates from polymer matrices, either. The temperature rose at the electromagnet surface at a rate of 8°C/h for the first 30 min after the magnet was turned on. The rate of BSA release from a polymer matrix without an embedded magnet adjacent to the electromagnet face did not change over this time period and for 7 h afterward (40).

g. In Vivo Studies. Using inulin as a marker, the preceding effects observed *in vitro* (response time, response duration, amplitude) were also observed *in vivo* (40).

Furthermore, implants composed of EVAc-embedded magnets and bovine zinc insulin were placed in diabetic rats for two months. After implantation the blood glucose level decreased due to diffusion of insulin from the polymer implant. When the diabetic rats were exposed to an oscillating magnetic field, the blood glucose levels were further lowered from 50 to 200 mg dL^{-1} below this basal level depending on the magnetic field conditions. These results were confirmed by radioimmunoassays. This phenomenon was not observed in (i) control diabetic rats receiving EVAc implants with insulin without a magnet, (ii) control normal rats receiving implants with a magnet but without insulin, or (iii) control diabetic rats not containing any implant. All these animals were exposed to the same manipulations as the experimental group of animals (41).

2. *Ultrasound Modulation*

It was also discovered that ultrasound could affect the release of substances from polymers. The ultrasound system has a potential advantage over many other systems in that no additional substance (e.g., a magnetic bead) is required in the polymeric matrix. Furthermore, in the case of ultrasound the polymer can be injected, and since it can be erodible there is no need for surgical removal. The application of ultrasound in humans, both for diagnostic and therapeutic purposes, has been extensively studied and is considered a safe practice.

Enhanced (up to 20 times baseline) polymer erosion and drug release were observed when bioerodible samples were exposed to ultrasound. The system's response to the ultrasonic triggering was also rapid (within 2 min) and reversible. This was determined by an on-line UV spectrophotometric response in a closed-loop detection system where the concentration of the releasing agent was continuously monitored (42).

The enhanced release was also observed in non-erodible systems exposed to ultrasound where the release is diffusion dependent. This was tested on EVAc copolymers loaded with BSA or insulin. The released insulin was also evaluated by HPLC. No significant difference was detected between insulin samples exposed to ultrasound and unexposed samples, suggesting that the ultrasound is not degrading the releasing molecules.

The effect of ultrasound on non-erodible polymers suggests that ultrasound also affects the diffusion of the releasing molecules in addition to polymer degradation. Support for this can be found when comparing release and degradation rates of erodible polymers, where the increase in the rate of drug release is more pronounced than that of the polymer degradation. As the drug release is dependent on both matrix degradation and diffusion, the study suggests that ultrasound affects both processes (42).

Experiments were also performed to evaluate whether the extent of enhancement could be regulated externally. By varying the ultrasound intensity, the degree of enhancement for both polymer degradation and drug release for the bioerodible and non-erodible systems could be altered 10-fold (42).

In vivo experiments were performed using *para*-aminohippuric acid (PAH) as a marker inside the polymers. Data of rats' PAH concentration in the urine after implantation showed that the PAH concentration in the urine was pronounced during the exposure and mainly in the timespan just after the exposure. The delay was presumably the diffusion time from the implantation site to the bloodstream and then the removal by the kidneys. When control animals were treated by the same procedure, i.e., placing the ultrasonic applicator head over the treated area with the power level of the ultrasound set to zero, no effect of the ultrasound could be detected (43). In addition, there was no difference in the rat skin histopathology between ultrasound-treated areas after an exposure of one hour at 5 W/cm^2 and untreated areas (43).

It was proposed that cavitation and acoustic streaming were responsible for this augmented degradation and release. In experiments conducted in a degassed buffer, where cavitation was minimized, the observed enhancement in degradation and release rates was much smaller. It was also considered that several other parameters (temperature and mixing effects) might be responsible for the augmented release due to ultrasound. However, experiments were conducted which suggested that these parameters were not significant. A temperature rise of only 2.5°C was recorded in samples during the triggering period. A separate release experiment done at 40°C instead of 37°C, however, showed that the rate increase was less than 10%. This suggests that the enhancement phenomena cannot be attributed to heat. To evaluate the ultrasound effect on the diffusion boundary layer, release experiments were performed under vigorous shaking. The increases of the release rates due to shaking were always below 20%. Therefore, the effect of ultrasound on the augmented release cannot be due to mixing only. Even though ultrasound may eliminate or diminish the diffusion boundary layer, that effect cannot be responsible for the 10- to 30-fold increase in release rates (42).

It was considered that if ultrasound was useful in augmenting drug release through polymers, it might also be useful in augmenting drug transport through skin. Three model substances and two animal models were used. The effect of therapeutic-range ultrasound (1 MHz) on skin permeation of D-mannitol, a highly polar sugar alcohol; inulin, a high molecular-weight polysaccharide; and physostigmine, a lipophilic anti-cholinesterase drug was studied in rats and guinea pigs. D-Mannitol and inulin are totally and rapidly excreted, once they have penetrated through the skin into the bloodstream, permitting direct *in vivo* monitoring. For evaluating skin penetration of physostigmine, the decrease of whole blood cholinesterase was measured. Ultrasound nearly completely eliminated the lag time usually associated with transdermal delivery of all these substances. Three to five minutes of ultrasound irradiation (1.5 W/cm^2 continuous wave or 3 W/cm^2 pulsed wave) increased the transdermal permeation of inulin and mannitol in rats by 5–20-fold within 1–2 h following ultrasound application. Ultrasound treatment also significantly increases ($p < 0.05$) the inhibition of cholinesterase during the first hour after application in both physostigmine-treated rats and guinea pigs: While in control guinea pigs, no significant inhibition of cholinesterase could be detected during the first two hours after application of physostigmine, the ultrasound-treated group showed a $15 \pm 5\%$ (mean $\pm$ SEM) decrease in blood cholinesterase one hour after ultrasound application. For physostigmine-treated rats the level of cholinesterase inhibition one hour after ultrasound application was $53 \pm 5\%$ in the treated groups and $35 \pm 5\%$ in the controls (44).

3. *Enzyme-Mediated Release*

An approach for feedback control of polypeptides incorporated within polymeric drug delivery systems was also developed. This approach is based on the observation that changes in pH can cause dramatic shifts in the solubility of polypeptide drugs; solubility is one of the prime determinants of release rate in any diffusion-, dissolution-, or osmosis-controlled release system. The system components involve an external trigger molecule and a polymer-bound enzyme that, in the presence of the trigger molecule, will cause acid or base to form. To test this concept, insulin was used as a drug and diabetic rats as the animal model. As a model system, an ethylene–vinyl acetate (EVAc) polymeric insulin delivery system capable of treating diabetic rats for more than 100 days was used. To establish feedback, two principles were used: that insulin solubility is pH-dependent and that, in the presence of glucose oxidase, glucose is converted to gluconic acid. Thus, when this enzyme is incorporated within a controlled-release polymer matrix, external glucose should theoretically reduce the pH in the polymer microenvironment. Since the isoelectric point of insulin is 5.3, when the polymer is exposed to the physiological pH of 7.4 a decrease in insulin solubility and release rate is expected. This undesired effect is overcome by using a modified insulin which contains more basic groups and thus has a higher isoelectric point. Tri-lysyl insulin with an isoelectric point of 7.4 was synthesized for this purpose (31). The feasibility of this enzyme-mediated feedback mechanism was investigated by three sets of experiments: (i) the effect of glucose on the pH in the microenvironment of the polymer, (ii) the effect of glucose on insulin release *in vitro*, and (iii) the effect of glucose on insulin release *in vivo*.

When polymer matrices containing insulin and glucose oxidase were exposed to buffer solutions containing 1000 mg/dL glucose, a decrease of nearly 0.5 pH units inside the matrix was recorded after 4 min; the pH then stabilized. The effect was reversible. The pH returned to its original value when the solution was replaced with fresh buffer containing no glucose. Control polymer matrices containing no enzyme did not show any changes in pH after exposure to glucose solutions (45).

The results of insulin release *in vitro* from different groups of polymer matrices before, during, and after glucose exposure over a one-month period were analyzed by the method of analysis of variances with repeated measurements. When polymer matrices containing enzyme and tri-lysyl or regular insulin were exposed to glucose, an average increase in release rate of tri-lysyl insulin of 19% ($p \leq 0.001$) and an average decrease in release rate of regular insulin of 29% ($p \leq 0.005$) was observed. Control polymers matrices containing either regular or tri-lysyl insulin with no enzyme showed no response to glucose ($p > 0.5$) (45).

Serum insulin levels in diabetic rats implanted with polymer matrices containing tri-lysyl insulin and enzyme showed a significant increase in serum insulin level ($p \leq 0.001$) during the infusion of glucose, compared to the insulin levels before glucose infusion. Similar to the previous results *in vitro*, a decrease ($p \leq 0.025$) in insulin release rate was observed when diabetic rats implanted with polymer matrices containing regular insulin and enzyme were infused with glucose. Control diabetic rats implanted with polymers containing no enzyme or with no polymer implanted showed no insulin response to glucose infusion ($p > 0.5$ in both cases) (45).

The preceding studies, as well as other studies on controlled release from numerous other laboratories are but examples of how polymers may be useful in controlling drug release. These delivery concepts may not only be of value in their own right, but will hopefully stimulate additional research in the release of polypeptides, the creation of new bioerodible polymers, and the design of pulsatile delivery systems.

II. Immobilized Enzyme Bioreactors

A second area of research involves reactors composed of enzymes immobilized to solid supports. Such systems offer a highly specific means of removing undesired substances from the bloodstream. By immobilizing the enzyme, the possibility of inducing an immune response is minimized. Three examples of using immobilized enzymes are now discussed.

A. Immobilized Heparinase

One system utilizes the enzyme heparinase to remove the anticoagulant heparin. Heparin is administered to patients undergoing treatment with an artificial kidney or pump oxygenator and has been cited as the drug responsible for the most deaths in otherwise healthy patients (46). The enzyme can be immobilized to various supports. In one example, heparinase is immobilized to cyanogen bromide–activated agarose (these are spherical beads containing hydroxyl groups which can be chemically activated), which is then placed in an arterial blood filter that serves as a reactor. The blood passes through the reactor, where the heparin is degraded to small fragments that have almost no anticoagulant activity (47).

In developing a reactor such as the one just described, it is important to understand important design parameters, such as the radial distribution of the enzyme within the catalyst particles, the kinetics of heparin degradation catalyzed by immobilized heparinase, the flow properties in the reactor, and the effect of *in vivo* factors such as blood proteins which bind to the substrate. These parameters and how they can be evaluated are now discussed.

1. Distribution of Enzyme within the Catalyst

The heparin degradation rate at any radial position inside the catalyst particle is proportional to the bound heparinase concentration at that position. If the immobilized enzyme concentration is not uniform, the conventional analysis of simultaneous diffusion and reaction within a porous catalytic particle must be modified. The reaction rate within the catalyst particle will have an explicit radial dependence introduced via the enzyme concentration, as well as a dependence on the substrate concentration.

The heparinase used in many studies has certain protein impurities, and thus using labeled enzyme to visually define the protein is not sufficient. These impurities do not cause a reaction with heparin or heparin degradation products. To determine the enzyme distribution for heparinase, one can analyze the kinetics of heparinase binding to the catalyst particle (in this case, an agarose bead). These catalyst particles contain functional groups which are activated with cyanogen bromide to produce highly reactive cyanate esters. In the presence of the enzyme, the NH_2 groups of the enzyme will bind to the cyanate esters, forming an enzymatically active catalyst. The enzyme distribution can be estimated by analyzing the binding rate dependence on both the enzyme and the functional group concentrations during an immobilization. A model of the immobilization process based on the experimentally derived binding kinetics can then be developed to predict the bound heparinase concentration as a function of the radial position in the catalyst particles.

The first step in characterizing the heparinase binding rate to the catalyst particles is to establish experimental conditions where neither enzyme denaturation or external mass transfer are important. This can be accomplished by controlling the duration of immobilization, the mixing rate, and the catalyst particle size. In the absence of diffusional limitations and enzyme denaturation effects, the disappearance of enzymatic activity from the bulk phase equals the rate at which the enzyme binds to the catalyst particle. The molar conservation equation for heparinase in the bulk phase is given by

$$V_F \frac{dC}{dt}\text{H} = W_a R(C_H, C_{c\equiv n}), \tag{6}$$

where V_F is the total volume of the fluid phase, C_H is the heparinase concentration in the bulk solution, $C_{c\equiv n}$ is the cyanate ester concentration, W_a is the weight of the catalyst particle, and $R(C_H, C_{c\equiv n})$ is the binding rate at the respective enzyme and ester concentrations.

The binding kinetics were studied as a function of heparinase concentration at two different cyanate ester concentrations. These cyanate ester groups were present in excess, and this remained constant throughout the experiment. At both ester levels, the disappearance of heparinase from the fluid phase was first-order and the binding constant depended on the cyanate ester concentration (48).

A model of the actual immobilization process with intact spherical catalyst particles was developed using the experimentally determined binding kinetics (48). The system was treated as a group of porous spheres suspended in a well-mixed solution of heparinase. The enzyme diffused through the porous network, where it reacted with the surface cyanate esters to produce the bound enzyme.

Normally, the immobilization of heparinase to agarose catalyst particles is terminated after 4–5 h because greater than 85% of the initial heparinase is bound (49). Based on a cyanate ester stability study, the cyanate ester concentration drops to only 88% of its initial value. For modeling purposes, the cyanate ester concentration was assumed constant. In addition, because of its small size relative to the large molecular weight cutoff (1.5×10^6 daltons) of the catalyst particle, cyanogen bromide (MW 106) should diffuse rapidly into the particle and uniformly activate the matrix.

The activated agarose was initially swollen, and it was assumed that convective effects due to pore swelling could be neglected. The conservation equations describing the situation within the catalyst spheres and the well-mixed fluid phase are

$$\frac{\partial C_F}{\partial} = \frac{D_e}{r^2}\frac{\partial}{\partial r}\left(\frac{r^2 \partial C_F}{\partial r}\right) - k_b C_F, \tag{7}$$

$$\frac{\partial C_I}{\partial t} = k_b C_F \qquad \text{(bound enzyme)}, \tag{8}$$

$$V_F \frac{dC_R}{dt} = \frac{3V_B \varepsilon}{r_0}\left(-D_e \left.\frac{\partial C_F}{\partial r}\right|_{r=r_0}\right) \qquad \text{(well-mixed fluid)}, \tag{9}$$

where V_F is the volume of the immobilization solution, V_B is the total volume of gel, ε is the porosity of the agarose gel, k_b is the binding constant of the enzyme to the agarose, C_R is the heparinase concentration in the well-mixed fluid, C_F is the free heparinase concentration inside the sphere based on the pore volume, C_I is the concentration of bound heparinase within the sphere based on the pore volume, t is time, and r is radial position within a spherical particle. Both C_F and C_I are functions of time and radial distance. The following boundary conditions were used:

$$r = 0, \qquad \frac{\partial C_F}{\partial r} = 0,$$

$$r = r_0, \qquad -\varepsilon D_e \frac{\partial C_F}{\partial r} = k_g\left(\frac{C_F}{K_p} - C_R\right).$$

K_p is a partition coefficient of the enzyme in agarose and k_g is a mass transfer coefficient. Although predictions can be made about the bound-enzyme profile, it is not possible to directly verify them experimentally because of the protein impurities in heparinase. However, it is possible to measure the bulk heparinase concentration during the course of an immobilization and compare it to the model predictions. A series of immobilizations were conducted using intact agarose spheres with different cyanate ester concentrations and the bulk heparinase concentration monitored.

An example of the experimental dimensionless bulk heparinase profile together with the model predictions is shown in Fig. 7. The agreement between the model and the experimental profiles was good, with no systematic devation.

The bound-enzyme profile under the normal immobilization conditions is given in Fig. 8 as a function of time and radial position. At each time, the profile was essentially uniform. At 4 h, which corresponded to the

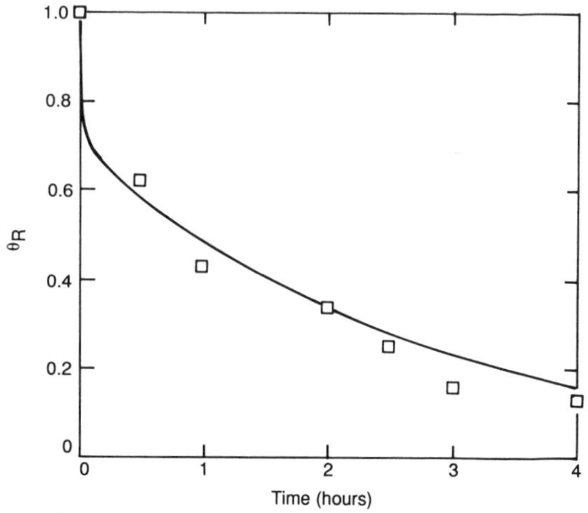

FIG. 7. Data and model predictions of dimensionless bulk heparinase concentration during course of enzyme immobilization at 4°C, pH 7.0. V_F = 6.8 mL, V_B = 3.6 mL, and $C_{c\equiv n}$ = 9.8 μmol/g. Each point is mean of three independent experiments, and all samples assayed in duplicate. Error bars are size of points. Line is model prediction [from Bernstein *et al.* (48)].

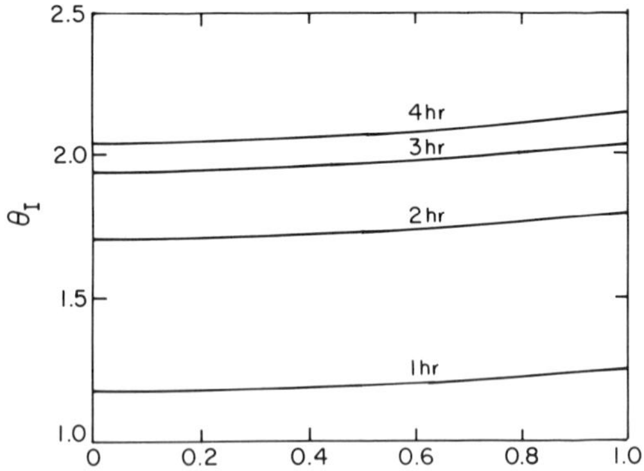

FIG. 8. Model predictions of dimensionless immobilized heparinase concentration at different times at 4°C, pH 7.0, $V_F = 7.0$ mL, $V_B = 3.5$ mL, and $C_{c\equiv n} = 25\ \mu$mol/g [from Bernstein *et al.* (48)].

termination of the immobilization, the difference between the centerline and surface concentrations was equal to 4.8% of the centerline value. These data predict a uniform heparinase concentration throughout the catalyst particles under typically used immobilization conditions.

2. *Kinetics of Heparin Degradation*

The rate of heparin degradation was studied in an agitated batch reactor. First the effect of agitation speed on the kinetics of immobilized heparinase was determined. The rates were measured at high enzyme loadings and at substrate concentrations less than the K_m (the K_m, also known as the Michaelis constant, is the substrate concentration at which the reaction rate is one-half its maximum) of the immobilized enzyme. At these conditions, the system is most sensitive to external diffusion limitations. However, at this stage the K_m of the immobilized enzyme was unknown. As a first approximation, the K_m value of the soluble enzyme, 0.11 mg/mL, was assumed. A bulk heparin concentration of 0.1 mg/mL was used, which corresponded to a heparin concentration of 0.036 mg/mL at the catalyst particle surface using the partitioning coefficient (50). At the end of the kinetic study, this concentration was verified to be less than the K_m of the immobilized enzyme. The heparinase loading was 230 units/mL, which corresponded to the highest enzyme loading used for the kinetic characterization.

The reaction rate as a function of agitation speed is shown in Fig. 9. The reaction rates increased with increasing agitation rate up to a speed of 140 rpm. In the range 140–170 rpm, the reaction rate enhancement

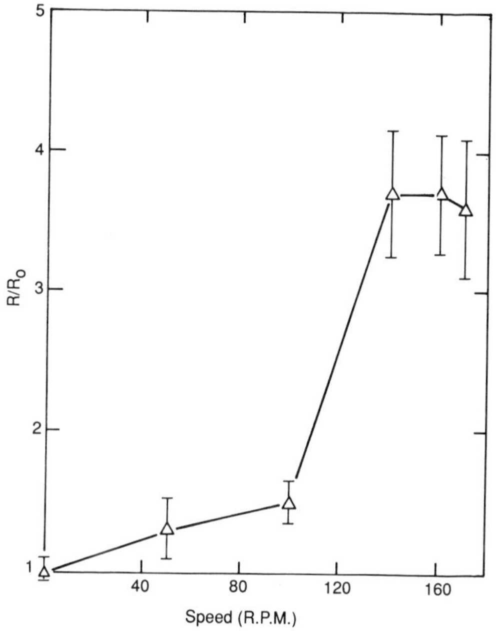

FIG. 9. Effect of agitation speed on rate of heparin degradation catalyzed by immobilized heparinase at $T = 37°C$, pH 7.4, $E = 230$ units/mL, and $C_b = 0.1$ mg/mL. Ratio of volume of fluid phase to volume of beads, 200:1. Each point is mean of 10 independent experiments [from Bernstein *et al.* (50)].

remained constant at a factor of 3.5. All further kinetic studies were conducted at an agitation speed of 140 rpm.

The intrinsic kinetic parameters of immobilized heparinase were obtained by investigating heparin degradation as a function of the system Thiele moduli at heparin concentrations far away from the zero-order regime. This was accomplished by increasing the enzyme loading at a constant particle diameter. The mean diameter of the agarose beads was 223 ± 25 mm ($N = 230$). Ten sets of beads with enzyme loadings in the range 9–230 units/mL were characterized at bulk heparin concentrations between 0.1 and 25 mg/mL. These corresponded to surface concentrations of 0.015–3.75 mg/mL. The reaction rates at surface heparin concentrations of 0.036 and 0.072 mg/mL were used for varying the Thiele moduli. Both concentrations were expected to be less than the K_m of the immobilized enzyme. As described earlier, rates at substrate levels less than the K_m were utilized because the system is most sensitive to internal diffusion under such conditions.

A plot of R/R_0 vs. E/E_0 is shown in Fig. 10 (R is rate, E is enzyme concentration, and the subscript 0 symbolizes the reference condition),

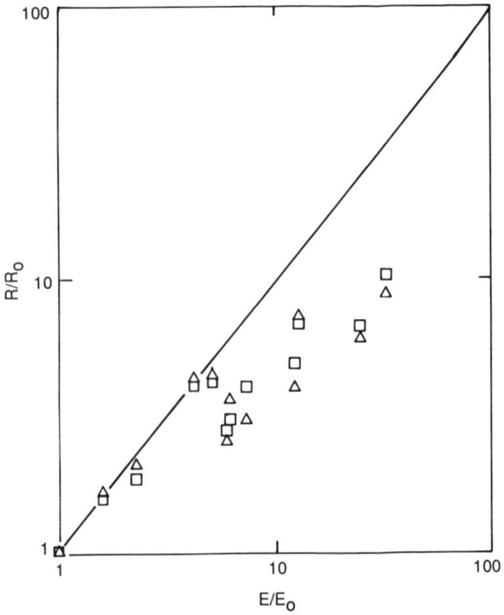

FIG. 10. Effect of immobilized enzyme concentration on initial rate of heparin degradation at T = 37°C, pH 7.4, and agitation speed 140 rpm. Ratio of volume of fluid phase to volume of beads, 200:1. Each point was the mean of four independent experiments. Error bars are the size of points. Line is the theoretical prediction for case of no internal diffusion (C_b = 0.1 mg/mL, C_b = 0.2 mg/mL) [from Bernstein *et al.* (50)].

where the reference loading was taken as the set of beads with the lowest enzyme concentration (9 units/mL). The reaction rate increased in proportion to the enzyme concentration up to loadings of 45 units/mL. Above this value, the reaction rates increased in proportion to the enzyme concentration to a fractional power (50).

For each of five sets of beads with enzyme loadings less than 45 units/mL, the reaction rate data were fitted to the Michaelis–Menten equations over the complete range of surface concentrations. The K_m value was equal to 0.15 ± 0.3 mg/mL.

The validity of both the immobilized K_m and the model of simultaneous diffusion and reaction was examined by comparing the experimental data with predictions. At each substrate concentration, an effectiveness factor, η, using the experimentally observed reaction rate and the K_m was calculated from

$$\eta = \frac{R_{obs}/V_{max}K_pC_b}{K_m + K_pC_b}. \tag{10}$$

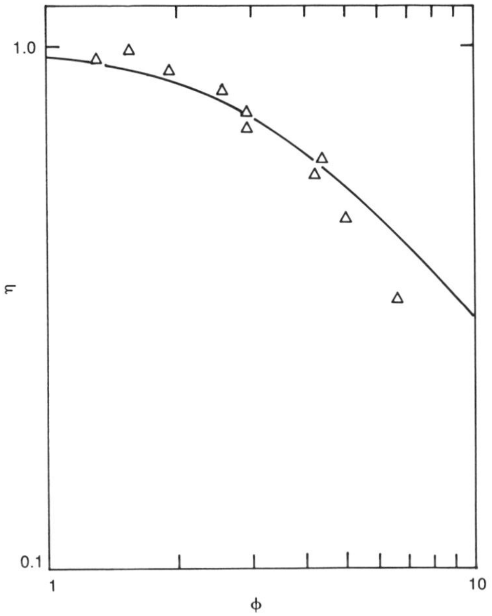

FIG. 11. Comparison of theoretical and experimental effectiveness factors as function of Thiele modulus at pH 7.4, $T = 37°C$, $\beta = 0.24$, and agitation speed 140 rpm. Line is theoretical prediction for effectiveness factor, and points are experimental data [from Bernstein *et al.* (50)].

For each bead set and heparin concentration, the experimentally determined effectiveness factor was compared to the predicted effectiveness factor. The Thiele modulus, Φ, was calculated from

$$\Phi^2 = r_0^2 V_{max}/D_e K_m, \tag{11}$$

where V_{max} is experimentally determined for the particular bead set, K_m is equal to 0.15 mg/mL, and D_e is the effective diffusion coefficient of heparin. The diffusivity of heparin in buffer was taken as 1.2×10^{-6} cm^2/s, and the effective diffusivity was calculated as

$$D_e = \Sigma K_r D/\gamma, \tag{12}$$

where γ is the tortuosity of the gel, Σ is porosity, and K_r accounts for hindered-diffusion effects. A typical theoretical η vs. Φ curve with the experimental data is shown in Fig. 11.

3. Mixing Properties

The RTD (residence time distribution) of the heparinase reactor was studied using a large-molecule (MW 2,000,000) blue dextran, which is

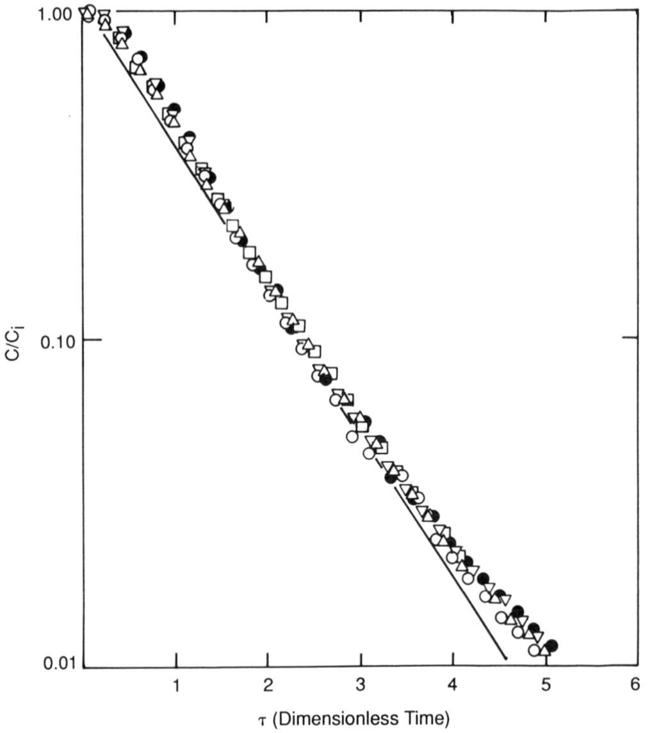

FIG. 12. Concentration profile of blue dextran in effluent of heparinase reactor during washout experiment. Inlet flow rate 120 mL/min. Concentration is normalized by initial concentration of dye in the reactor, and time is normalized by mean residence time in the reactor as determined by best fit to data. Line is theoretical prediction for washout of dye from CSTR [from Bernstein *et al.* (50)].

excluded from the beads. The concentration of blue dextran in the reactor effluent after clear fluid is infused into the reactor is shown in Fig. 12. The dashed line represents the exponential decay expected for ideal CSTR behavior. The data was well approximated by an exponential fit to an effluent fraction of 0.01.

The heparinase reactor was modeled as an ideal CSTR for which a steady-state mass balance for heparin is given by

$$Q(C_e - C_i) = V_b R_e, \tag{13}$$

where Q is the volumetric flow rate, C_i and C_e are the inlet and outlet heparin concentrations, V_b is the volume of catalyst, and R_e is the overall rate of heparin degradation per volume of catalyst evaluated at the outlet conditions. Experimental *in vitro* data were consistent within 10% of predictions made using this model (50).

4. In Vivo Considerations

To extend the model to *in vivo* situations, one must understand the physiological events which can affect heparin concentration and other parameters. In particular, heparin binds a blood protein, antithrombin. Thus, two forms of heparin must be considered, free and bound. The process is represented by the following reversible chemical reaction:

$$\text{heparin} + \text{antithrombin} \longleftrightarrow [\text{heparin–antithrombin}]. \qquad (14)$$

The degradation of heparin by the reactor is a multistep process. Heparin and the heparin–antithrombin complex must first diffuse from the bulk phase to the surface of the immobilized enzyme particle. The two species diffuse into the agarose particles where they encounter immobilized heparinase. The heparin–antithrombin complex is assumed to be sterically inhibited from binding to immobilized heparinase, and under these conditions only unbound heparin is enzymatically degraded. As unbound heparin is consumed, heparin dissociates from the heparin–antithrombin complex to generate more free heparin. The breakdown of heparin is given by the following chemical reaction:

$$\text{heparin} \longrightarrow n \text{ product}, \qquad (15)$$

where n is the number of moles of product generated.

The breakdown of heparin results in a distribution of low molecular-weight fragments ranging in size from a disaccharide to an octasaccharide (51). Except for the disaccharides, the other products can bind to antithrombin with affinities that depend on their molecular weight. Of these, only the octasaccharides bind to antithrombin to any significant degree, and this is the only product which must be considered in the modeling. The octasaccharide–antithrombin binding process is represented by the following reversible chemical reaction:

$$\text{octasaccharide} + \text{antithrombin} \longleftrightarrow [\text{octasaccharide–antithrombin}]. \qquad (16)$$

As octasaccharide products are generated, they compete for the binding site on the antithrombin molecule as well as diffuse out of the catalyst particles. Heparin is displaced from antithrombin by the octasaccharide product, and the concentration of unbound heparin available for degradation is increased.

Within the particle, molar conservation equations are written for heparin (H),* octasaccharide (P), antithrombin (A), the heparin–antithrombin complex (AH) and the octasaccharide–antithrombin complex (AP). The

* The letters in parentheses refers to the subscript notation used for the model formulation.

transport of species j within the catalytic particle is assumed to occur by diffusion only. Steady-state conservation equations for each species are written as follows:

$$\nabla^2[D_H C_H] - R_1 - R_2 = 0, \tag{17}$$

$$\nabla^2[D_A C_A] - R_2 - R_3 = 0, \tag{18}$$

$$\nabla^2[D_{AH} C_{AH}] + R_2 = 0, \tag{19}$$

$$\nabla^2[D_P C_P] + aR_1 + R_3 = 0, \tag{20}$$

$$\nabla^2[D_{AP} C_{AP}] + R_3 = 0, \tag{21}$$

where D_i is the effective diffusivity of species i within the particle, a is the number of moles of octasaccharide produced per mole of heparin, C_i is the concentration of species i per volume of fluid/plasma at position r, R_1 is the volumetric production rate of heparin by Reaction (14), R_2 is the volumetric production rate of heparin by Reaction (15), R_3 is the volumetric rate of octasaccharide product formation by Reaction (16), and

$$\nabla^2[\ ] = \frac{1}{r^2}\frac{d}{dr}\left(r^2\frac{d}{dr}[\ ]\right). \tag{22}$$

The reaction rates are based on the total gel volume. The kinetics of heparin degradation [Reaction (14)] follow Michaelis–Menten kinetics (52):

$$R_1 = \frac{V_{max} C_H}{C_H + K_m}, \tag{23}$$

where K_m is the Michaelis constant, C_H is the heparin concentration, and V_{max} is the reaction rate at substrate saturation. The reaction rate V_{max} is given by

$$V_{max} = k_{cat} E(t), \tag{24}$$

where k_{cat} is the catalytic constant and $E(t)$ is the concentration of immobilized heparinase at time t.

To test the model predictions, the single-pass clearance of heparin was determined as a function of time in three different sheep. For each experiment, the volume of beads, the initial enzyme loading, the animal's antithrombin level, the hematocrit, the inlet heparin concentration, and the half-life of the enzyme were used to generate model predictions for the clearance of heparin as a function of time.

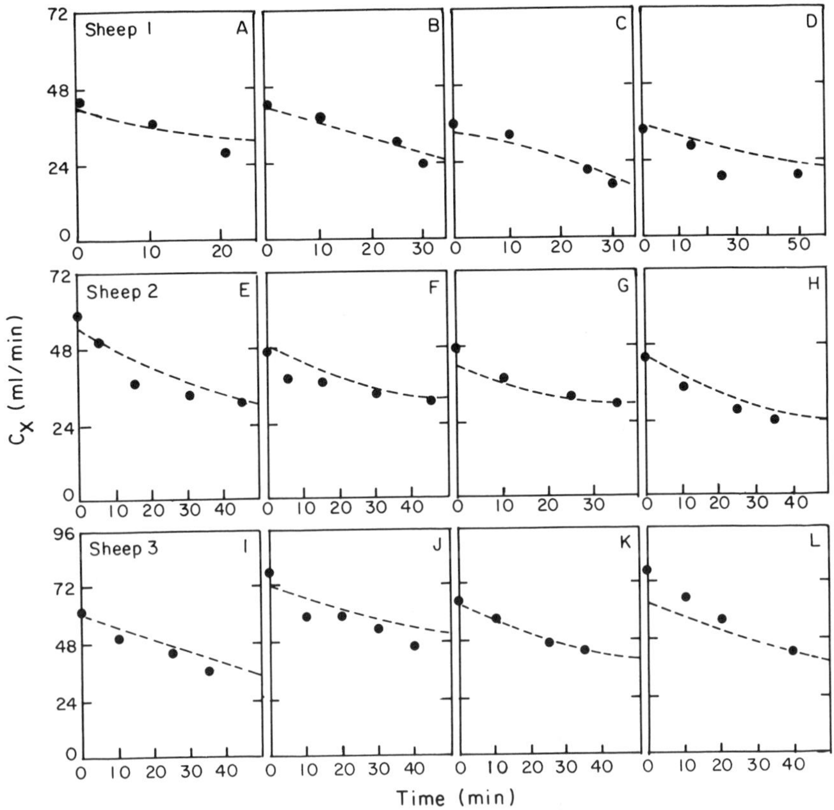

FIG. 13. Clearance of heparin by the heparinase filter at a blood flow of 120 mL/min as a function of time. Four experiments were conducted for each animal. Broken lines represent the model predictions; the closed circles are the experimentally determined clearances. Each point is the mean of three measurements, and the standard deviations are within the size of the symbols in all cases [from Bernstein and Langer (47)].

Two control experiments determined that essentially no heparin was non-specifically removed from the extracorporeal circuit. Four experiments were then conducted on each of the three animals, and the model predictions are shown together with the experimental data in Fig. 13. In all cases, the model clearances were within a few percent of the experimentally determined values (47).

Several other reactors for immobilized heparinase have been designed (53, 54). The initial reactor (47) caused no more blood damage than conventionally used extracorporeal devices such as the artificial kidney machine (54a). By controlling the mode of immobilized enzyme bead suspension, all blood damage can be essentially eliminated (54). The FDA has already approved a new diagnostic based on heparinase, and the reactor is in advanced animal trials.

B. Immobilized Bilirubin Oxidase

In a second example, a small blood filter containing immobilized bilirubin oxidase to reduce serum bilirubin concentrations was developed for potential application in the treatment of neonatal jaundice.

Twenty percent of all human newborns accumulate enough bilirubin to stain their skin, resulting in jaundice. Bilirubin binds to cellular and mitochondrial membranes, causing cell death in a variety of tissues; clinically, bilirubin toxicity may lead to mental retardation, cerebral palsy, deafness, seizures, or death.

In mild cases, jaundiced infants are treated by phototherapy. However, since only 15% of total body bilirubin can be photoisomerized through the skin, phototherapy does not control cases of severe jaundice. In those cases, infants undergo exchange transfusion, which requires staged removal of the infant's blood and its replacement with bilirubin-free adult blood. This procedure may result in hypoglycemia, hypocalcemia, acidosis, coagulopathies, graft-versus-host disease, transmission of infectious diseases (for example, hepatitis or acquired immune deficiency syndrome), or death. Although these treatments have reduced the occurrence of bilirubin toxicity, the risks associated with exchange transfusion remain a serious problem. Chromatography has been tested as a technique to replace exchange transfusions. Numerous resins have been used to adsorb bilirubin; however, they removed not only bilirubin but also essential compounds such as thyroxine.

The use of highly specific enzymes was proposed to remove bilirubin from the bloodstream. More than 50 enzymes were tested, and an enzyme from *Myrothecium verrucaria*, bilirubin oxidase, which catalyzes the oxidation of bilirubin with O_2, was chosen. The initial product of the enzymatic reaction is biliverdin, which is much less toxic than bilirubin. The stability of bilirubin oxidase was greatly enhanced by immobilization: At physiological temperature and pH, free bilirubin oxidase lost half of its activity in 12 h, whereas the half-life of the immobilized enzyme was 60 h.

To determine the effectiveness of the immobilized enzyme in blood, a column containing 5 g of agarose with the active enzyme was tested. Control columns contained the same amount of either untreated agarose or agarose containing denatured bilirubin oxidase. For the experiments *in vivo*, Gunn rats on lipid-free or regular diets were used. For the experiments *in vitro*, a blood reservoir of human umbilical-cord blood was used.

The experimental columns, both *in vitro* and *in vivo*, cleared 90–95% of the bilirubin in the blood. Control columns had no effect on serum bilirubin concentrations. Serum bilirubin concentrations in the treated rats and reservoirs fell less rapidly than effluent concentrations, presumably because of mixing with untreated blood. In a series of six experiments *in vitro*, serum bilirubin concentration in the blood reservoir decreased on the average by 61% within 30 min. In a series of six experiments *in vivo*, serum bilirubin concentration in the rats decreased by 50% within 30 min and remained low even after the enzyme treatment, indicating that a short period of exposure rapidly lowers the bilirubin level in rats (Fig. 14) (55).

Blood sampled after the trials revealed no statistically significant change in platelet or white blood cell counts and a 20% decrease in hematocrit in both experiments and controls. The decrease in hematocrit could be eliminated by changing the size of the agarose beads (56). The electrolyte balance was unaffected, and the concentrations of calcium, phosphorus, albumin, blood urea nitrogen, creatinine, uric acid, cholesterol, triglyceride, and liver enzyme remained within normal limits. The glucose concentration increased during the experiments, as expected in a postoperative, restrained animal.

Recently it was discovered that oral administration of this bilirubin oxidase preparation can prevent bilirubin absorption in jaundiced Gunn rats.

One major concern in developing an oral enzymatic therapy is the retention of enzyme activity with passage through the gastrointestinal tract, especially the acidic pH environment of the stomach. To be useful the enzyme must retain its activity to act in the near-neutral pH environment of the small intestine. Thus, immobilized bilirubin oxidase was

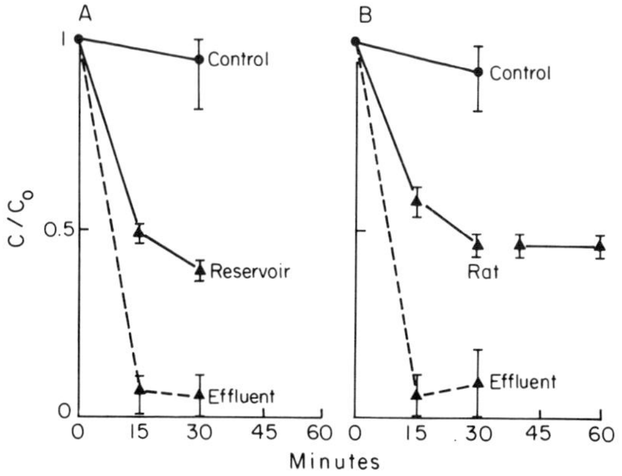

FIG. 14. Enzymatic clearance of bilirubin from blood [from Lavin *et al.* (55)].

incubated for 1 h at 37°C in acidic pH and the subsequent enzymatic activity measured at pH 7.4.

Results show that immobilized bilirubin oxidase incubated at pH 3.2 and 1.4 still retained greater that 90% of its original activity. In contrast, free soluble enzyme lost more than 80% of its activity at pH 3.2 and more than 95% of its activity at pH 1.4. These results indicate that the immobilized enzyme has a greatly increased stability that may survive the harshly acidic environment of the stomach.

To test the concept of oral bilirubin oxidase, as controls, 11 rats were fed either regular rat chow ($n = 2$), chow supplemented with lyophilized agarose beads ($n = 3$), chow supplemented with lyophilized agarose beads containing immobilized bilirubin oxidase which had been heat-denatured ($n = 4$), or chow supplemented with lyophilized agarose beads which had been activated with tresyl chloride and quenched with β-mercaptoethanol ($n = 2$). Agarose quenched with β-mercaptoethanol was examined because the effectiveness of agar in binding bilirubin has been directly correlated to its sulfur content. The results for the four groups were not significantly different ($p > 0.10$) and were considered as one control group ($n = 11$) (57).

In the experimental animals, each received active immobilized bilirubin oxidase (0.1 mg enzyme/day). Results were divided into two groups, depending on the rat's initial bilirubin/serum albumin molar ratio (abbreviated as B/RSA). In the experimental group, rats with a B/RSA ratio > 0.35 were designated treated high bilirubin:RSA ratio (this is what would be expected in humans with jaundice); rats with a B/RSA ratio < 0.35 were designated treated low bilirubin:RSA ratio. For the treated high bilirubin:RSA ratio group plasma bilirubin declined from an initial value of 11.3 mg/dL to 7.1 mg/dL after the 4-day treatment period, and further to 6.3 mg/dL at Day 8, before rebounding to 9.1 mg/dL at Day 20. The treated low bilirubin:RSA Ratio group and the control group demonstrated little change in plasma bilirubin.

Histological results revealed no damage to the intestinal tract which had been in contact with the immobilized enzyme preparation. Tissues studied included the kidney, thyroid, stomach, duodenum, pancreas, jejunum, ileum, cecum, colon, and rectum.

C. Removal of Low-Density Lipoprotein–Cholesterol

In a final example, the use of enzymes to remove low–density lipoprotein (LDL) cholesterol was explored. Although plasma cholesterol may be reduced by drugs, diet, and direct removal of LDL from the blood, drug therapy may have side effects which limit its use. Moreover, many familial hypercholesterolemic patients are resistant to diet and drug therapy. Plasmapheresis, the direct removal of the patient's high cholesterol plasma and replacement with donor albumin, although a successful therapy, is expensive and removes a wide range of circulating proteins in addition to LDL. Alternative extracorporeal techniques have been developed to improve LDL specificity and to lower cost. Removal of LDL can be accomplished with columns of heparin–agarose, dextran sulfate cellulose, or antibody–agarose, or by LDL precipitation at acidic pH. However, the limited capacity of the adsorbents makes these techniques cumbersome and very expensive. Therefore, enzymes that could modify plasma LDL were explored, in the hopes that a modified LDL could be removed by an individual's own metabolic processes. After searching for many enzymes, it was discovered that phospholipase A_2 has this ability. The feasibility of reducing plasma cholesterol by PLA_2 treatment was first tested by injecting rabbits intravenously with $[^{125}I\text{-}]PLA_2$-LDL. Clearance rates and biodistributions were determined in three animal models: New Zealand white rabbits (NZW), New Zealand rabbits that were cholesterol fed and therefore had high cholesterol levels (HNZW), and Watanabe rabbits, which possess an LDL receptor deficiency which make them an excellent model for patients with coronary heart disease (WHHL). Human $[^{125}I\text{-}]$LDL was used as a control. The results indicated that PLA_2-LDL was degraded 17, 10, and 6 times faster than native LDL in NZW, WHHL, and HNZW rabbits, respectively (58).

The biodistribution of injected PLA_2-LDL per organ in both WHHL and NZW rabbits was also studied. PLA_2-LDL accumulated to a greater extent in the liver than native LDL ($P < 0.002$); in NZW rabbits, the percent injected doses of radioactivity for the liver (mean $\pm$ s.e.m.) were 36 ± 4 and 19 ± 2, respectively for the modified and native LDL; in WHHL rabbits, the numbers were 26 ± 3 and 12 ± 1, respectively. A significant increase in radioactivity (10–20%) was also seen in the adrenals, kidneys, bile, and urine.

PLA_2-LDL was tested for atherogenicity by measuring its distribution in rabbits with ballooned healing aortic lesions, a well-characterized model of atherosclerosis. The contents of iodinated native LDL or PLA_2-LDL in the walls of the ballooned and healing abdominal aorta were, respectively, 4.6 ± 0.8 and 3.4 ± 0.5 percent of the plasma concentration. The data suggest that, in this model, PLA_2-LDL was less atherogenic than native LDL.

Having demonstrated that PLA_2-LDL was rapidly removed from the blood pool, an extracorporeal circuit containing an immobilized PLA_2 reactor was then designed.

The effectiveness of the treatment was verified *in vivo* using HNZW rabbits (average initial plasma cholesterol concentration ranging from 300 to 500 mg/dL). The reactors contained 1.5–3 g (wet weight) of agarose–enzyme conjugate, or agarose as a control. In this case a plasma separator was used so that the blood cells were not exposed to the enzyme, because PLA_2 may react with cell membrane components. Between 33 and 95% of the plasma phospholipids were modified after a 60–90 min treatment with the PLA_2 reactor. In contrast, control experiments with NZW and HNZW rabbits showed no phospholipid modification. The average decreases in plasma cholesterol concentrations were 13–40%, at the end of the 90 min treatments. In contrast, in the control studies, no significant drops in plasma cholesterol were observed ($p < 0.05$) (58).

Blood samples at the end of treatment revealed no significant net change in red blood cell counts, white blood cell counts, platelets, or hematocrit. The concentrations of albumin, uric acid, bilirubin, and liver enzymes remained within the normal range. Plasma free hemoglobin levels were less than 0.2 g/dL. The level of high-density lipoproteins showed no significant change with treatment (58).

Each of these three examples show how enzymes can be used to very specifically remove undesired substances from the body. Many of the principles in reactor design, described earlier, may also be applied to the use of immobilized antibodies as well.

III. Tissue Engineering

A. Introduction

Cell transplantation has been proposed as a strategy to achieve organ replacement or tissue repair for a variety of therapeutic needs, including diseases of the liver, pancreas, and other tissues. In cell transplantation, donor tissue is dissociated into individual cells or small groups of cells, which may then be attached to or encapsulated in a support matrix, and transplanted to the patient to restore lost tissue function. A number of approaches to cell transplantation have been explored.

One approach to achieve this goal is based on the following observations: (i) Every tissue undergoes constant remodeling because of attrition and renewal of consituent cells. (ii) Isolated cells will tend toward forming appropriate tissue structure *in vitro* under appropriate conditions. For example, capillary endothelial cells will form tubular structures when placed on a properly adhesive substratum *in vitro* (59) and mammary epithelial cells *in vitro* on the appropriate substratum will form acini which secrete milk (60). (iii) Although isolated cells have the capacity to remodel and form tissue structures, they can do so only to a limited degree when placed as a suspension into the midst of mature tissue. (iv) Tissue, in general, cannot survive if the constituent cells are more than a few hundred microns from the nearest capillaries because of the inability of cells in the center of the tissue mass to obtain oxygen and nutrients and eliminate waste. Based on these observations, an approach to tissue generation was proposed involving attaching isolated cells to a polymeric support structure which would have suitable surface chemistry for guiding the reorganization and growth of the cells; the support was configured so that the cells could survive by diffusion once the cell–polymer matrix was implanted (61). Ideally, the cell–polymer matrix would become vascularized if necessary in concert with expansion of the cell mass following implantation, and both these processes could be influenced if desired by release of appropriate growth factors at the site.

B. Materials and Matrix Structures for Transplant Devices

Several criteria define the ideal material for a cell transplantation matrix. (i) The material should be biocompatible, in the sense that it does not provoke a connective tissue response which will impair the function of the new tissue; (ii) it should be resorbable, to leave a completely natural tissue replacement (this is important, because it could avoid some of the problems that occur in long-lasting polymers such as those used in breast implants); (iii) it should be processable into a variety of shapes and structures which retain their shape once implanted; and (iv) the surface should interact with transplanted cells in a way which allows retention of differentiated cell function and which promotes cell growth if such growth is desired.

From the perspective of biocompatibility, degradability, and processability, synthetic polymers have many advantages over complex natural polymers such as collagen. One class of polymers in particular, polyesters in the family of polylactic acid (PLA), polyglycolic acid (PGA), and copolymers of lactic and glycolic acids (PLGAs), most closely meets the listed criteria. These polymers have been approved by the FDA for *in vivo* use, and methods were developed to process them into a variety of configurations. These polymers degrade by hydrolysis to yield natural metabolic intermediates, and the resorption rate can be varied from months to years by varying the relative ratio of the monomers.

1. Cartilage Cell Transplantation

It was demonstrated that the preceding approach is feasible for generating cartilage in animals when the matrix is constructed from a resorbable material. Initial experiments were carried out using bovine chondrocytes. Chondrocytes were harvested using collagenase digestion of hyaline cartilage from the articular surfaces of newborn calf shoulders (62).

In vitro, the behavior of the chondrocytes on the polymer fiber matrices was evaluated for up to 6 months. The gross morphologic appearance of chondrocytes was monitored using phase contrast microscopy, and the evolution of tissue-like structure was assessed using histologic sectioning and staining for cells and for components of the extracellular matrix. The chondrocytes were observed to adhere to the polymer fibers in multiple layers, proliferate, and retain a rounded configuration. Hematoxylin and eosin (H & E) staining of the experimental specimens *in vitro* demonstrated a basophilic matrix after 2 weeks. Aldehyde fuschin–alcian blue staining, and safranin 0 stains of the same specimens, indicated the presence of sulfated glycosaminoglycans (GAGs). In contrast, histologic evaluation using H & E or safranin 0 staining showed no evidence of chondrocytes or chondroitin sulfate in the *in vitro* control matrices (62).

In vivo experiments were conducted using male nude mice as transplant recipients. Chondrocytes were cultured on the polymer matrices for up to 10 days before they were implanted subcutaneously. Mice were sacrificed at intervals of time up to 9 months, and the implants were excised. Matrices which contained chondrocytes were progressively replaced by cartilage, until only cartilage with very little evidence of polymer remained. The cartilage formed retained the approximate shape and dimensions of the original cell–polymer complex as it matured. The wet weights of the specimens increased gradually until Day 49, after which time they remained stable, averaging 60–70 mg. Histologic examination of these specimens using hematoxylin and eosin stains revealed evidence of cartilage formation in over 90% of the experimental implants, with all specimens having been implanted for at least 28 days appearing very similar to normal cartilage. An early mild inflammatory response was noted. Aldehyde fuschin–alcian blue staining of these specimens suggested the presence of sulfated GAGs. Type II collagen, considered indicative of cartilage formation, was demonstrated in specimens implanted 49 days or more but was not found in earlier specimens. Neither control implants, or injected cells demonstrated evidence of cartilage formation (62).

2. *Liver Cell Transplantation*

Several facets of liver cell transplantation were studied. First was an *in vitro* characterization of cell–substrate interactions. Hepatocytes cultured under standard tissue culture conditions typically die, de-differentiate, or revert to fetal phenotype in less than a week. In contrast, hepatocytes cultured on complex extracellular matrix (ECM) substrates can maintain a highly differentiated phenotype for months. These findings suggest that the use of the proper attachment substrate might facilitate development of functional grafts for cell transplantation. The goal was to identify the features of the substrate which are important for maintaining cell function, and to incorporate these features into the polymer matrix used for transplantation. The problem was approached from two perspectives: (i) characterizing the interactions of liver cells with specific ECM proteins; and (ii) characterizing the interactions of liver cells with polymers of interest for cell transplantation.

a. Hepatocyte Interactions with ECM Substrata. The ECM substrata generally used to maintain hepatocytes in a highly differentiated state *in vitro* were complexes composed of many different types of macromolecules. Besides being poorly defined, they also suffer from batch-to-batch variations and are of limited engineering use because of their poor structural properties. The only large-scale source of these proteins is tumor tissue, which may not be suitable for clinical implantation. While the mechanism by which the ECM controls hepatocyte function is unclear, much can be learned by varying the coating density of purified ECM molecules on otherwise non-adhesive plates. This approach was used to study the effects of purified ECM molecules on hepatocyte function.

Initial results show that hepatocyte shape and function can be finely controlled by varying the coating density of any one of a variety of different, naturally occurring ECM molecules (laminin, fibronectin, type IV collagen, or type I collagen) on non-adhesive bacteriologic plates. Hepatocytes cultured on low ECM densities (≤ 1 ng/cm^2) attached, and exhibited a round morphology. Hepatocytes on high ECM densities (≥ 1000 ng/cm^2) attached, but spread extensively to achieve an epithelium-like morphology. Hepatocyte spreading increased in proportion to the ECM coating density. Hepatocytes on low ECM densities maintained high secretion rates for albumin, transferrin, and fibrinogen (plasma proteins produced by differentiated hepatocytes) that were near *in vivo* levels. In contrast, secretion rates for all three of these differentiation markers decreased by 50–100% when the ECM density was raised and hepatocyte spreading was promoted (63). These results indicate that hepatocytes can be switched between programs of growth and differentiation simply by modulating the ECM coating density.

b. Cell–Polymer Interactions. The results obtained with substrates coated with ECM proteins, as well as other published results (64), suggest that cell shape may be an important determinant of function. In addition to using coatings of ECM proteins to control cell shape, the physicochemical properties of an uncoated polymer surface may be modulated to alter cell shape and affect cell physiology (65). As a first step in understanding how the surface chemistry of the PLA and PLGA polymers might be altered to affect cell behavior, the interactions of hepatocytes with several formulations of PLA and PLGA polymers representing a range of degradation times and polymer physical properties were characterized. Solvent-cast films of the following polymers were used: poly-(L-lactide) (PLLA), a crystalline polymer, poly(D,L-latide co-glycolide) with an 85:15 lactide: glycolide ratio (PLGA 85:15), an amorphous polymer; and a 50:50 blend of the two polymers. The behavior of cells on the polymer films was compared to the behavior of cells on type I collagen–coated polystyrene culture dishes using serum-free medium for attachment and culture.

Three criteria were used to assess the interactions of hepatocytes with the polymer films: initial degree of adhesion to the substrate; cell longevity on the substrate; and retention of hepatospecific function, as measured by albumin secretion, by cells maintained on the substrate. Cells adhered to films of PLGA 85:15 and to the blend of PLLA and PLGA 85:15 to the same degree as to controls at cell concentrations below 50,000 cells/cm^2, but adhesion was inhibited at higher cell concentrations. Adherence of hepatocytes to PLLA films was negligible. Because hepatocytes can form a confluent monolayer after spreading at a concentration of 30,000 cells/cm^2, this inhibition may not be a constraint in seeding matrices at cell concentrations high enough for transplantation (66).

The observation that cells adhered to the substrates equally as well as to the controls in a cell concentration range suitable for seeding transplant devices prompted a study of cell growth and retention of differentiated function on the polymer films. Culture was carried out for 5 days. Of the polymer substrates tested, only the blend of PLLA and PLGA 85:15 was suitable for maintenance of cells in culture; the number of cells attached to the blend substrate was similar to that for controls over 5 days, while cells detached from the other polymer substrates after 2–4 days. On the polymer blend substrate, hepatocytes exhibited similar rates of DNA synthesis to the cells on the collagen controls, a substrate which is optimal for DNA synthesis in hepatocytes obtained from adult rats (63). The ability of the substrates to allow retention of hepatospecific function was assessed by measuring the rate of albumin secretion into the culture supernate. On collagen substrata, both our research group and others (63, 68) observed a significant decline in the rate of albumin secretion over 5 days; the decline is typically 50–60% (63). On the polymer blend substrate, however, a 50% increase was observed in the rate of albumin secretion over the first 3 days to a level in the range of that reported for normal rat liver *in vivo* (69), and this rate was maintained for the remaining time in culture (63). While the suitability of this substrate for maintaining the survival and function of hepatocytes *in vivo* remains to be demonstrated, the results are significant because they offer the possibility that a simple substrate, unmodified by exogenous peptides or proteins, may fulfill the criteria for cell transplantation.

c. *In Vivo Behavior of Transplanted Hepatocytes.* The results of the *in vitro* experiments provided a basis for designing a matrix for *in vivo* transplant experiments. Because the adherence of hepatocytes to most formulations of lactide/glycolide copolymers was very good (the exception was poly-L-lactide), a fibrillar PGA mesh, which had no specialized functional groups on the surface, was initially studied. This matrix also seemed ideal for other reasons described earlier.

After resolving the issue of matrix design, the next step was to determine a desirable anatomical location. Several considerations were used in determining possible implant sites. The first is the size of the implant and the requirement that it be placed in juxtaposition to well-vascularized tissue. A transplant matrix constructed as a porous sheet-like structure could be at most 200 mm thick, based on estimates of nutrient transport limitations (66). The size of a device required to replace about 5% of the mass of an adult liver would then be about 0.5 m^2. Surgical trauma must be avoided when implanting the device, because such trauma produces fibrin clots and hematoma formation around the wounded area, which creates a poor environment for cell survival. Also, the implant may behave better if supplied by the portal circulation rather than the systemic, because the portal circulation contains potential hepatotrophic factors. For these reasons, the mesentery—the vascularized membrane which secures the intestines—was selected as the best potential site (Fig. 15).

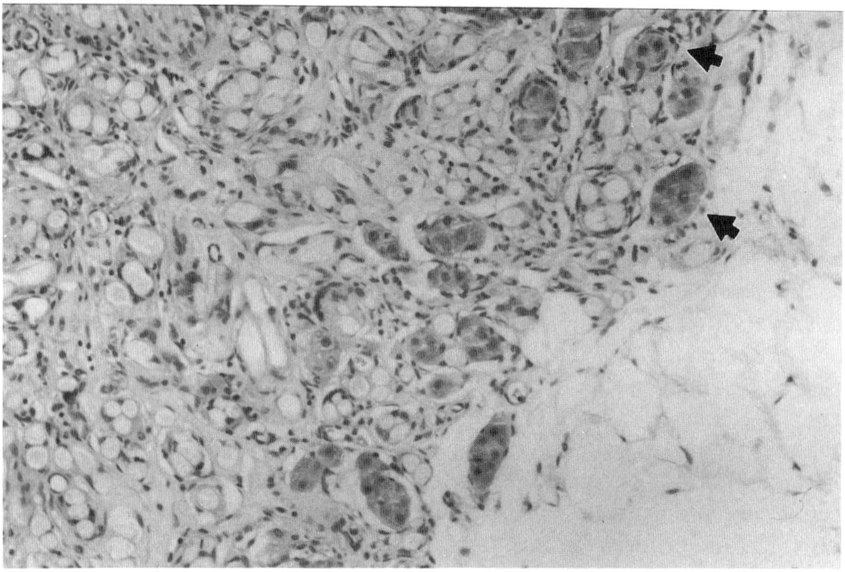

FIG. 15. Histologic appearance of hepatocytes transplanted between syngenic Fischer rats 9 weeks after transplantation into the mesentery using the PGA mesh. Hepatocytes are located in small islands (arrows) predominantly at the interface of the host tissue. Connective tissue surrounding the polymer fibrils can be seen in the lower right [from Cima *et al.* (66)].

The rat was used as an experimental model for studying hepatocyte transplantation, because several inbred strains exist, and among them are good models for metabolic deficiency states representative of human liver diseases. For evaluating the success of transplants by routine histology (H & E staining) and immunostaining for hepatospecific function such as albumin secretion, syngeneic male Fisher rats were used. Typically cells are isolated using collagenase perfusion of the liver *in situ*, seeded onto the PGA mesh to give a cell concentration 1–10% of that in normal liver tissue, cultured for up to 24 h, and then implanted into the recipient animal.

Time course studies from the time of implantation to six months after implantation show that there is a loss of viable cells within the first six hours after implantation, which is relatively constant and appears not to be related to the site selected. After one week, clusters of hepatocytes remain and blood vessels begin to grow into the graft. Clusters are most abundant adjacent to native tissue and become less abundant as they approach the center of the graft. The cells appear normal histologically. Immunohistochemical staining for the presence of albumin, a marker of liver-specific function, has shown that the surviving cells retain differentiated function up to six months.

An additional test of function of the transplanted cells is demonstrating their ability to replace a liver function which is damaged or missing in the recipient of the transplant. For this test, model transplants from healthy Wistar rats to the enzyme-deficient Gunn rat were used. The Gunn rat lacks UDP glucuronyl transferase, the enzyme to conjugate bilirubin, and the Wistar rat is a convenient donor because it is genetically similar and can conjugate bilirubin. Success of the transplant can be measured both by lowering of blood bilirubin and by the presence of conjugated products of bilirubin in the bile. Using the Gunn rat model, cell masses equivalent to 1–25% of the native liver were transplanted. Decreases in serum bilirubin levels up to 50% occurred, and appearance of conjugated bilirubin products in the native bile up to 9 weeks post-transplantation were observed, indicating metabolic activity by the transplanted cells.

IV. Conclusions

The preceding three topics of research—drug delivery systems, immobilized enzyme bioreactors, and tissue engineering—are areas of chemical engineering research that can potentially affect human life. These specific research topics presented are largely our own research and represent but a small portion of the broad area of how chemical engineering can be used to address important medical problems. Numerous other laboratories are conducting important research not only on drug delivery systems, immobilized enzymes, and tissue engineering, but on other areas of biomedical engineering as well. With advances in biology and medicine occurring more and more at a molecular level, the depth and range of these research topics should grow, and chemical engineering, above all of the other engineering disciplines, should take on an increasingly dominant role in biomedical engineering.

Acknowledgments

This research was supported by NIH grants GM 25810 and 26698. This article was adapted from Dr. Langer's Professional Progress Award Lecture at the 1991 AIChE Meeting in Los Angeles.

References

1. Stannett, V. T., Koros, W. J., Paul, D. R., Lonsdale, H. K., and Baker, R. W., *Adv. Poly. Sci.* **32**, 71 (1979).
2. Langer, R., and Folkman, J., *Nature (London)* **263**, 797 (1976).
3. Gimbrone, M. A., Jr., Contran, R. S., Leapman, S. B., and Folkman, J., *J. Natl. Cancer Inst. (U.S.)* **52**, 413 (1974).
4. Davis, B. K., *Proc. Natl. Acad. Sci. U.S.A.* **71**, 3120 (1974).
5. Langer, R., Brem, H., and Tapper, D., *J. Biomed. Mater. Res.* **15**, 267 (1981).
6. Rhine, W., Hsieh, D. S. T., and Langer, R., *J. Pharm. Sci.* **69**, 265 (1980).
7. Bawa, R., Siegel, R., Marasca, B., Karel, M., and Langer, R., *J. Controlled Release* **1**, 259 (1985).
8. Balazs, A. C., Calef, D. F., Deutch, J. M., Siegel, R. A., and Langer, R., *Biophys. J.* **47**, 97 (1985).
9. Siegel, R. A., and Langer, R., *J. Colloid Interfac. Sci.* **109**, 426 (1986).
10. Brown, L., Wei, C., and Langer, R. *J. Pharm. Sci.* **72**, 1181 (1983).
11. Hsieh, D., Rhine, W., and Langer, R. *J. Pharm. Sci.* **72**, 17 (1983).
12. Cohen, J., Siegel, R., and Langer, R., *J. Pharm. Sci.* **73**, 1034 (1984).
13. Sefton, M. V., Brown, L. R., and Langer, R., *J. Pharm. Sci.* **73**, 1859 (1984).
14. Cohen, S., Yoshioka, T., Lucarelli, M., Hwang, L. H., and Langer, R., *Pharm. Res.* **8**, 713 (1991).
15. Brown, L., Siemer, L., Muñoz, C., Edelman, E., and Langer, R., *Diabetes* **35**, 692 (1986).
16. Murray, J., Brown, L., Klagsbrun, M., and Langer, R., *In Vitro* **19**, 743 (1983).
17. Levy, R. J., Wolfrum, J., Schoen, F., Hawley, M., Lund, S. A., and Langer, R., *Science* **228**, 190 (1985).
18. Langer, R., Hsieh, D. S. T., Brown, L., and Rhine, W., *in* "Better Therapy with Existing Drugs: New Uses and Delivery Systems" (A. Bearn, ed.), p. 179. Merck & Company, Biomedical Information Corporation, New York, 1981.
19. Langer, R. S., and Folkman, J., *in* "Polymeric Delivery Systems, Midland Macromolecular Monograph" (R. J. Kostelnik, ed.), Vol. 5, p. 175. Gordon & Breach, New York, 1978.
20. Lee, A., and Langer, R. *Science* **221**, 1185 (1983).
21. During, M. J., Freese, A., Sabel, B. A., Saltzman, W. M., Deutch, A., Roth, R. H., and Langer, R., *Ann. Neur.* **25**, 351 (1989).
22. Leong, K. W., Simonte, V., and Langer, R., *Macromolecules* **20**, 705 (1987).
23. Domb, A., and Langer, R., *J. Polym. Sci.* **25**, 3373 (1987).
24. Domb, A., Ron, E., and Langer, R., *Macromolecules* **21**, 1925 (1988).
25. Leong, K. W., Brott, B. C., and Langer, R., *J. Biomed. Mater. Res.* **19**, 941 (1985).
26. Mathiowitz, E., and Langer, R., *J. Controlled Release* **5**, 13 (1987).
27. Mathiowitz, E., Saltzman, M., Domb, A., Dor, P., and Langer, R., *J. Appl. Polym. Sci.* **35**, 755 (1988).
28. Domb, A., and Langer, R., *Macromolecules* **19**, 189 (1988).
29. Brem, H., Mahaley, M. S., Vick, N. A., Black, K. L., Schold, S. C., Burger, P. C., Friedman, A. H., Ciric, I. S., Eller, T. W., Cozzens, J. W., and Kenealy, J. N., *J. Neurosurg.* **74**, 441 (1991).
30. Kohn, J., and Langer, R., *J. Am. Chem. Soc.* **109**, 817 (1987).

31. Preis, I., and Langer, R., *J. Immunol. Methods* **28**, 193 (1979).
32. Niemi, S., Fox, J., Brown, L., and Langer, R., *Lab. Anim. Sci.* **35**, 609 (1985).
33. Kohn, J., Niemi, S. M., Albert, E. C., Murphy, J. C., Langer, R., and Fox, J. G., *J. Immunol. Methods* **95**, 31 (1986).
34. Kohn, J., and Langer, R., *Biomaterials* **7**, 176 (1986).
35. Laurencin, C. T., Koh, H. J., Neenan, T. X., Alcock, H. R., and Langer, R., *J. Biomed. Mater. Res.* **21**, 1231 (1987).
36. Hsieh, D. S. T., Langer, R., and Folkman, J., *Proc. Natl. Acad. Sci. U.S.A.* **78**, 1863 (1981).
37. Edelman, E., Kost, J., Bobeck, H., and Langer, R., *J. Biomed. Mater. Res.* **19**, 67 (1985).
38. Kost, J., Noekker, R., Kunica, E., and Langer, R., *J. Biomed. Mater. Res.* **19**, 935 (1985).
39. McCarthy, M., Soong., D., and Edelman, E., *J. Controlled Release* **1**, 143 (1984).
40. Edelman, E., Brown, L., and Langer, R., *J. Biomed. Mater. Sci.* **21**, 339 (1987).
41. Kost, J., Wolfrum, J., and Langer, R., *J. Biomed. Mater. Res.* **21**, 1367 (1987).
42. Kost, J., Leong, K., and Langer, R., *Proc. Natl. Acad. Sci. U.S.A.* **86**, 7663 (1989a).
43. Kost, J., Leong, K., and Langer, R., *Makromol. Chem. Macromol. Symp.* **19**, 275 (1988).
44. Levy, D., Kost, J., Meshulam, Y., and Langer, R., *J. Clin. Invest.* **83**, 207 (1989).
45. Ghodsian, F. F., Brown, L., Mathiowitz, E., Brandenburg, D., and Langer, R., *Proc. Natl. Acad. Sci. U.S.A.* **85**, 2403 (1988).
46. Porter, J., and Fick, H., *JAMA, J. Am. Med. Assoc.* **237**, 879 (1977).
47. Bernstein, H., and Langer, R., *Proc. Natl. Acad. Sci. U.S.A.* **85**, 8751 (1988).
48. Bernstein, H., Yang, V. C., and Langer, R., *Biotechnol. Bioeng.* **30**, 239 (1987).
49. Bernstein, H., Yang, V. C., Cooney, C. L., and Langer, R., *in* "Methods in Enzymology" (K. Mosbach, ed.), Vol. 137, p. 515. Academic Press, San Diego, 1988.
50. Bernstein, H., Yang, V. C., and Langer, R., *Biotechnol. Bioeng.* **30**, 196 (1987).
51. Linhardt, R. J., Grant, A., Cooney, C. L., and Langer, R., *J. Biol. Chem.* **257**, 7310 (1982).
52. Yang, V. C., Linhardt, R. J., Bernstein, H., Cooney, C. L., and Langer, R., *J. Biol. Chem.* **260**, 1849 (1985).
53. Comfort, A. R., Albert, E., and Langer, R. *Biotechnol. Bioeng.* **34**, 1374 (1989).
54. Freed, L. E., Vunjak-Novakovic, G. V., Drinker, P. A., and Langer, R., *Ann. Biomed. Eng.* **21**, 57 (1993).
54a. Bernstein, H., Yang, V. C., and Langer, R., *Kidney. Int.* **30**, 196 (1987).
55. Lavin, A., Sung, C., Klibanov, A., and Langer, R., *Science* **230**, 543 (1985).
56. Mullon, C., Saltzman, W., and Langer, R., *Bio/Technology* **6**, 927 (1988).
57. Soltys, P., Mullon, C.J.-P., and Langer, R., *Artif. Organs* **16**, 331 (1992).
58. Labeque, R., Mullon, C.J.-P., Ferreira, J.-P.M., Lees, R. S., and Langer, R., *Proc. Natl. Acad. Sci. U.S.A.* **90**, 3476 (1993).
59. Folkman, J., and Haudenschild, C., *Nature (London)* **288**, 551 (1980).
60. Bissell, M. J., and Barcellos-Hoff, M. H., *J. Cell Sci.* **8**, 327 (1987).
61. Vacanti, J. P., Morse, M. A., Saltzman, W. M., Domb, A. J., Perez-Atayde, A., and Langer, R., *J. Pediat. Surg.* **23**, 3 (1988).
62. Vacanti, C. A., Langer, R., Schloo, B., and Vacanti, J. P., *J. Plast. Reconstr. Surg.* **88**, 753 (1991).
63. Cima, L., Ingber, D., Vacanti, J., and Langer, R., *Biotechnol. Bioeng.* **38**, 145 (1991).

64. Ben-Ze'ev, A., Robinson, G., Bucher, N. L. R., and Farmer, S., *Proc. Natl. Acad. Sci. U.S.A.* **85**, 1 (1988).
65. Folkman, J., and Moscona, A., *Nature (London)* **273**, 345 (1978).
66. Cima, L., Vacanti, J., Vacanti, C., Ingber, D., Mooney, D., and Langer, R., *J. Biomech. Eng.* **113**, 143 (1991).
67. Sudhakaran, P., R., Stamatoglou, S., and Hughes, R., *Exp. Cell Res.* **167**, 505 (1986).
68. Guguen-Guillouzo, C., Clement, B., Bafet, G., Beaumont, C., Morel-Chany, E., Glaise, D., and Guillouzo, A., *Exp. Cell Res.* **143**, 47 (1983).
69. Friedman, J. M., Chung, E. Y., and Darnell, J. E., Jr., *J. Mol. Biol.* **179**, 37 (1984).

DIFFUSION AND PROBABILITY IN RECEPTOR BINDING AND SIGNALING

J. J. Linderman,* P. A. Mahama,[†] K. E. Forsten,[‡] and D. A. Lauffenburger[§]

*Department of Chemical Engineering
University of Michigan
Ann Arbor, Michigan 48109

[†]Department of Chemical Engineering
University of Toledo
Toledo, Ohio 43606

[‡]Department of Chemical Engineering
Virginia Polytechnic Institute
and State University
Blacksburg, Virginia 24061

[§]Department of Chemical Engineering
University of Illinois at Urbana-Champaign
Urbana, Illinois 61801

ADVANCES IN CHEMICAL ENGINEERING, VOL. 19

I. Introduction

A central goal of many chemical engineers, bioengineers, cell biologists, molecular biologists, and biotechnologists today is to understand and manipulate cell behavior in terms of molecular properties. All may be interested, as an example, in learning how cell proliferation and/or cellular production of a particular protein product are affected by properties that directly reflect molecular structure, such as the affinity of a key regulatory component for its site of action. At the same time, these investigators may also desire to know the effect of properties that are less related to molecular structure, such as the cellular concentrations of the key regulatory component and its site of action. In both cases, what is needed is an ability to know how a change in any such properties may influence a particular cell function.

Great advances have been made toward this goal by the application of tools from molecular cell biology. Specific cellular constituents can be isolated, identified, and genetically or synthetically altered. Amounts of a particular component can be manipulated by expression levels or by microinjection. Molecular structures can be modified by site-directed mutagenesis or covalent chemistry. These tools provide an opportunity for investigating the effect of a molecular alteration and for developing technologies based on it. A major portion of effort by the pharmaceutical industry, for example, is aimed at constructing drugs that mimic, replace, or interfere with natural compounds which regulate cell function. For reproducible success in such efforts, as well as those directed toward other applications, reliable prediction of the consequences of changes in molecular properties will be vital.

Moreover, this predictive capability must be as quantitative as possible. Information such as that illustrated schematically in Fig. 1 would be of great assistance to analysis and design of molecular-based processes for manipulation of cell function, whether in scientific or industrial (health care, bioprocessing) applications. This figure shows that the dependence of a cell function (e.g., proliferation, secretion, movement) on a particular molecular property may be relatively insensitive or highly sensitive, and further that the dependence may not be monotonic. In order to decide how best to alter relevant molecular properties to bring about a desired cell behavior, we must be able to predict the corresponding relationships as accurately as possible.

Though there has been tremendous progress in the identification of molecular components involved in cell functions, this is only a beginning step in the process of understanding. It is not sufficient to study compo-

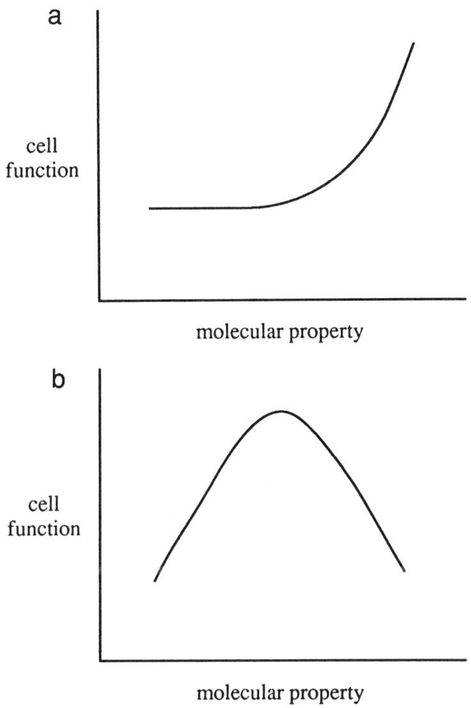

FIG. 1. Schematic relationship between a cell function and a molecular property. As examples, the property may be affinity, valency, concentration, or a rate constant, and the cell function may be proliferation, contraction, secretion, motility, or adhesion. (a) The sensitivity of a cell function to a particular molecular property may vary from insensitive to highly sensitive. (b) The cell response may not simply be an increasing or decreasing function of a particular molecular property.

nent molecules by themselves; quantitative integration of molecular parts will ultimately be required to understand the cellular whole. As Maddox (1992) writes in *Nature*, "...the neglect of quantitative considerations [in molecular biology] may well be a recipe for overlooking problems inherently of great importance." It is particularly in the quantitation of cell functions and their dependence of molecular properties that chemical engineers may play a role, for many of the tools used now to describe diffusion and reaction in non-biological situations may find applicability in this new arena.

Our aim in this article is to describe some mathematical approaches and models now being used to quantitatively understand the links between molecular properties and cell function. To narrow the scope of molecular components to be considered, we limit our attention to cell surface

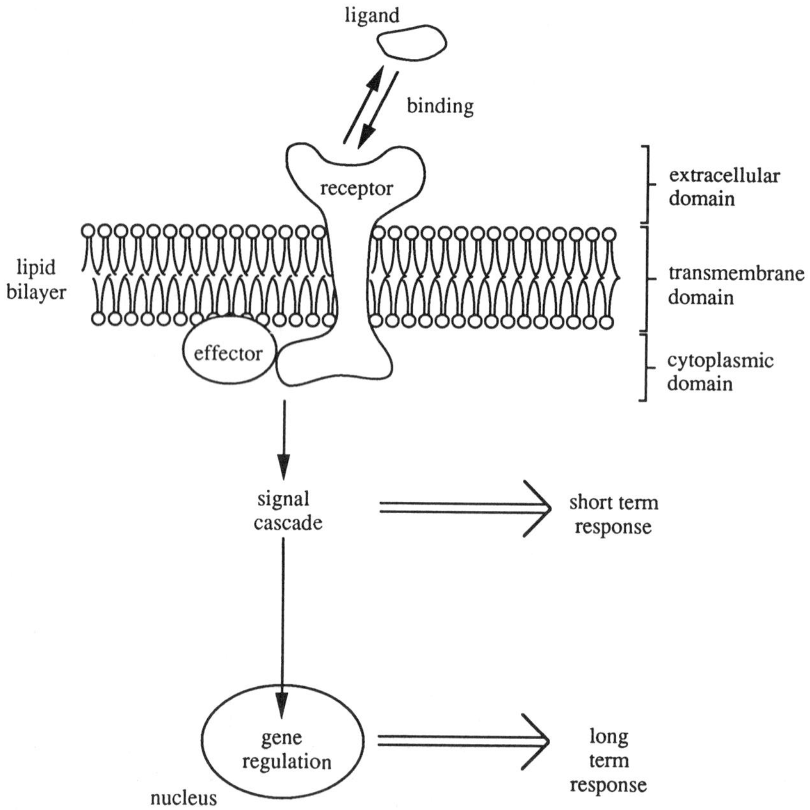

FIG. 2. Schematic structure of cell receptors and levels of complexity in receptor signaling. Bound receptors may initiate a cascade of intracellular reactions that lead to short- and/or long-term responses.

receptors. Receptors, as shown in Fig. 2, possess an extracellular domain for binding ligands (e.g., growth factors, hormones, adhesion molecules), a transmembrane domain, and an intracellular or cytoplasmic domain. We choose to focus on receptors for two reasons. First, receptor-driven cell behavior is now known to be extremely important—for example, growth, secretion, contraction, motility, and adhesion are all receptor-mediated cell behaviors. Receptors are uniquely able to direct such cell behavior by virtue of their ability to sense the environment, through binding of ligands, and their ability to transmit this signal to the cell interior, through interaction of their intracellular domains with enzymes and proteins within the cell. Second, receptors and their ligands are ideal candidates for manipulation. For example, cell and molecular biologists can now alter the structure of a receptor and its ligand, thereby modifying association and dissociation rate constants and signaling capabilities. This sort of manipulation provides a straightforward tool for the testing of hypotheses as to the role these molecular properties play in directing cell function.

As illustrated in Figs. 2 and 3, receptor-mediated cell functions are highly complicated phenomena. Receptor signaling induced by ligand binding is itself a process with multiple aspects, and these events are only a subset of the many concurrent dynamic events involving receptors. Following Fig. 2, the first step is the binding of ligands to receptors at the cell surface. Bound receptors can activate various intracellular enzymes and entire cascades of intracellular reactions. Some of these reactions trigger short-term (on the order of milliseconds to minutes) responses. Long-term (on the order of hours or more) responses, such as those requiring protein synthesis, involve additional molecular interactions. Each step is characterized by parameters such as rate constants and concentrations which are in principle measurable and alterable. At the same time, as shown in Fig. 3, the receptor population is undergoing events of coupling with other cell surface molecules, internalization, recycling, degradation, and synthesis—the whole pathway termed trafficking.

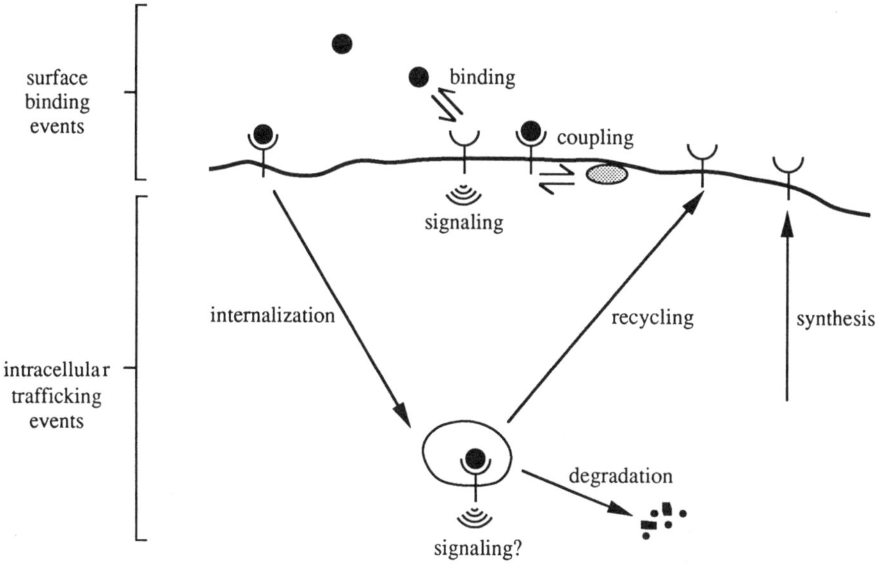

FIG. 3. Levels of complexity in receptor state and location. Receptors may be unbound, bound, or coupled with other membrane-associated molecules. Receptors and their ligands may be internalized and routed through intracellular compartments. Both receptors at the cell surface and receptors inside the cell may have signaling capabilities, although these capabilities are likely to be a function of the receptor state and location.

In this article, we will focus on the role of receptors in binding and signaling. In particular, we will examine approaches for dealing with two physical aspects which may affect such processes: molecular transport (primarily diffusion) and probabilistic effects due to relatively small numbers of molecules. These effects may be particularly important in describing cell receptor phenomena. For example, the interaction of two cell surface molecules, e.g., two receptors or a receptor and a membrane-associated signal transducing molecule, is likely to be diffusion-limited. Probabilistic effects are likely to be important because of the small number of molecules involved in many relevant reactions. In Section II, we will discuss the relevant background for these topics. We will review analytical approaches to both topics in Sections III and IV. Finally, in Section V we will apply these ideas to understanding two aspects of receptor/ligand binding and signal transduction. Computer simulation methods will be highlighted in these applications.

Readers interested in a more comprehensive treatment of cell receptor phenomena as outlined in this introduction are referred to the recently published book by Lauffenburger and Linderman (1993).

II. Background

A. Receptor/Ligand Binding Fundamentals

We will consider here only the simplest possibility, reversible binding between a free (not bound by ligand) receptor R and a free ligand L to form a receptor/ligand complex C, as illustrated in Fig. 2 or written as

$$R + L \underset{k_r}{\overset{k_f}{\rightleftarrows}} C.$$

We assume that the ligand and receptor are both monovalent. Because monovalent receptors and ligands by definition have only one binding site, no additional receptors or ligands of the same type can bind to the complex. The relevant rate constants are the association rate constant, k_f, and the dissociation rate constant, k_r. For typical units of the free receptor number, R[#/cell], free ligand concentration L[M], and receptor/ligand complex number C[#/cell], the units of k_f and k_r are M^{-1} $time^{-1}$ and $time^{-1}$, respectively. (Henceforth throughout this article, appropriate units for model variables and parameters will be listed in the Notation section.) We will use italic symbols (e.g., R, L, and C) to denote numbers and concentrations of receptor and ligand species. Although receptors might be expressed in terms of concentration (moles/volume solution) or density (#/cell surface area), it is best for most purposes to express the receptor number as simply #/cell. Knowledge of the cell surface area or number of cells per volume solution can be used to convert R into density or concentration units when desired.

Thermodynamic principles dictate that the free receptor and complex numbers and ligand concentration are related at chemical equilibrium through the equilibrium dissociation constant $K_D = k_r/k_f$:

$$C = \frac{RL}{K_D}. \tag{1}$$

A small value of K_D, corresponding to a large value of the equilibrium association constant, $K_A = k_f/k_r = 1/K_D$, indicates a high affinity of the receptor for the ligand. The values of K_D for various systems fall within a wide range, with 10^{-12} M near the high-affinity end [the avidin/biotin bond with $K_D = 10^{-15}$ M (Green, 1975), is an extreme exception] to 10^{-6} at the low-affinity end. Sample values of K_D and the rate constants k_f and k_r, typically measured by analyzing the time course of radio- or fluorescent-labeled ligand binding or dissociation (Limbird, 1986; Hulme, 1992), can be found in Table I.

Let ligand be present in the extracellular medium at initial concentration L_0, receptors be present on the cell surface at constant number R_T, and cells be present at concentration n [#/volume medium]. We will assume here that the medium is well mixed, so that the ligand is available at uniform concentration from a macroscopic point of view.

The most common (and simplest) approach is to describe receptor/ligand binding from a deterministic approach, assuming no significant role for probabilistic events. The deterministic equation describing the time rate of change of the receptor/ligand complex density C as a function of the free receptor number R and the ligand concentration L is

$$\frac{dC}{dt} = k_f RL - k_f C. \tag{2}$$

If we restrict our attention to situations in which the cohort of surface receptors is unchanged, the total surface receptor number R_T is constant. If we also assume that the total amount of ligand is unchanged, the following conservation laws apply at all times:

$$R_T = R + C, \tag{3a}$$

$$L_0 = L + \left(\frac{n}{N_{Av}}\right)C, \tag{3b}$$

TABLE I

SAMPLE RECEPTOR/LIGAND BINDING PARAMETERS[a]

Receptor	Ligand	Cell type	R_T (#/cell)	k_f (M^{-1} min^{-1})	k_r (min^{-1})	K_D (M)	$t_{95\%}$ ($L_0 = K_D$) (min)	Reference
Transferrin	Transferrin	HepG2	5×10^4	3×10^6	0.1	3.3×10^{-8}	15	Ciechanover *et al.* (1983)
Fc_γ	2.4G2 Fab	Mouse macrophage	7.1×10^5	3×10^6	0.0023	7.7×10^{-10}	650	Mellman and Unkeless (1980)
Chemotactic peptide	FNLLP	Rabbit neutrophil	5×10^4	2×10^7	0.4	2×10^{-8}	3.7	Zigmond *et al.* (1982)
Interferon	Human interferon-α_2a	A549	900	2.2×10^8	0.072	3.3×10^{-10}	20	Bajzer *et al.* (1989)
TNF	TNF	A549	6.6×10^3	9.6×10^8	0.14	1.5×10^{-10}	11	Bajzer *et al.* (1989)
β-adrenergic	Hydroxybenzylpindolol	Turkey erythrocyte	—	8×10^8	0.08	1×10^{-10}	19	Rimon *et al.* (1980)
α_1-adrenergic	Prazosin	BC3H1	1.4×10^4	2.4×10^8	0.018	7.5×10^{-11}	83	Hughes *et al.* (1982)
Insulin	Insulin	Rat fat cells	1×10^5	9.6×10^6	0.2	2.1×10^{-8}	7.5	Lipkin *et al.* (1986)
EGF	EGF	Fetal rat lung	2.5×10^4	1.8×10^8	0.12	6.7×10^{-10}	7.5	Waters *et al.* (1990)
Fibronectin	Fibronectin	Fibroblasts	5×10^5	7×10^5	0.6	8.6×10^{-7}	2.5	Akiyama and Yamada (1985)
FC_ε	IgE	Human basophils	—	3.1×10^6	0.0015	4.8×10^{-10}	1000	Pruzansky and Patterson (1986)
IL-2 (heavy chain)	IL-2	T lymphocytes	2×10^3	2.3×10^7	0.015	6.5×10^{-10}	100	Smith (1988b)
IL-2 (light chain)			1.1×10^4	8.4×10^8	24.0	2.9×10^{-8}	0.06	
IL-2 (heterodimer)			2×10^3	1.9×10^9	0.014	7.4×10^{-12}	110	

[a]Shown are the measured number of receptors per cell R_T, the association rate constant k_f, the dissociation rate constant k_r, and the equilibrium dissociation, constant $K_D = k_r/k_f$. The time required to reach 95% of equilibrium receptor binding when no bound receptors are initially, present, $t_{95\%}$, is calculated from $t_{95\%} = -\ln(0.05)/[k_r(1 + L_0/K_D)]$ for the case of $L_0 = K_D$. HepG2 = human hepatoma cell line; 2.4G2 Fab = Fab portion of 2.4G2 antibody against receptor; FNLLP = *N*-formylnorleucylleucylphenylalanine; A549 = human lung alveolar carcinoma; TNF = tumor necrosis factor; hydroxybenzylpindolol is an antagonist to the receptor; EGF = epidermal growth factor; IgE = immunoglobulin E; IL-2 = interleukin 2; prazosin is an antagonist to the receptor; BC3H1 = smooth muscle-like cell line; RBL = rat basophilic leukemia cell line.

where N_{Av} is Avogadro's number. Use of these two conservation laws together with Eq. (2) allows us to describe the system with a single ordinary differential equation:

$$\frac{dC}{dt} = k_{\mathrm{f}}[R_{\mathrm{T}} - C]\left[L_0 - \left(\frac{n}{N_{\mathrm{Av}}}\right)C\right] - k_{\mathrm{f}}C. \tag{4}$$

Because this equation follows only cell-associated ligand that is bound to cell surface receptors, this formulation assumes that nonspecific binding of ligand to the cell surface has been already corrected for [Munson and Rodbard (1980), Hulme (1992), and Lauffenburger and Linderman (1993)].

In the limiting case of $(n/N_{\mathrm{Av}})C \ll L_0$, we may neglect ligand depletion (or accumulation, for dissociation experiments) in the medium and instead assume that the ligand concentration remains constant at its initial value, L_0. Equation (4) then simplifies to

$$\frac{dC}{dt} = k_{\mathrm{f}}[R_{\mathrm{T}} - C]L_0 - k_{\mathrm{r}}C. \tag{5}$$

With imposition of an initial condition $C(t = 0) = C_0$ we obtain the transient solution, $C(t)$:

$$C(t) = C_0 \exp\{-(k_{\mathrm{f}}L_0 + k_{\mathrm{f}})t\} + \left(\frac{k_{\mathrm{f}}L_0R_{\mathrm{T}}}{k_{\mathrm{f}}L_0 + k_{\mathrm{r}}}\right)$$
$$\times\left[1 - \exp\{-(k_{\mathrm{f}}L_0 + k_{\mathrm{r}})t\}\right]. \tag{6}$$

The number of receptor/ligand complexes at equilibrium, C_{eq}, is in this case identical to the steady-state value at which $dC/dt = 0$ and is asymptotically approached for $t \gg (k_{\mathrm{f}}L_0 + k_{\mathrm{r}})^{-1}$:

$$C_{\mathrm{eq}} = \frac{R_{\mathrm{T}}L_0}{K_{\mathrm{D}} + L_0}. \tag{7}$$

Alternatively, in dimensionless form, we define the dimensionless number of complexes u,

$$u = C/R_{\mathrm{T}}, \tag{8}$$

and the dimensionless time τ,

$$\tau = k_{\mathrm{r}}t, \tag{9}$$

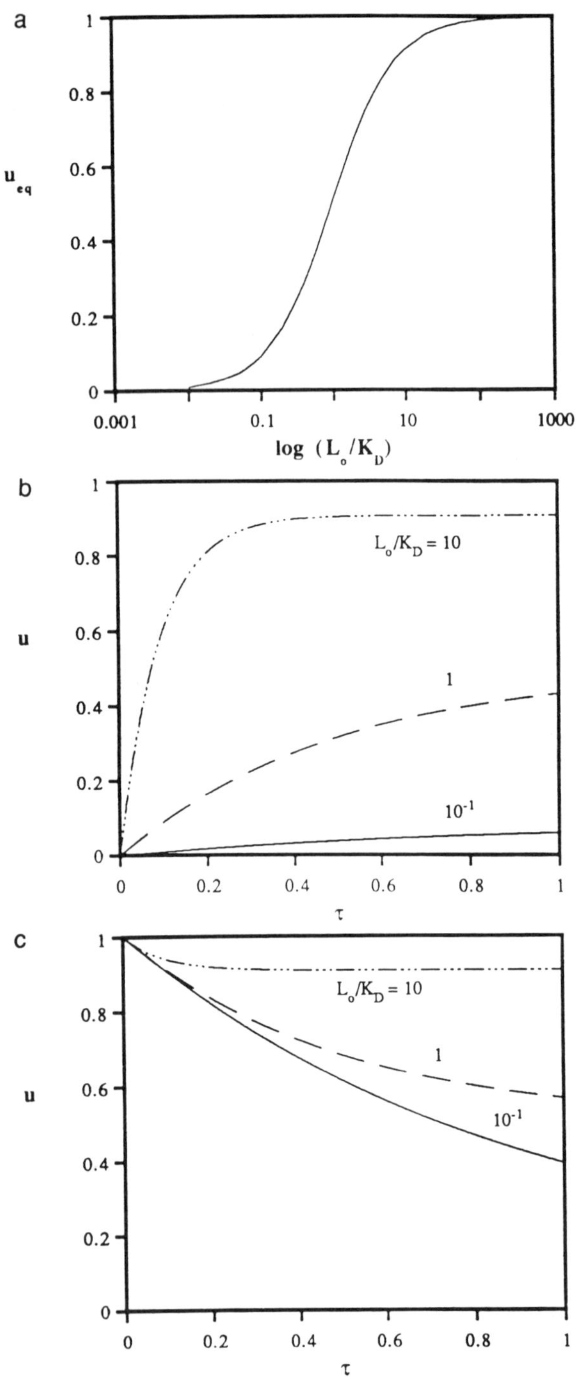

a
1
0.8
0.6
0.4
0.2
0
u_{eq}
0.001
0.1
10
1000
log (L_o/K_D)
b
u
$L_o/K_D = 10$
1
10^{-1}
0
0.2
0.4
0.6
0.8
1
τ
c
u
$L_o/K_D = 10$
1
10^{-1}
0
0.2
0.4
0.6
0.8
1
τ

and Eq. (5) becomes

$$\frac{du}{d\tau} = (1-u)\frac{L_0}{K_D} - u, \tag{10}$$

with solution

$$u(t) = u_0 \exp\left\{-\left(1 + \frac{L_0}{K_D}\right)\tau\right\} + \frac{(L_0/K_D)}{1 + (L_0/K_D)} \times \left[1 - \exp\left\{-\left(1 + \frac{L_0}{K_D}\right)\tau\right\}\right], \tag{11}$$

$$u_{eq} = \frac{(L_0/K_D)}{1 + (L_0/K_D)}. \tag{12}$$

In Fig. 4a, the dimensionless equilibrium number of complexes u_{eq} is plotted as a function of the dimensionless ligand concentration L_0/K_D. It is convenient to note that $u_{eq} = C_{eq}/R_T = 0.5$ when $L_0/K_D = 1$; in other words, half of the receptors are bound by ligand at equilibrium when the ligand concentration is equal to the value of K_D.

Figure 4b depicts the transient solution $u(\tau)$ for a sample association "experiment" when the initial condition is $u_0 = C_0/R_T = 0$. The dimensionless half-time $\tau_{1/2}$ for this transient, defined as the value of τ needed to yield half the change from $u_0 = 0$ to u_{eq}, is given by $\tau_{1/2} = 0.69/[1 + (L_0/K_D)]$. In this case, binding deviates from its equilibrium value by less than 5% after roughly three half-times, or $t \sim 2/(k_r[1 + (L_0/K_D)])$. Figure 4c shows a sample dissociation "experiment" starting with the initial condition $C_0/R_T = 1$; i.e., all receptors are initially bound.

We have neglected here many considerations that may complicate analyses of receptor/ligand binding: nonspecific binding, depletion of ligand concentration, cooperativity, multiple receptor states and interconversion between those receptor states, crosslinking of receptors by multivalent ligands, and trafficking (internalization/recycling) of receptors and

---

FIG. 4. Transient and equilibrium binding of ligand to cell surface receptors for the case of ligand concentration L approximately constant and equal to L_0. The fraction of total surface receptors bound, u, is shown. (a) The equilibrium value, u_{eq}, is plotted as a function of the logarithm of the ratio L_0/K_D. (b), (c) u is plotted as function of scaled time τ for several values of the ratio L_0/K_D. The initial value and time course of u in (b) correspond to an association experiment. The initial value and time course of u in (c) correspond to a dissociation experiment.

ligands through the cell. These and other complexities are discussed in detail elsewhere (Lauffenburger and Linderman, 1993).

B. Probabilistic Issues

In our discussion of simple receptor/ligand binding, we assumed that all cells have R_T receptors and behave identically. In other words, the unique solution to Eqs. (4), (5), or (10) was presumed to describe each and every cell in the system under study. In reality, of course, this solution represents the mean behavior of the system, and individual cells may show some deviations from the mean behavior. In addition to deviations from the mean behavior caused by, for example, slightly different numbers of receptors on individual cells (Mahama and Linderman, 1994a), these deviations may be due to the probabilistic, or stochastic, nature of the system.

When there are very large number of molecules present in a chemically reacting system, a great number of reaction events will occur in a small amount of time, allowing us to mathematically describe the overall rate of change of complex number in an average sense. For instance, we can follow the change in the mean number per cell of receptor/ligand complexes, C, with time for simple receptor/ligand binding by using Eqs. (4), (5), or (10). There are no explicit considerations of probability in these equations, and they are known as deterministic differential equations. Their solution uniquely determines the dynamics of the receptor/ligand binding process they model, giving the exact number of complexes and free receptors and concentration of ligand at any instant in time. In truth, however, these exact numbers are only the mean behavior expected in this situation and hence will be accurate only in that sense. In principle, receptor/ligand binding experiments should show fluctuations around a mean. As the number of participating molecules decreases, the greater the relative magnitude of these probabilistic, or stochastic, deviations (e.g., McQuarrie, 1963). It must be emphasized that these deviations have nothing to do with biochemical heterogeneity of a system, but rather arise inherently as a statistical process in a perfectly homogeneous system.

Although the probabilistic nature of a chemically reacting system may be interesting in the abstract, for most traditional applications of chemical reaction models the number of molecules present is usually so great that a deterministic model is entirely adequate. However, in cell biology, when we are concerned with the rates of reactions within a given cell, the number of molecules available for any given reaction may be comparatively small, with corresponding opportunity for relatively significant probabilistic fluctuations. Relevant examples may include the observation of probabilistic distributions of microtubule lengths (Mitchison and Kirschner, 1984), bacterial chemotactic response trigger molecules (Spudich and Koshland, 1976), and ion channel openings (Faber *et al.*, 1992). In considering cell receptors, we note that sometimes there are as few as 100 to 10,000 of a particular type present on a cell surface. Further, it has become apparent that cell behavior can be influenced in an exquisitely sensitive way to very small levels of signal through intracellular amplification cascades (Taylor, 1990).

In addition, modern techniques for following receptor/ligand binding and events triggered by binding are often able to give us information at the level of single cells. For example, flow cytometry allows data on thousands of individual cells to be collected in a matter of seconds. Many researchers now follow single-cell behavior, such as increases in intracellular ion concentrations, adhesion to surfaces, and migration paths, by video microcopy. In these data, differences between cells likely to be the result of stochastic effects are indeed observable.

For these reasons, then, an ability to quantitatively model and analyze receptor/ligand binding from a probabilistic viewpoint will turn out to be quite useful. In at least a few applications so far, probabilistic models of receptor/ligand binding have provided excellent interpretations of cell behavior. In Section III, we will examine mathematical approaches to dealing with these probabilistic effects and estimating their impact. In Section V, we will discuss the applications of probabilistic models to cell receptor binding and signaling.

C. Diffusion

Diffusion plays an important role in receptor binding and signaling. Ligand molecules present in solution must first reach receptors before binding can occur. The distance over which diffusion or, more generally, molecular transport takes place depends on the source of the ligand. Endocrine ligands, or hormones, must travel through the bloodstream to reach their target cells. Paracrine ligands such as epidermal growth factor (EGF) are secreted by source cells and then diffuse to target cells within the same tissue. Autocrine ligands such as interleukin-2 (IL-2) and platelet-derived growth factor (PDGF) are those for which the source and target cell are the same, so that the ligand acts on the cell that released it and, presumably, on similar cells nearby. Typical ligand diffusion coefficients are on the order of 10^{-7} to 10^{-5} cm^2/s. Depending on factors such as the ligand diffusivity, number of receptors, and intrinsic receptor/ligand binding kinetics, the binding of solution ligands to cell surface receptors may be transport- or reaction-limited. This situation is analyzed in detail in Sections IV, B and IV, D and a model for autocrine ligand binding is presented in Section V, A.

Furthermore, receptors and other proteins are known to diffuse in the plasma membrane. Such mobility is an important physical aspect to modeling receptor-mediated phenomena, for receptor diffusion may allow receptor coupling with another receptor, cytoskeletal elements, and other membrane-associated components. For example, a receptor to which a bivalent ligand is bound may diffuse close to a second, unbound receptor, allowing the ligand to simultaneously bind (or crosslink) both receptors. As a second example (analyzed in Section V, B), receptors may interact with and thus activate membrane-associated molecules or "effectors" such as GTP-binding proteins (G-proteins). G-proteins then in turn act on other molecules in the cell, and thus play the role of transmitting the external message of a bound ligand into an intracellular message and an eventual cellular response (Taylor, 1990; Birnbaumer, 1992). The importance of receptor mobility to such interactions was originally termed the "mobile receptor hypothesis" (Jacobs and Cuatrecasas, 1976; Jans, 1992). The idea is that receptors and "effectors" are separate entities that couple only when they "find" each other via diffusion, an event often termed collision coupling. We note that these sorts of coupling processes can significantly alter the equilibrium and kinetic binding properties of a receptor with its ligand (Lauffenburger and Linderman, 1993).

Typical values of the receptor translational diffusion coefficient D_R in cell membranes found by fluorescence recovery after photobleaching (FRAP) (Axelrod *et al.*, 1976; Edidin *et al.*, 1976), post-electrophoresis relaxation (PER) (Poo *et al.*, 1979), and single-particle tracking (Sheetz and Elson, 1993) methods fall in the range 10^{-11} to 10^{-9} cm^2/s. Using this range, we can estimate the time t for receptor traverse across a cell surface from $t \sim d^2/4D_R$, where d is the distance to be traveled. For a cell radius of 5 μm, $d \sim 5\pi$ μm, and thus $t \sim$ 10 minutes to 17 hours. The mobile fraction of receptors, the fraction of receptors that is able to freely diffuse on the cell surface, often falls between 0.1 and 1 (Gennis, 1989); some receptors are apparently constrained by linkages to the cytoskeleton or other cellular components.

A theoretical prediction for the receptor translational diffusion coefficient D_R based on viscous interactions of proteins with membrane lipids was derived by Saffman and Delbruck (1975). In their hydrodynamic model, a solitary cylindrical protein (i.e., a protein at infinite dilution) of radius s embedded in a membrane of thickness h and viscosity η_m, surrounded on both (extracellular and intracellular) sides by a solution of viscosity η_s, is predicted to have a translational diffusion coefficient given by

$$D_R = \left[\frac{K_B T}{4\pi\eta_m h}\right](-\gamma_E + \ln\theta), \tag{13}$$

where K_B is Boltzmann's constant, γ_E is Euler's constant, and $\theta = \eta_m h/\eta_s s$ is a ratio of membrane to solution viscosities (assumed $\gg 1$ for this derivation to hold). A value of approximately $D_R \sim 10^{-8}$ cm^2/s is obtained for the set of parameter values $K_B T = 4 \times 10^{-14}$ g-cm^2/s^2 (at 37°C), $h = 10$ nm, $s = 2$ nm, $\eta_m = 2$ g/cm-s, and $\eta_s = 0.01$ g/cm-s. This estimate is roughly one to three orders of magnitude greater than typical experimentally measured values for D_R, though a few membrane proteins —notably rhodopsin on photoreceptor cells (Wey and Cone, 1981)—possess diffusivities very close to the theoretical limit.

There are several possible explanations for this discrepancy, as reviewed by Gennis (1989) and Sheetz (1993). Receptor diffusion would be restricted by immobile and mobile obstacles (Saxton, 1990); however, in most cases these barriers do not appear to be present in sufficient density to restrict receptor diffusion to this extent. Alternatively, receptor diffusion may be slowed by the interaction of receptors with cytoskeletal components or other membrane-associated macromolecules. This could also account for the existence of a fraction of receptors deemed to be immobile on typical experimental time scales ($D_R < 10^{-12}$ cm^2/s). Experimental support for this explanation is provided by measurements of much larger values of D_R, close to the theoretical estimate, for LDL receptors on cell membrane regions known to be absent of cytoskeletal connections (Barak and Webb, 1982) and for bacteriorhodopsin in reconstituted lipid vesicles (Peters and Cherry, 1982). The interaction of receptors with membrane-associated molecules has also been suggested as the reason why even fairly small receptor oligomers exhibit a diffusivity more than an order of magnitude lower than their subunit monomers (Menon *et al.*, 1986; Baird *et al.*, 1988), for such an interaction would depend strongly on the number of receptors in the aggregate. [Note that Eq. (13) predicts only a weak (logarithmic) dependence on the size of the aggregate.] In fact, the extracellular, transmembrane, and/or intracellular domains of membrane receptors may each interact with other macromolecules present in the local extracellular environment (Wier and Edidin, 1988; Sheetz, 1993). Compilation of diffusion measurements for membrane proteins with different structural features may permit development of general rules governing mobility (Zhang *et al.*, 1991). Sheetz (1993) suggests that Eq. (13) may need to be revised to include the separate effects of the external, bilayer, and internal viscous fluid.

An alternative and very recent explanation for the poor correspondence of Eq. (13) with experimental measurements of D_R has been offered by Bussell *et al.* (1992, 1994a, b). They argue that hydrodynamic interactions *between* proteins may be important even at low protein concentrations, and show that inclusion of these hydrodynamic interactions together with excluded area (obstacle) effects mentioned earlier quantitatively account for experimental data.

Measurements of the mobility of membrane-associated components, particularly those associating with the cytoplasmic side of the lipid bilayer and positioned to interact with the intracellular domain of the receptor, are few (Bruckert *et al.*, 1992; Kwon and Neubig, 1992; Kwon, 1992). Measurements of the diffusivity of membrane-associated "effectors" (see Fig. 2), for example, will be important in determining the role of diffusion in receptor/effector coupling and signal transduction.

III. Probabilistic Formulation of Receptor / Ligand Binding

For purposes of instruction, we wish to construct a probabilistic formulation of the simple case considered in Section II, A, that of receptor/ligand binding in the absence of significant ligand depletion and nonspecific binding effects. We will consider two distinctly different sources of fluctuations: (1) fluctuations in local ligand concentration, and (2) fluctuations in receptor/ligand binding processes.

A. Fluctuations in Ligand Concentration

We will examine first fluctuating ligand concentration, for it is the ligand concentration that cell surface receptors detect. Although the bulk ligand concentration L is typically known and may, for most purposes, be considered constant, the actual ligand concentration very near a particular cell will vary with time because of the random, thermal fluctuations of molecular diffusion (see Fig. 5). It is, of course, this latter ligand concentration that the cell actually "samples" with surface receptors. Thus, random fluctuations in the ligand concentration near a cell may result in deviations in the number of bound receptors from the mean behavior predicted by deterministic models.

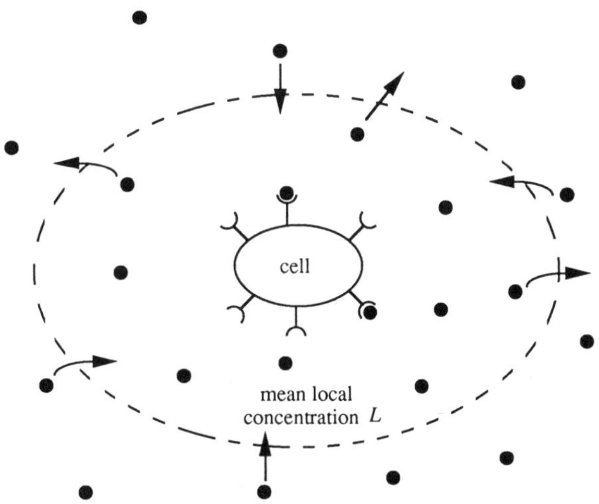

$$V \sim \left[\left(\frac{D_L}{k_r} \right)^{1/2} \right]^3$$

FIG. 5. Variation in the ligand concentration around an individual cell. The cell samples only the ligand concentration in its local environment of approximately volume V.

For simplicity, we will examine only the effect of these fluctuations on the equilibrium number of bound receptors. Consider the equilibrium solution of the kinetic equation for simple ligand binding to cell surface receptors [Eq. (7)]. If there are random, thermal fluctuations δL of ligand concentration in the volume of medium accessible to receptor binding, these will lead to corresponding fluctuations in the equilibrium number of complexes C_{eq} according to

$$\delta C_{eq} = \frac{dC_{eq}}{dL} \delta L = \frac{R_T K_D}{(K_D + L)^2} \delta L, \tag{14}$$

where δC_{eq} is the standard deviation in C_{eq} as a result of a δL, the standard deviation in the value of L (Tranquillo, 1990). The relative magnitude of these fluctuations in receptor binding is given by

$$\frac{\delta C_{eq}}{C_{eq}} = \left[1 + \left(\frac{L}{K_D} \right) \right]^{-1} \frac{\delta L}{L}. \tag{15}$$

Equation (15) dictates, for example, that at a mean or bulk ligand concentration of $L = K_D$, a 10% fluctuation in local ligand concentration (i.e., the ligand concentration that the cell detects) translates into a 5% fluctuation in equilibrium receptor occupancy.

In order to use Eq. (15) to calculate the expected effect of fluctuations in ligand concentration on equilibrium receptor binding, we need to estimate a value for the term $\delta L/L$. Estimates for thermal fluctuations in local ligand concentration can be easily obtained (Tranquillo and Lauffenburger, 1987a). The magnitude of $\delta L/L$ is approximately

$$\delta L/L = (N_{\text{Av}} LV)^{-1/2}, \tag{16}$$

where V is the "sampling volume" of medium accessible to ligand binding and the product $N_{\text{Av}} LV$ is simply the expected number of ligand molecules in the sampling volume if there were no such fluctuations. To specify the volume V, we assume that $V \sim l^3$, where l is a characteristic system dimension. The average distance or length that a diffusing molecule will travel in a time period t_{sample} is $l \sim (D_{\text{L}} t_{\text{sample}})^{1/2}$, where D_{L} is the translational diffusion coefficient of the ligand. A estimate for t_{sample} is given by k_{r}^{-1} for receptor/ligand binding, since that is the mean time period between receptor binding events at steady state when $L = K_{\text{D}}$. Hence, $V \sim (D_{\text{L}}/k_{\text{r}})^{3/2}$. To determine the value of $\delta L/L$ at $L = K_{\text{D}}$, then, we simply substitute this estimate for V into Eq. (16) to find $\delta L/L = [(k_{\text{r}}^{3/2})/(N_{\text{Av}} K_{\text{D}} D_{\text{L}}^{3/2})]^{1/2}$. For the parameter value ranges of $D_{\text{L}} = 10^{-7}$ to 10^{-5} cm^2/s, $k_{\text{r}} = 10^{-4}$ to 10^{-1} s^{-1}, and $K_{\text{D}} = 10^{-10}$ to 10^{-6} M, we find that $\delta L/L \sim 10^{-7}$ to 10^{-1}, or 10^{-5}% to 10%. The high end of this range should be achieved only rarely, for ligands with high affinity but large dissociation rate constant and low diffusivity. Most commonly, the lower, negligible end of the range will be applicable. Thus, fluctuations in ligand concentration are unlikely to contribute significantly to deviations from mean or deterministic equilibrium receptor binding. In other words, the "signal" of extracellular ligand concentration that the cell must detect is unlikely to vary significantly as a result of thermal fluctuations.

B. Fluctuations in Kinetic Binding Processes

The second and more likely source of deviations in the number of bound receptors from the mean behavior predicted by deterministic models is fluctuating reaction kinetics. Stated another way, the "signal" of ligand concentration analyzed earlier may be relatively constant, but the "detector" of surface receptors may contribute random errors caused by the probabilistic nature of the binding event. The rate constant for a chemical reaction represents the time-probability that the reaction will occur for any particular reactant molecule. For instance, when we write k_r with units of time^{-1} to characterize the rate constant for dissociation of a receptor/ligand complex into its component receptor and ligand molecules, that rate constant can be alternatively interpreted as the probability per unit time that a single complex will, in fact, dissociate. In other words, as the time interval Δt gets small, at most one dissociation event will occur on a particular receptor, and the probability of that event is approximately $k_r \Delta t$. A similar situation exists for the association step, where $k_f L$ actually represents the probability per unit time (at a given ligand concentration) that a receptor will bind a ligand to form a complex. See Fig. 6 for an illustration of this concept. These fluctuations can be analyzed using a probabilistic, so-called "population balance," model for receptor/ligand complexes in place of the deterministic model [Eq. (4), (5), or (10)]. An excellent background text for this approach is Gardiner (1983).

Consider the association and dissociation events that might occur during a short time interval Δt. If we choose this time interval to be small enough, at most one event of each type can take place. Let $P_j(t)$ represent the probability that there are j complexes on a cell at time t. We can then write a kinetic equation describing changes in the number of complexes during Δt, given that there are C complexes present at time t:

$$\begin{aligned} P_C(t + \Delta t) - P_C(t) = {} & k_f L[R_T - (C - 1)]P_{C-1}(t)\,\Delta t \\ & -k_f L[R_T - C]P_C(t)\,\Delta t - k_r C P_C(t)\,\Delta t \\ & +k_r(C + 1)P_{C+1}(t)\,\Delta t. \end{aligned} \tag{17}$$

In this equation, the first and second terms on the right-hand side represent the probability that there were $C - 1$ and C complexes, respectively, present at time t and one binding event occurred during Δt; the third and fourth terms represent the probability that there were C and $C + 1$ complexes, respectively, present at time t and one dissociation event occurred. (Terms of higher order in Δt are neglected based on our assumption that the time interval is sufficiently short that at most one event can happen.) In the limit $\Delta t \sim 0$, this discrete-time equation can be rewritten as a differential equation:

$$\begin{aligned} \frac{dP_C}{dt} = {} & k_f L[R_T - (C - 1)]P_{C-1} + k_r(C + 1)P_{C+1} \\ & -\{k_f L[R_T - C] + k_r C\}P_C, \qquad C = 1, 2, 3, \ldots, (R_T - 1). \end{aligned} \tag{18a}$$

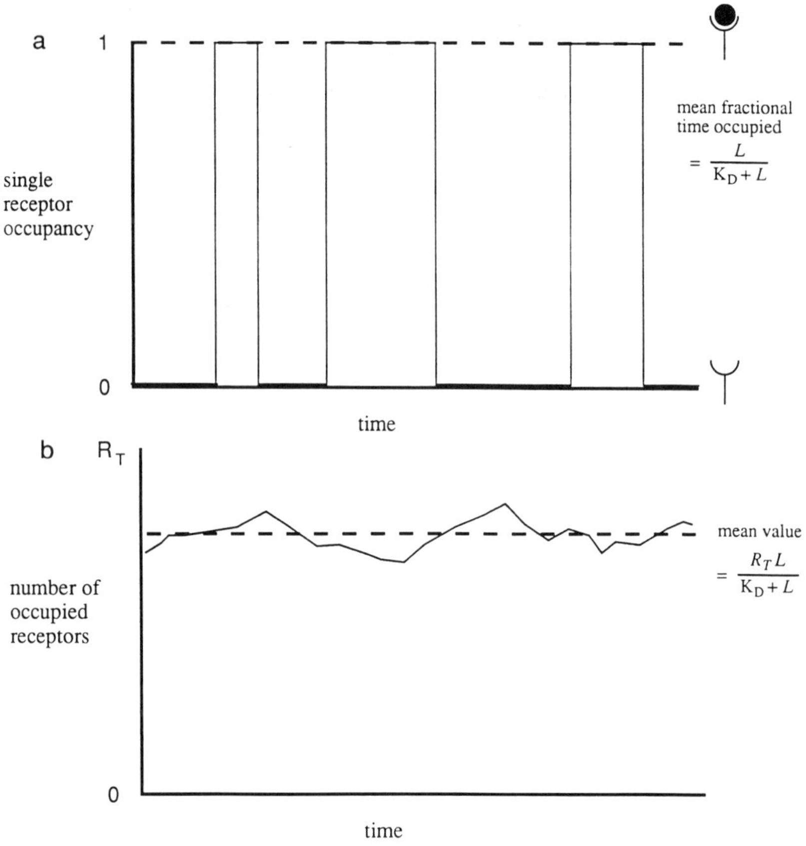

FIG. 6. Variation in equilibrium receptor occupancy. (a) A fictional history of the occupancy of a single receptor is shown. The state of the receptor jumps between 0, unbound, and 1, bound. The mean fraction of time that a particular receptor is occupied is given by $L/(K_D + L)$. (b) The actual number of receptors bound on a single cell following a long exposure to a constant ligand concentration is plotted as a function of time. The mean or deterministic prediction for the equilibrium number of bound receptors is $R_T L/(K_D + L)$.

Note that there are $(R_T - 1)$ such equations, for $C = 1, 2, 3, \ldots, (R_T - 1)$. For $C = 0$ and $C = R_T$, the corresponding equations are slightly different:

$$\frac{dP_0}{dt} = -k_f L R_T P_0 + k_r P_1, \tag{18b}$$

$$\frac{dP_{R_T}}{dt} = k_f L P_{R_T - 1} - k_r R_T P_{R_T}. \tag{18c}$$

This set of equations is termed the Master Equation. When the ligand concentration L remains constant, Eqs. (18a)–(18c) form a system of $(R_T + 1)$ coupled linear ordinary differential equations, and as such can be solved analytically for the various transient probabilities, $P_C(t)$. A possible set of initial conditions, those describing the case when no receptors are bound at time 0, is $P_C(0) = 0$ for $C \neq 0$ and $P_C(0) = 1$ for $C = 0$.

One method of solving Eqs. (18a–c) is to transform the system of ordinary differential equations into a single partial differential equation which can be more easily solved. An approach for doing this is to define a generating function, $G(s, t)$:

$$G(s,t) = \sum_{C=0}^{R_T} s^C P_C(t), \tag{19}$$

where s is a dummy variable (Bharuca-Reid, 1960). We next multiply each of our original equations [Eqs. (18a–c)] by s^C, sum the equations, and then recognize that the terms of containing P_C can be written as functions of G and its derivatives. This procedure yields the single partial differential equation

$$\frac{\partial G}{\partial t} = (1 - s)\left\{[k_f L s + k_r]\frac{\partial G}{\partial s} - [k_f L R_T]G\right\}. \tag{20}$$

The initial condition on P_C given earlier [$P_C(0) = 0$ for $C \neq 0$ and $P_C(0) = 1$ for $C = 0$) gives rise to the initial condition on G:

$$G(s,0) = \sum_{C=0}^{R_T} s^C P_C(0) = 1. \tag{21}$$

The requirement that all probabilities must sum to one can be shown to correspond to the boundary condition on G:

$$G(1,t) = \sum_{C=0}^{R_T} P_C(t) = 1. \tag{22}$$

An alternative method for converting the large set of ordinary differential equations as in Eqs. (18a–c) to a single partial differential equation involves a Taylor series expansion of P_C (see, for example, Gardiner, 1983). An example of this procedure relevant to receptor/ligand phenomena is provided by Tranquillo and Lauffenburger (1987b) for simulation of cell migration paths.

The solution $G(s, t)$ of Eq. (20), once found, can then be used to recover all of the individual probabilities from the formulas

$$P_0(t) = G(0, t), \tag{23a}$$

$$P_C(t) = \frac{1}{C!}\left[\frac{d^C G}{ds^C}\right]_{s=0}. \tag{23b}$$

Typically, one is most interested in the expected or mean value of C, denoted $\langle C \rangle$, and the variance σ_c^2. Expressions for these quantities can be found from the generating function $G(s, t)$, once the solution to Eq. (20) is known. $\langle C \rangle$ and σ_c^2 are defined and related to the generating function by

$$\langle C \rangle = \sum_{C=0}^{R_\mathrm{T}} C P_C = \left[\frac{\partial G}{\partial s}\right]_{s=1}, \tag{24a}$$

$$\sigma_C^2 = \sum_{C=0}^{R_\mathrm{T}} (C - \langle C \rangle)^2 P_C = \left[\frac{\partial^2 G}{\partial s^2} + \frac{\partial G}{\partial s} - \left(\frac{\partial G}{\partial s}\right)^2\right]_{s=1}. \tag{24b}$$

Using the approach outlined earlier, we examine first the steady-state solution to Eq. (20), the same as equilibrium in this case, arising from setting $\partial G/\partial t = 0$. This solution, obtained by direct integration, is given by

$$G(s) = \left[\frac{s + \dfrac{k_\mathrm{r}}{k_\mathrm{f} L}}{1 + \dfrac{k_\mathrm{r}}{k_\mathrm{f} L}}\right]^{R_\mathrm{T}}. \tag{25}$$

Using this solution together with Eqs. (24a, b), we can find that at equilibrium

$$\langle C_\mathrm{eq} \rangle = \frac{R_\mathrm{T} L}{K_\mathrm{D} + L}, \tag{26a}$$

$$(\sigma_C^2)_\mathrm{eq} = \frac{R_\mathrm{T} L K_\mathrm{D}}{(K_\mathrm{D} + L)^2}. \tag{26b}$$

Notice that $\langle C_\mathrm{eq} \rangle$ is identical to C_eq given by the solution to the deterministic model [Eq. (7)]; this is a general result for linear equations. The interesting and important observation is that the statistical variance expected at equilibrium binding is proportional to the total number of cell receptors, R_T. The root-mean-square deviation, $\delta C_{eq} = (\sigma_c)_{eq}$, is equal to $[(R_T L K_D)^{1/2}/(K_D + L)]$.

Using this expression for δC_{eq} together with Eq. (26a) permits us to write a simple expression for the expected relative root mean square fluctuation in equilibrium complex number due to stochastic effects in binding:

$$\frac{\delta C_{eq}}{C_{eq}} = \left(\frac{K_D}{LR_T}\right)^{1/2}. \tag{27}$$

Calculated values of $\delta C_{eq}/C_{eq}$ are plotted in Fig. 7 as a function of L/K_D and R_T. At $L = K_D$, the expected mean fluctuation in receptor occupancy at equilibrium will be $\delta C_{eq}/C_{eq} = R_T^{-1/2}$. When $R_T = 10^4$ receptors/cell, then statistical fluctuations with average magnitude equal to 1% of equilibrium receptor/ligand complex number can be expected around the mean complex number. Such small fluctuations are difficult to measure experimentally, but they may have significant consequences for cell behavior. A central example is chemotaxis, in which cells can bias the spatial orientation of their movement in the direction of chemotactic attractant concentration gradients. Zigmond (1977) has shown experimentally that relative concentration gradients of about 1% across cell dimensions are sufficient to induce noticeable directional bias in neutrophil

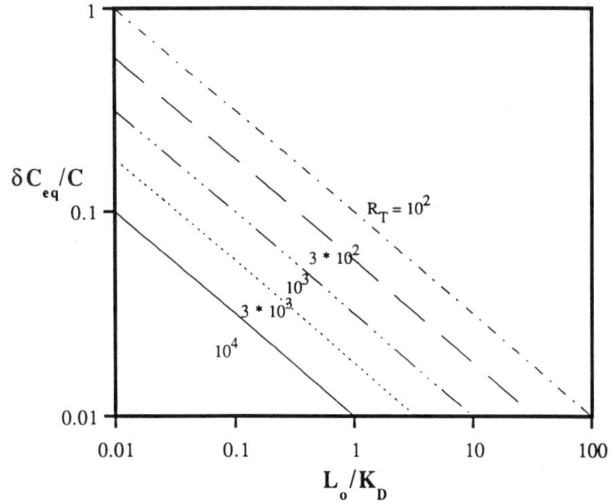

FIG. 7. Relative root mean square fluctuation in the equilibrium number of complexes on a cell. The plot shows the prediction of the probabilistic model for homogenous receptor/ligand binding. Note that fluctuations become more significant as the number of receptors or the ratio of L to K_D decreases.

leukocytes when $L \sim K_D$ for a peptide attractant and with $R_T \sim 10^4$ peptide receptors/cell. Thus, statistical fluctuations in receptor binding may be of the same order of magnitude as the apparent gradient signal. In other situations, such as receptor binding in small interfacial contact zones during cell adhesion, the number of receptors involved may be even smaller, so that the significance fluctuations can be expected to be greater still.

Next, consider the transient solution of Eq. (20) with initial and boundary conditions given by Eqs. (21) and (22). The solution for $G(s, t)$ can be obtained by the method of characteristics (see Rhee *et al.*, 1986). The mean and variance of C can be found again by using Eqs. (24a, b) (McQuarrie, 1963):

$$\langle C(t) \rangle = \frac{R_T L}{K_D + L}\left[1 - e^{-(k_f L + k_r)t}\right], \tag{28a}$$

$$\left(\sigma_C^2\right) = \frac{R_T L}{(K_D + L)^2}\left[Le^{-(k_f L + k_r)t} + K_D\right]\left[1 - e^{-(k_f L + k_r)t}\right]. \tag{28b}$$

Note that Eq. (28a) is the same as the transient solution to the deterministic binding equation with $C_0 = 0$ [Eq. (6)].

It should be clear that treatment of probabilistic aspects of receptor/ligand binding is mathematically much more complicated than the deterministic, or mean, behavior analyses given in Section II. Furthermore, for understanding receptor-driven cell behavior it may also be necessary to investigate the stochastic behavior not only of receptor/ligand binding, but also of later events, such as receptor coupling to signal transducing molecules. In addition to the analytical techniques mentioned here and discussed at length in Bharuca-Reid (1960), Gardiner (1983), Doraiswamy and Kulkarni (1987), and Goel and Richter-Dyn (1974), one can also use computer simulation techniques to model stochastic events. In these simulations, for example, the motion of individual particles can be simulated by choosing random numbers from a specified distribution. Examples of such simulations are discussed in Section V.

Of course, a probabilistic modeling approach ought to be applied only when it is strongly suspected that interpretation of experimental behavior requires it. It is our belief that probabilistic models will prove to be of increasing utility in the near future as experimental assays for cell function become more commonly designed to generate data on individual cells. Examples include models of cell orientation and migration paths (Tranquillo *et al.*, 1988; Dickinson and Tranquillo, 1993), cell detachment from surfaces due to fluid shear flow (Cozens-Roberts *et al.*, 1990a, b), and cell rolling along surfaces (Hammer and Apte, 1992).

IV. Diffusion Effects

As described in Section II, simple binding of a ligand molecule to a receptor is generally treated as a reversible, one-step process. However, it is well known in chemical reaction kinetics that the binding of two molecules is really a two-step process, requiring first the molecular transport of the individual molecular species, R and L, with transport rate constant k_+ before intrinsic chemical reactions of binding interactions can occur (see Fig. 8). We will consider the transport mechanism to be molecular diffusion, because diffusive transport dominates convective transport at cellular and subcellular length scales (Weisz, 1973). The chemical reaction step itself is then characterized by the intrinsic association rate constant k_{on} and intrinsic dissociation rate constant k_{off}. Thus, the values of k_f and k_r that are measured in kinetic experiments are really combination rate constants which include both the transport and reaction effects, and our analysis will allow us to determine the relative contributions of each. By the analyses presented in this section, we can examine how the individual rate constants k_+, k_{on}, and k_{off} contribute to the overall observed rate constants k_f and k_r. In this way, we can gain a quantitative understanding of how the diffusion coefficient D can affect binding kinetics. We will also learn that diffusion effects can cause the binding parameters k_f and k_r to be not constants, but instead functions of the number of available free receptors, R; this phenomenon can arise because diffusion is highly affected by geometry.

We will consider the interplay of diffusion and intrinsic binding interactions in three types of situations: (1) binding of ligand to receptor when

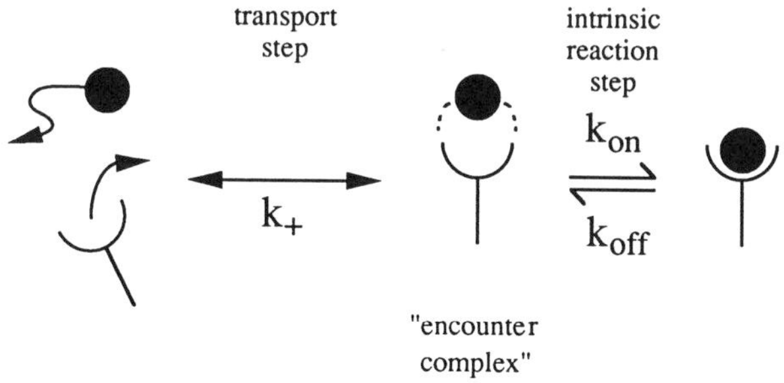

FIG. 8. Separation of an overall binding or dissociation event into two steps. The intrinsic binding step is characterized by rate constants k_{on} and k_{off}, which are determined by receptor and ligand molecular properties. The transport step is characterized by rate constant k_+ and is influenced by diffusion and geometric considerations. The state in which receptor and ligand are close enough to bind but have not yet done so is sometimes termed the encounter complex.

both are free in solution; (2) binding of ligand to receptor when the former is free in solution and the latter is on a cell surface; and (3) interaction between a receptor and an accessory molecule when both are on a cell surface (in this latter case, the binding parameters k_f and k_r are replaced by the coupling parameters k_c and k_u). These cases are illustrated in Fig. 9 and will now be examined in order.

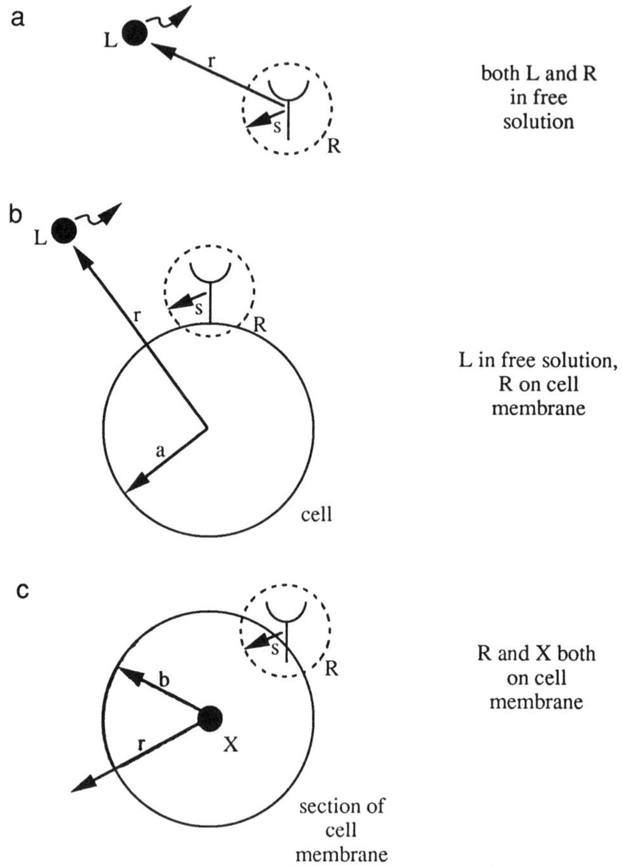

FIG. 9. Receptor binding in three geometric situations. (a) Binding of ligand to receptors free in solution. (b) Binding of ligand to cell surface receptors. (c) Binding of cell surface molecules (X) to cell surface receptors. The radius of an encounter complex is s, the cell radius is a, a typical distance between molecule X and a receptor R is b, and r is the radial position.

A. Ligand Binding to Solution Receptors

We will begin by looking at the binding of ligand to receptor when both are free in solution (Fig. 9a) and will follow the approach by Shoup and Szabo (1982). Our aim is to obtain expressions for the overall forward and reverse rate constants, k_f and k_r, as they depend on diffusion coefficients and free receptor number. In order to accomplish this, we will calculate the rate at which a ligand molecule would be expected to bind to a receptor molecule by the two-step diffusion and intrinsic reaction process.

A steady-state diffusion equation is written for the concentration of ligand molecules, $L(r)$, around a single receptor molecule placed at the origin of a spherical coordinate system:

$$D\frac{1}{r^2}\frac{d}{dr}\left(r^2\frac{dL}{dr}\right) = 0, \tag{29}$$

where D is the sum of the ligand and receptor diffusivities, $D = (D_L + D_R)$. The ligand concentration L varies with distance form the receptor, but very far away it is just equal to the bulk ligand concentration L_0. This provides one boundary condition:

$$r \to \infty, \qquad L \to L_0. \tag{30a}$$

The rate at which ligand molecules are bound by a receptor is equal to the intrinsic reaction rate constant k_{on} times the ligand concentration at the receptor surface, L evaluated at $r = s$; s is often termed the encounter radius. At steady state, this must be equal to the ligand diffusion rate (moles/time) to the receptor surface (the diffusive flux multiplied by the surface area, again evaluated at $r = s$). This provides the second boundary condition needed for Eq. (29):

$$4\pi s^2 D\frac{dL}{dr}\bigg|_{r=s} = k_{on}L(s). \tag{30b}$$

The solution to Eq. (29) with these boundary conditions [Eqs. (30a, b)] is

$$L(r) = \frac{-k_{on}sL_0}{4\pi Ds + k_{on}}\left(\frac{1}{r}\right) + L_0. \tag{31}$$

The overall flux of molecules to the receptor is given by $k_f L_0$ and is equal to $4\pi s^2 D(dL/dr)_{r=s}$. Thus, the overall or observable association rate constant k_f is determined as

$$k_f = L_0^{-1} 4\pi s^2 D \left[\frac{dL}{dr} \right]_{r=s} = k_{on} L(s) L_0^{-1}, \tag{32}$$

giving

$$k_f = \frac{4\pi D s k_{on}}{4\pi D s + k_{on}}. \tag{33}$$

The quantity $4\pi Ds$ appearing in Eq. (33) is worthy of further examination. Consider the situation in which binding events occur much more rapidly than diffusion, such that all ligand reaching the receptor can be assumed to disappear instantaneously. To describe this situation using the classical diffusion theory of Smoluchowski (1917), Eq. (29) is solved with the boundary condition $L = 0$ at $r = s$ replacing the boundary condition Eq. (30b). The solution can then be used in Eq. (32) to find that the overall rate constant in this situation is equal to $4\pi Ds$. Because this rate constant describes the situation in which diffusion is playing the limiting role, we identify the value $4\pi Ds$ with the rate constant k_+. Thus, Eq. (33) can be rewritten as

$$k_f = \frac{k_+ k_{on}}{k_+ + k_{on}} = \left(\frac{1}{k_+} + \frac{1}{k_{on}} \right)^{-1}, \tag{34a}$$

with

$$k_+ = 4\pi D s. \tag{34b}$$

The form of this equation suggests an appealing interpretation: the overall "resistance" to binding, $1/k_f$, is the sum of the two individual "resistances" of diffusion ($1/k_+$) and intrinsic reaction ($1/k_{on}$) in series. This expression is the key result that enables us to assess the relative contribution of the diffusion, or transport, step to the overall forward rate constant for isolated receptors and ligands binding in solution. Note that if $k_{on} \gg k_+$, then $k_f \sim k_+ = 4\pi Ds$, and the binding is termed diffusion-limited. On the other hand, if $k_{on} \ll k_+$, then $k_f \sim k_{on}$, and the binding is termed reaction-limited.

Typical values for k_+ can be easily estimated for receptor/ligand binding in free solution. Using the parameter ranges $D = 10^{-7}$ to 10^{-5} cm^2/s and $s = 1$ to 10 nm, we obtain $k_+ \sim 1 \times 10^{-13}$ to 1×10^{-10} cm^3/s. Because the initial problem we solved [Eq. (29)] is based on the diffusion of a single ligand molecule to a receptor, the units on k_+ (also k_{on} and k_f) are more accurately $(\#/cm^3)^{-1}$ s^{-1}. We can thus change the units of our calculated k_+ by multiplying by Avogadro's number and converting from cm^3/mole to M^{-1} to give $k_+ \sim 6 \times 10^7$ to 6×10^{10} M^{-1} s^{-1}. Most values of k_f measured in free solution are less than this range, so pure diffusion-control of isolated receptor/ligand binding reactions is not common. Thus, for receptors and ligands in free solution, the experimentally measured value of the overall forward rate constant k_f is usually a reasonable estimate for the intrinsic binding rate constant k_{on}.

As an aside, we note that the derivation of $k_+ = 4\pi Ds$ assumes that the molecules are uniformly reactive, i.e., there are no spatial orientation restrictions. For macromolecules such as ligands and receptors, this is not really true. A number of investigators have tackled this problem (see the review by Berg and von Hippel, 1985), with the finding that if the reactive site has radius s' which is small compared to s, then a good approximation is $k_+ = 4Ds'$. This result is not surprising, for it is the rate constant for diffusion to a disk of radius s' lying on an infinite plane. A more detailed expression is $k_+ = 2\pi Ds\{\sin^2(\theta_R/2)[(1/2)^{1/2} + (3/8)^{1/2}]\}$, where θ_R is the angle circumscribing the reactive portion of the receptor. Note that when $\theta_R = \pi/2$, the relation $k_+ \sim 4Ds$ is obtained. These alternative expressions for k_+, as well as others depending on the specific geometric situation, may be substituted as appropriate for k_+ in the equations that follow. It should also be mentioned at this point that a more sophisticated computational approach to this issue is the application to Brownian dynamic simulations incorporating molecular structure and intermolecular interactions for the reacting species (e.g., see McCammon, 1991).

Shoup and Szabo (1982) define the "capture probability" γ,

$$\gamma = \frac{k_{on}}{k_{on} + k_+}, \tag{35}$$

which is the probability that closely associated receptor and ligand actually bind to become a true receptor/ligand complex. With this, Eq. (34a) can be rewritten in the elegant form

$$k_f = \gamma k_+. \tag{36}$$

Thus, γ essentially quantifies the extent to which receptor/ligand association is rate-limited by the reaction step. As γ approaches 0, association is severely reaction-limited, while as γ nears 1, binding is almost purely diffusion-limited.

The overall reverse rate constant, k_r, can be found by similar means. Expressed in its clearest form, the result is

$$k_r = (1 - \gamma)k_{off}. \tag{37}$$

Hence, the overall dissociation rate constant is the product of the complex dissociation rate constant and the "escape probability" (equal to $1 - \gamma$).

B. Ligand Binding to Cell Surface Receptors

The preceding analysis has been devoted to receptor/ligand binding in free solution. In this paper, on the other hand, we are mainly interested in binding of ligands to receptors restricted to two-dimensional cell membranes. Beginning with the seminal contribution by Berg and Purcell (1977), investigators have developed various approaches for this desired extension of the analysis (e.g., DeLisi and Wiegel, 1981; Brunn, 1981; Zwanzig, 1990). In the context of our current presentation, the approach by Shoup and Szabo (1982) discussed earlier is most direct. Consider a spherical cell of radius a with receptors of radius s, as shown in Fig. 9b. Equation (34a) can be applied after two important modifications. First, the forward transport rate constant for ligand molecules diffusing to the cell surface is

$$(k_+)_{\text{cell}} = 4\pi Da, \tag{38}$$

because the relevant radius is now a and not s. The diffusion coefficient D is equal to $(D_\text{L} + D_{\text{cell}})$, or, because $D_{\text{cell}} \ll D_\text{L}$, $D \sim D_\text{L}$. The diffusion of receptors on the cell surface is neglected because $D_\text{R} \ll D_\text{L}$. Second, the effective forward reaction rate constant for the entire cell is

$$(k_{\text{on}})_{\text{cell}} = Rk_{\text{on}}, \tag{39}$$

for a cell possessing R free surface receptors, where k_{on} is the individual receptor intrinsic association rate constant. Thus, by Eq. (34a), the rate constant for ligand binding by the entire cell is

$$(k_\text{f})_{\text{cell}} = \frac{(k_+)_{\text{cell}} Rk_{\text{on}}}{(k_+)_{\text{cell}} + Rk_{\text{on}}}. \tag{40}$$

As shown explicitly by Goldstein (1989), the overall forward rate constant for ligand association with a free receptor on a cell surface, on our usual per receptor basis, is simply found by dividing Eq. (40) by the number of free receptors, R, to obtain

$$k_\text{f} = \frac{(k_+)_{\text{cell}} k_{\text{on}}}{(k_+)_{\text{cell}} + Rk_{\text{on}}}. \tag{41}$$

Because the interaction of isolated receptors and ligands in solution is typically close to a reaction-limited situation (as seen in the previous section), k_{on} is essentially the association rate constant that would be experimentally measured for an isolated receptor in free solution if there were no chemical effects of removing the receptor from its cell membrane lipid environment.

Recalling from Eq. (36) the relationship between k_f and the capture probability γ, we see from Eq. (40) that for this present case of cell surface receptors, the capture probability for the entire cell is

$$\gamma_{\text{cell}} = \frac{Rk_{\text{on}}}{(k_+)_{\text{cell}} + Rk_{\text{on}}}. \tag{42}$$

[Compare this expression to Eq. (35) for an isolated receptor in free solution.] We now use Eqs. (37) and (42) to evaluate the overall reverse rate constant for dissociation of a ligand molecule from cell surface receptors (Goldstein, 1989):

$$k_r = \frac{(k_+)_{\text{cell}} k_{\text{off}}}{(k_+)_{\text{cell}} + Rk_{\text{on}}}. \tag{43}$$

A striking consequence of Eqs. (41) and (43) is that the overall rate constants for ligand association to and dissociation from cell surface receptors, k_f and k_r, are not, in fact, constants in general, but rather may be functions of the free receptor number R. k_f, k_r, and $(k_f)_{\text{cell}}$ as functions of R are illustrated in Fig. 10. Notice from this figure that the *per receptor* rate constants k_f and k_r decrease as R increases. The diminuation in k_f is caused by the spatial restriction of receptors onto the cell surface, where they can compete with one another for ligand molecules. As increase in R reduces the dissociation rate constant k_r by increasing the probability that ligand dissociation from one receptor results in binding to a neighboring receptor, rather than escape from the cell surface entirely (Goldstein, 1989). The implications of these changing rate constants on the kinetics of receptor/ligand binding are discussed more fully in Section IV, D.

Another consequence of these equations is that the rate constant for ligand capture by the entire cell, $(k_f)_{\text{cell}}$, approaches a significant fraction of its maximum value, $(k_+)_{\text{cell}} = 4\pi Da$, for small cell surface area coverage by receptors. This can be seen from the diagonal line on Fig. 10, which converts the quantity $Rk_{\text{on}}/(k_+)_{\text{cell}}$ to an equivalent value of ϕ, the fractional surface coverage of cell surface area by receptors ($\phi = R\pi s^2/4\pi a^2$), for a typical set of parameter estimates. For the estimates used in Fig. 10, for example, a fractional surface coverage of only 0.2 (20%) gives approximately 50% of the maximal rate of ligand binding to cells.

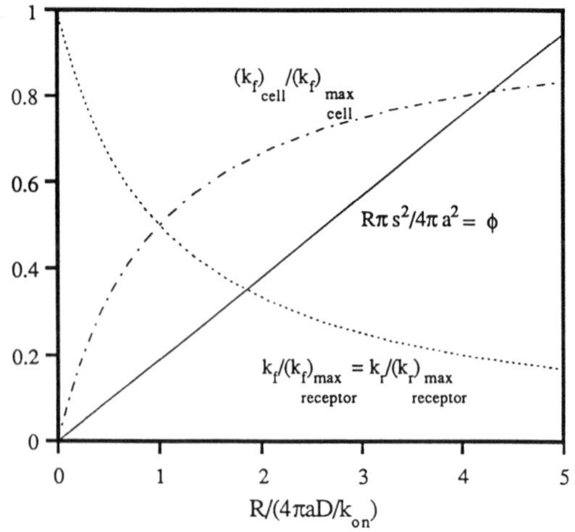

FIG. 10. Variation of the per receptor association and dissociation rate constants, k_f and k_r, with the number of free receptors. Although the assumption is typically made that k_f and k_r are constants, this is not strictly true when diffusion effects are significant [see Eqs. (41) and (43)]. $(k_f)_{max\,rec}$ and $(k_r)_{max\,rec}$, the maximum values of k_f and k_r, are given by k_{on} and k_{off}. The per cell association rate constant $(k_f)_{cell}$ also varies with the number of free receptors [see Eq. (40)]; the maximum value $(k_f)_{max\,cell}$ is given by $(k_+)_{cell}$. ϕ is the fractional surface coverage of cell area by receptors. For calculation of ϕ, $s = 10$ nm, $a = 10$ μm, $k_{on} = 10^7$ M^{-1} s^{-1}, and $D = 10^{-6}$ cm^2/s.

A rigorous experimental verification of these theoretical results has appeared (Erickson *et al.*, 1987). These investigators quantitatively varied cell surface receptor number by binding different amounts of monoclonal anti-DNP IgE antibodies to Fc receptors on rat basophilic leukemia (RBL) cells. These IgE molecules then served as (bivalent) receptors for the monovalent hapten ligand 2,4-dinitrophenyl (DNP)-aminocaproyl-L-tyrosine, or DCT, so that ligand binding to cells possessing a range of values for R_T could be explored. The critical result is shown in Fig. 11, a plot comparing the value of the rate constants $(k_f)_{cell}$ and k_f as determined from their kinetic data to the theoretical predictions of Eqs. (40) and (41). Excellent agreement exists for realistic values of D and a. Furthermore, the value of k_{on} estimated from this comparison, $k_{on} = 1.1 \times 10^8$ M^{-1} s^{-1}, is very close to the value measured for the binding of DCT to isolated IgE molecules in free solution, as expected.

A different sort of check on the diffusion-limitation theory has been performed by Northrup (1988), who reported Brownian dynamics computer simulations of ligand diffusing to cell surface receptors. His calculations were aimed at the special case in which the intrinsic binding rate constant takes on a diffusion-limited value; that is, $k_{on} = 4Ds$ (which

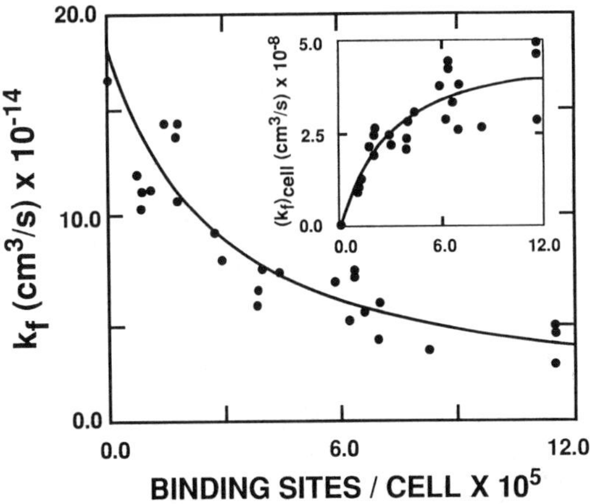

FIG. 11. Experimental data and model fit on the variation of the per receptor and per cell association rate constants with the total number of receptors. Reproduced from the *Biophysical Journal*, Erickson *et al.* (1987), vol. 52, pp. 657–662, by copyright permission of the Biophysical Society.

arises for diffusion of ligand to a disk of radius s) (Berg and Purcell, 1977). In this limiting case, $(k_f)_{cell} = 4\pi DaRs/(Rs + \pi a)$ (Berg and Purcell, 1977; Shoup and Szabo, 1982). Northrup found that the computer simulations yielded a binding rate constant in close agreement with this expression at low receptor surface coverages (ϕ), but greater than this expression by about 5% when ϕ increased to about 0.25. This is certainly a minor discrepancy, given the uncertainty in experimental binding measurements, but it represents a real effect. At significant receptor surface coverages, interference among ligand concentration fields around neighboring receptors arises. Such interference is neglected in the theory described earlier in this section; rather, receptors are assumed to act independently, each possessing its own isolated ligand concentration field. As shown by Northrup, interference among receptor fields acts further to deplete the ligand concentration near a receptor and enhance the effective per receptor binding rate.

Zwanzig (1990) has presented a theoretical analysis of this enhancement, finding that the denominator of Eqs. (40) and (41) becomes $[(k_+)_{cell} + Rk_{on}](1 - \phi)$. Hence, as receptor coverage ϕ increases, the overall binding rate constant increases as a result of the interference effect. For any particular type of receptor, however, ϕ is typically much less than 1%, so that this correction will usually be negligible. The Brownian dynamics approach may also be used to assess the effect of cell surface receptor distribution on the rate constants (Northrup, 1988); receptors dispersed uniformly on the cell surface will exhibit less interaction than those clustered or aggregated on the cell surface (Goldstein and Wiegel, 1983; Goldstein, 1989). Finally, the effect of an autocrine ligand, source on receptor binding can be assessed using a Brownian dynamics approach (see Section V, A).

C. Receptor Coupling with Membrane-Associated Molecules

We now turn to interactions between two molecules both associated with the cell surface. As mentioned briefly in Section II, C, such interactions include receptor crosslinking by a multivalent ligands, receptor coupling with cytoskeletal components, and receptor interactions with effectors such as G-proteins. The effect of molecular diffusion on the rate constants for such interactions between two surface-bound species can be analyzed in a fashion analogous to that for diffusion of free solution ligand to cell surface receptors. In this new case, the coupling and uncoupling rate constants, k_c and k_u, will replace the forward and reverse binding rate constants, k_f and k_r. Thus we note that the interaction of the two species—which we will denote as R and X—is a two-step process, requiring first diffusive transport with rate constant k_+ before coupling with rate constant k_{on} can occur. The overall coupling reaction rate constant, k_c, depends on k_+ and k_{on}. We will find that the overall uncoupling reaction rate constant, k_u, will depend on the intrinsic uncoupling rate constant k_{off} as well as the diffusion rate constant k_+.

Before we begin, a note on units is in order. For the two-dimensional reactions we are now considering, it is typical to write the rate constants k_c, k_+, and k_{on} in the units of cm^2/s, or, more accurately, $(\#/cm^2)^{-1}\ s^{-1}$ (recall that for the three-dimensional reactions considered in the last section, we used the units of cm^3/s or, more accurately, $(\#/cm^3)^{-1}\ s^{-1}$). For comparison of the magnitudes of the rate constants for the different geometries, however, it would be convenient to be able to convert the two-dimensional rate constants to an effective three-dimensional rate constant. To do this, we will multiply the two-dimensional rate constants by the membrane thickness h to give an estimated local volume for cell surface components. In all cases, the units of $(\#/cm^3)^{-1}\ s^{-1}$ can be easily converted to $M^{-1}\ s^{-1}$. Finally, we mention that the units of $(\#/cell)^{-1}$ s^{-1} may also be used for k_c. These units can easily be converted to $(\#/cm^2)^{-1}\ s^{-1}$ by multiplying by the surface area/cell.

Different methods for deriving the diffusion rate constant k_+ are applied by Adam and Delbruck (1968), Berg and Purcell (1977), and Keizer (1985), with similar, though not identical, results. Here we will use an approach closely following that for the case of ligand in solution binding to surface receptors (Section IV, B) and based on the work of Shoup and Szabo (1982). A steady-state diffusion equation is first written for the concentration of receptors, $n_R(r)$ [#/area], around a single membrane-associated X molecule placed at the origin of a circle (Fig. 9c):

$$D\frac{1}{r}\frac{d}{dr}\left(r\frac{dn_R}{dr}\right) = 0. \tag{44}$$

D is the sum of the diffusivities of R and X in the membrane. One boundary condition represents reaction between R and X at the encounter radius s:

$$2\pi sD\frac{dn_R}{dr}\bigg|_{r=s} = k_{on}n_R(s). \tag{45a}$$

A second boundary condition cannot be specified at infinite r, for then Eq. (44) would have no solution. [An alternative approach, analyzing a non–steady-state situation, is offered by Torney and McConnell (1983).] Instead, a "bulk" membrane receptor concentration, n_{Rb}, can be imposed at a distance $r = b$:

$$r = b, \qquad n_R = n_{Rb}, \tag{45b}$$

where b is one-half the mean distance between species X molecules. If X is the number of species X available for interaction and A is the surface area of the cell, then b can be specified from the approximate relation $X\pi b^2 = A$, so that

$$b = (A/\pi X)^{1/2}. \tag{46}$$

For example, if $X = 10^4$ #/cell on a cell possessing 300 μm^2 surface area, then $b \sim 0.1$ μm or 100 nm. It is essential to point out that as interactions proceed dynamically, the value of b will vary as the number of available X molecules changes.

The solution of Eqs. (44) and (45a, b) for the concentration profile of receptors, $n_R(r)$, around the species X molecule is

$$n_R(r) = n_{Rb}\left[1 - \frac{k_{on}\ln(b/r)}{2\pi D + k_{on}\ln(b/s)}\right]. \tag{47}$$

The overall or observable coupling rate constant, k_c, is determined from

$$k_c = n_{Rb}^{-1}2\pi sD\left[\frac{dn_R}{dr}\right]_{r=s} = k_{on}n_R(s)n_{Rb}^{-1}, \tag{48}$$

yielding

$$k_c = \frac{2\pi D k_{on}}{2\pi D + k_{on}\ln(b/s)}. \tag{49}$$

Following the analogy to the case of receptor/ligand binding in solution, k_c can be expressed in terms of rate constants for the diffusive step, k_+, and the coupling step, k_{on}:

$$k_c = \left(\frac{1}{k_+} + \frac{1}{k_{on}}\right)^{-1}, \tag{50a}$$

where the diffusive rate constant is now elucidated by comparing Eq. (50a) to Eq. (49):

$$k_+ = \frac{2\pi D}{\ln(b/s)}. \tag{50b}$$

Other approaches yield similar forms, except that a constant, C, is subtracted from the $\ln(b/s)$ term in the denominator of Eq. (50b). Adam and Delbruck (1968) obtained $C = \frac{1}{2}$, Berg and Purcell (1977) found $C = \frac{3}{4}$, and Keizer (1985) found $C = 0.231$. For typical values of $\ln(b/s)$ of roughly 2 to 5, these corrections do not change the estimated value of k_+ by more than a factor of 2. Note that whatever the precise expression, k_+ varies with b and thus with the number of species X molecules available for interaction with receptors.

As before, when $k_{on} \gg k_+$, then $k_c \sim k_+$, and the coupling is diffusion-limited. When $k_{on} \ll k_+$, $k_c \sim k_{on}$, and coupling is reaction-limited. Let us examine some typical numerical values in this context. For membrane proteins, D is generally in the range 10^{-10} to 10^{-9} cm^2/s. Using $s = 1$ to 10 nm, and $b = 100$ nm, we find that k_+ falls in the range 1×10^{-10} to 3×10^{-9} cm^2/s. To convert k_+ to the same units as k_{on}, we multiply by Avogadro's number and, to give an estimated local volume for cell surface components, by a membrane thickness h of approximately 10 nm. Our value for k_+ is then approximately 6×10^4 to 2×10^6 M^{-1} s^{-1}. In contrast to the situation for reactions in free solution, these values —especially the lower end of the range—are much smaller than typical values for the intrinsic reaction rate constant k_{on} (which might be estimated from the binding of ligand to solution receptors).

Therefore, we can expect that coupling reactions between two membrane-associated species will commonly be diffusion-limited. This result is in contrast to that for receptor/ligand binding in solution, which will not typically be diffusion-limited, and to that for ligand binding to cell surface receptors, which will be diffusion-limited only for unusually large receptor concentrations. Diffusion-limitation of membrane-associated species interactions on the one hand simplifies parameter estimation, since $k_c \sim k_+$ and knowledge of k_{on} is not necessary. On the other hand, diffusion-limitation means that k_c is not a pure constant, but will vary as the concentration of reacting species changes during the process.

To obtain the overall uncoupling rate constant, k_u, we can again make use of the "capture probability" γ [see Eq. (35)], such that $k_c = \gamma k_+$. Recall that γ quantifies the extent to which receptor/ligand association is rate-limited by the reaction step. As γ approaches 0, association is severely reaction-limited, while as γ nears 1, binding is almost purely diffusion-limited. k_u is thus given by

$$k_u = (1 - \gamma)k_{off}. \tag{51}$$

Hence, the overall uncoupling rate constant is the product of the intrinsic dissociation rate constant and the "escape probability" (equal to $1 - \gamma$).

There are further considerations to the modeling of the diffusion-limited coupling of two membrane-associated molecules. Using standard mass-action kinetics, we would typically describe the rate of coupling as $k_c RX$, where R and X are the concentrations of the two molecules to be coupled and k_c is the coupling rate constant. Such a formulation assumes that the membrane is "well-mixed," or that there are no local concentration gradients of R or X. This may not be the situation if molecules are crowded into some parts of the cell membrane, for molecules may diffuse more slowly in concentrated environments (Saxton, 1990) or may be unable to physically squeeze into these areas (Ryan *et al.*, 1988). Mounting evidence suggests that the cell membrane may be far from uniform, and may consist of many "microdomains" (Sheetz, 1993; Rodgers and Glaser, 1993). Furthermore, the interaction of two molecules may result in a depletion zone nearby, a situation far from well-mixed. One method of modeling this situation is to explicitly follow the movement and interactions of individual molecules by using computer simulations. The application of such computer simulations to the case of receptor signaling through G-protein activation is detailed in Section V, B.

D. Analysis of Cell Receptor Binding Data

Let us now explore the analysis of receptor binding data using these theoretical treatments of diffusion effects in receptor phenomena. An important remark concerning diffusion-limitation of binding is that, when present, it affects the kinetic rate constants but not the equilibrium constant or the Scatchard plot (Scatchard, 1949) of the equilibrium data. This can be seen by evaluating $K_D = k_r/k_f$ using Eqs. (41) and (43) for k_f and k_r, respectively, in the case of ligand binding to cell surface receptors to obtain $K_D = k_{off}/k_{on}$; the same is true for the cases of ligand binding to solution receptors or receptors coupling with membrane molecules. Diffusion limitations can, however, affect steady-state, non-equilibrium processes, as well as transient phenomena (Lauffenburger and Linderman, 1993).

First, let us consider possible complications in analyzing experimental receptor/ligand binding data when diffusion limitations are present. A key criterion for diffusion-limited binding of ligand to isolated receptors, according to Eq. (34a), is the value of the quantity ρ_{rec} relative to 1, where

$$\rho_{rec} = \frac{k_{on}}{k_+}. \tag{52}$$

The key criterion for diffusion-limited binding of ligand to cell surface receptors, following Eq. (41), is the value of the quantity ρ_{cell} relative to 1, where

$$\rho_{cell} = \frac{Rk_{on}}{(k_+)_{cell}}. \tag{53}$$

When $\rho \ll 1$, there is no limitation of association or dissociation by ligand diffusion, so $k_f = k_{on}$ and $k_r = k_{off}$ are constants, as had been assumed in our analyses in previous sections. However, as ρ becomes comparable to 1, diffusion begins to have an influence on the rates of these processes. For the case of ligand binding to cell surface receptors when ρ is comparable to 1, the rate constants k_f and k_r are functions of R and, through $(k_+)_{cell}$, the diffusion coefficient.

As an example of the use of ρ, consider EGF binding to its fibroblast receptor, following Wiley (1988). The value of k_{on} determined for this system is about 3×10^6 M^{-1} s^{-1}. An estimate for k_+, using $k_+ = 4\pi Ds$, $D_L = 1.5 \times 10^{-6}$ cm^2/s, $D = 2D_L$, and $s \sim 1$ nm, is 2×10^9 M^{-1} s^{-1}. Therefore, $\rho_{rec} \sim 0.001 \ll 1$. Hence, in free solution EGF binding to its receptor would not be diffusion-limited to any noticeable degree. An estimate for $(k_+)_{cell} = 4\pi Da$, using $D = D_L$ and $a = 5$ μm, is 6×10^{12} M^{-1} s^{-1}. For normal human fibroblasts with $R_T \sim 10^4$ receptors/cell, $\rho_{cell} \sim 0.005 \ll 1$. Clearly, this is purely reaction-limited behavior as well. In contrast, for A431 cells (an epidermoid carcinoma cell line) with $R_T > 10^6$ receptors/cell, $\rho_{cell} > 0.5$, allowing diffusion to play a significant role. For this cell type, according to Eqs. (41) and (43), the rate constants for EGF association and dissociation should be dependent on receptor occupancy through the effect of receptor occupancy on R, the free receptor number. Indeed, Wiley found this to be the case experimentally, observing an effect of receptor occupancy on EGF dissociation rates from A431 cells but not from normal fibroblasts.

When ρ_{cell} is not negligible compared to 1, then one must go back to the beginning and modify Eq. (5) for simple receptor/ligand binding, using Eqs. (41) and (43) in place of the simple constants k_{f} and k_{r}, respectively. When ligand depletion can be considered negligible, the appropriately altered form of Eq. (5) is

$$\frac{dC}{dt} = \left[1 + \frac{k_{\text{on}}(R_{\text{T}} - C)}{4\pi aD}\right]^{-1} \{k_{\text{on}}L_0R_{\text{T}} - (k_{\text{on}}L_0 + k_{\text{off}})C\}, \quad (54\text{a})$$

where we have used $(k_+)_{\text{cell}} = 4\pi aD$ and the receptor conservation relation $R_{\text{T}} = R + C$. Alternatively, in dimensionless form using the variables $\tau = k_{\text{off}}t$ and $u = C/R_{\text{T}}$, this equation becomes

$$\frac{du}{dt} = [1 + \rho_{\text{cell}}(1 - u)]^{-1}[\lambda_0 - (1 + \lambda_0)u], \quad (54\text{b})$$

where $\rho_{\text{cell}} = R_{\text{T}}k_{\text{on}}/4\pi Da$, $\lambda_0 = L_0/K_{\text{D}}$, and $K_{\text{D}} = k_{\text{off}}/k_{\text{on}}$. This equation, though nonlinear, possesses an implicit analytical solution for $u(t)$ for an association experiment with initial condition $u(0) = 0$:

$$\left(\frac{\rho_{\text{cell}}}{1 + \lambda_0}\right)u + \left[\frac{\rho_{\text{cell}}\lambda_0 - (1 + \rho_{\text{cell}})(1 - \lambda_0)}{(1 + \lambda_0)^2}\right]\ln\left|1 - \frac{(1 + \lambda_0)}{\lambda_0}u\right| = \tau. \quad (55)$$

Example computations from this expression, for parameters representing the EGF/A431 cell system, are graphed in Fig. 12a as transient $u(\tau)$ curves. Notice that increasing ρ_{cell} above unity markedly reduces the binding rate, as expected. Quantitative effects of this diffusion limitation can best be discovered by comparison with predictions for pure reaction limitation, following Eq. (6) or (11). In that case, equivalent to setting $\rho_{\text{cell}} = 0$, a plot of $\ln[u_{\text{eq}} - u(\tau)]$ versus τ gives a straight line with slope equal to $-(1 + \lambda_0)$. Figure 12b shows the transient curves from Fig. 12a replotted in this fashion. Clearly, values of ρ_{cell} larger than about 1 cause significant deviation of this slope from its limiting value and noticeable nonlinear behavior.

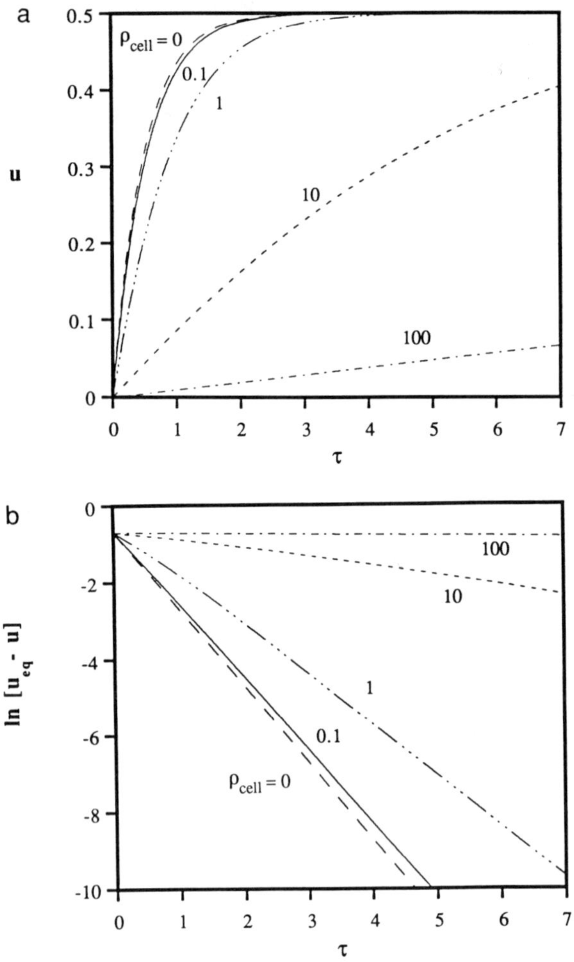

FIG. 12. Binding of ligand to cell surface receptors. (a) The scaled number of bound receptors u is plotted as a function of the scaled time τ. (b) The logarithm of the difference between the equilibrium and transient number of bound receptors, $\ln[u_{eq} - u]$, is plotted versus τ. Note that the curves vary with the value of ρ_{cell}, which measures the degree to which binding is diffusion-limited. When ρ_{cell} is small, the rate constants k_f and k_r are true constants. When ρ_{cell} is large, binding becomes diffusion-limited and the variation of k_f and k_r with time significantly affects the number of bound receptors.

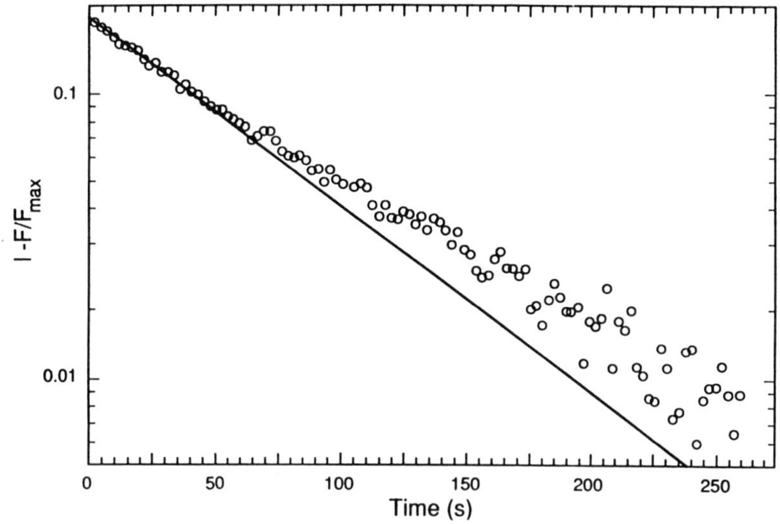

FIG. 13. Dissociation of DCT from IgE antibodies anchored on the surfaces of rat basophilic leukemia (RBL) cells. The rate of dissociation slows with time because of an increase in the number of free receptors. The effect is noticeable because ρ_{cell} is not $\ll 1$, and therefore k_r is not constant. Reproduced from the *Biophysical Journal*, Goldstein *et al.* (1989), vol. 56, pp. 955–966, by copyright permission of the Biophysical Society.

This type of observation is, in fact, made by Goldstein *et al.* (1989) in experimental studies of DCT dissociation kinetics from an IgE antibody anchored as a surface receptor on RBL cells. For their system, $D = 5 \times 10^{-6}$ cm^2/s, $a = 4$ μm, $R_T = 6 \times 10^5$ #/cell, and $k_{on} = 4.8 \times 10^7$ M^{-1} min^{-1}. These values yield $\rho_{cell} \sim 2$ when all receptors are available for binding (i.e., $R = R_T$), predicting that substantial diffusion-limitation effects should arise during transient association and/or dissociation experiments. Measurements showed a slowing of the effective dissociation rate of DCT from RBL cells as the number of free receptors increased during the dissociation experiment (see Fig. 13), as predicted. Goldstein and co-workers thus quite properly used the equivalent of Eq. (54a) to analyze their data. We should point out that the main focus of this paper was to examine the effects of competing receptors in solution on ligand binding to cell surface receptors, a more complicated situation which we will not address here.

Turning to receptor processes on cell membranes (case c of Fig. 9), we could infer the degree of diffusion limitation from a ratio analogous to that in Eq. (52), where k_+ is given by Eq. (50b). Unfortunately, values for an intrinsic reaction rate constant, k_{on}, are extremely difficult to determine for interactions between membrane-associated species. Indeed, measurements of coupling and uncoupling rate constant, k_c and k_u, are themselves rare at the present time. Mayo *et al.* (1989) determine values for overall coupling and uncoupling rate constants between EGF/EGF–receptor complexes and a hypothesized membrane-associated component on fibroblast membranes at 4°C to be $k_c = 8 \times 10^{-5}$ $(\#/\text{cell})^{-1}\ \text{s}^{-1}$ and $k_u = 8 \times 10^{-5}\ \text{s}^{-1}$. To convert k_c to more familiar units, we multiply by Avogadro's number and by an estimated local volume for cell surface components (the product of cell surface area A and a membrane thickness h of roughly 10 nm). Using $A = 1.3 \times 10^3\ \mu\text{m}^2$ for a cell of 10 μm radius, we obtain $k_c = 6 \times 10^5\ \text{M}^{-1}\ \text{s}^{-1}$. An estimate for k_+ based on Eq. (49b) and an estimate of b from Eq. (45c) can be calculated, using $X = 2.4 \times 10^4$ #/cell for the number of membrane-associated coupling species (as determined by Mayo *et al.* from comparison between their model and experimental binding data) on cells with 10 μm radius, $s = 3$ nm, $D = 1 \times 10^{-10}\ \text{cm}^2/\text{s}$, and $h = 10$ nm. These values yield $k_+ \sim 1 \times 10^5\ \text{M}^{-1}\ \text{s}^{-1}$. Though these are clearly crude estimates, we see that k_c and k_+ are of the same order of magnitude. While k_c seems to be greater than k_+, this is not possible; our conclusion is that k_c may be very nearly approaching its diffusion-limited value, as expected.

Goldstein *et al.* (1981) have used a related analysis to examine data for congregation of LDL receptors in endocytic clathrin-coated pits. Their question was whether passive diffusion of receptors is sufficient to account for congregation rates in coated pits, or whether receptor transport by membrane convective flow is necessary. We can estimate a value for the diffusion rate constant, k_+, for movement of receptors to a coated pit. Using Eq. (50b), but with $s = 0.05\ \mu$m being the coated pit radius and $b = 1\ \mu$m the average spacing between pits, we obtain $k_+ \sim 6 \times 10^{-10}$ cm^2/s for $d = 3 \times 10^{-10}\ \text{cm}^2$ s. Goldstein *et al.* found that $k_c = 3 \times 10^{-10}$ cm^2/s was a reasonable lower bound on the rate constant for receptor/coated-pit coupling, as determined from experimental data on LDL internalization (Brown and Goldstein, 1976). Thus, k_+ is of roughly the same magnitude as the value given by Goldstein *et al.* for k_c. The conclusion, then, would be that passive receptor diffusion should be sufficient to provide the observed rate of receptor congregation in coated pits. Goldstein *et al.* came to the same finding with a more detailed treatment. A later analysis by Keizer (1985) using a statistical mechanics approach reinforces this conclusion. Readers interested in pursuing further analysis of effects of membrane convective flow on receptor transport are referred to a few treatments of this phenomenon (Goldstein and Wiegel, 1988; Goldstein *et al.*, 1988; Echavarria-Heras, 1988).

V. Applications

The analyses presented in Sections III and IV rely on analytical techniques to investigate the roles of probability and diffusion in receptor phenomena. We turn now to an alternative approach, the use of computer simulation techniques, in the context of two particular applications. In the first subsection (Section V, A), we describe simulation of the three-dimensional motion of a single ligand molecule as it diffuses toward a receptor. The technique used is formally termed Brownian dynamics simulation (BDS) and involves following the trajectory of a molecule whose motion is dictated by any intermolecular forces present together with a stochastic term representing collisions with solvent molecules. The stochastic term is calculated with the use of a random-number generator. While the BDS technique has primarily been used to examine individual molecular interactions within a solvent environment (Ermak and McCammon, 1978; McCammon *et al.*, 1986; Northrup *et al.*, 1984, 1986), diffusion-controlled binding of exogenous ligand to cell receptors has been investigated by Northrup (1988). Here we show the use of this technique to examine the capture of autocrine ligand by a cell's own surface receptors.

In the second subsection (Section V, B), we describe the two-dimensional motion and collisions of dozens of receptors and effectors that results in activated effectors and thus the initial stages of signal transduction. For simplicity, receptors and effectors are constrained to move on a lattice; the random motion of each is determined by choosing random numbers according to a Monte Carlo scheme, yielding a dynamic computer simulation.

A. Autocrine Growth Factor Binding

As mentioned earlier, ligand diffusion must occur before binding to receptors can take place. In our earlier analysis (Section IV, B), we considered the binding of solution ligands to membrane receptors. In this case, ligand was assumed to be present at a uniform concentration in the medium surrounding a cell. In the case of autocrine ligands, however, the situation is somewhat different. Autocrine ligands are secreted by cells which also express the corresponding receptor, as shown schematically in Fig. 14. This advantageous source location for the autocrine ligand should facilitate receptor/ligand binding and, hence, lead to qualitatively different regulatory behavior. For example, in autocrine systems cell proliferation rates increase with increasing initial cell densities, as shown both

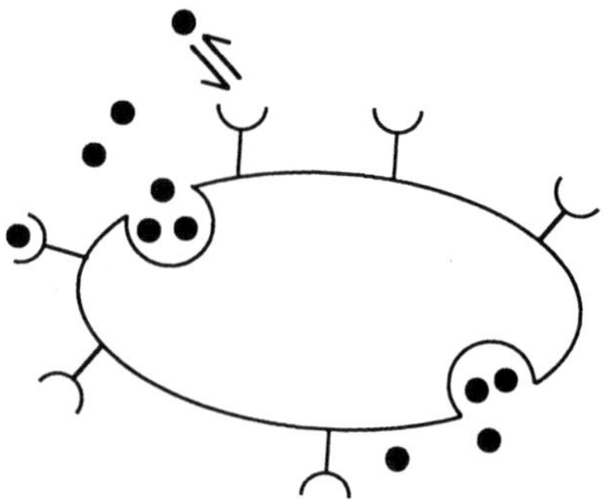

FIG. 14. Receptor binding of autocrine ligands. Autocrine ligands are secreted by the same cells which express receptors for them.

experimentally (Earle *et al.*, 1951; Hu *et al.*, 1985) and theoretically (Lauffenburger and Cozens, 1989).

Autocrine stimulation is recognized as an important elment in many normal and abnormal response systems (Sporn and Roberts, 1992; Sporn and Todaro, 1980). Autocrine ligand IL-2 secretion and binding are essential for a proper immune cell response (Cantrell *et al.*, 1988; Robb *et al.*, 1981; Smith, 1988a, b). A number of malignant cell lines have been shown to secrete autocrine growth factors and, through self-secretion, escape exogenous control (Cuttitta *et al.*, 1985; Imanishi *et al.*, 1989; Kawano *et al.*, 1988). While physiologically important, analysis and understanding of this mechanism and the cells themselves have been plagued by subtle complications arising from the proximal ligand source.

The secretion of autocrine ligand results in a competition between immediate cell surface receptor binding and diffusive transport to the bulk fluid phase. Accurate determination of autocrine secretion rates is thus generally compromised by the self-binding phenomena characteristic of these cells. Recent experimental work by Claret *et al.* (1992) has indeed shown that blockage of the receptor is essential for proper secretion measurement. Inhibition of receptor/ligand binding via addition of molecules such as anti-ligand or anti-receptor antibodies can also provide a level of exogenous control; however, theoretical work indicates that the concentration of inhibitor required to interrupt the autocrine ligand/receptor interaction is a strong function of the rate of both ligand secretion and receptor synthesis and may be much greater than anticipated from single binding affinity considerations (Forsten and Lauffenburger, 1992a, b). Further, studies examining the kinetics of the ligand binding and resulting cell behavioral responses are confounded because of the endogenous secretion.

These sorts of difficulties in interpreting and understanding experiments in autocrine systems can be alleviated by an understanding of what fraction of ligand is bound by the secreting cell and what fraction escapes to the medium, i.e., a capture probability for the ligand. In order to do this, Forsten and Lauffenburger (1994a) calculated this capture probability as a function of cell surface receptor density using BDS method. We will summarize their approach and findings.

A homogeneous distribution of receptors on the cell surface is assumed. Because of the difference in characteristic length scales between the ligand and the cell itself, curvature of the cell surface can be ignored. If periodic boundary conditions are used, a single receptor's unit area is representative of the entire surface of the cell. The receptor itself is modeled here as a 10 Å radius hemisphere, and a 10 Å radius sphere approximates the ligand (Fig. 15).

The receptor is assumed to be immobile. The position of the ligand molecule at each time step is determined using the Ermak–McCammon algorithm (Ermak and McCammon, 1978):

$$S_i = S_i^0 + R_i, \tag{56}$$

where S_i^0 represents the present position in the ith direction, S_i represents the next location of the ligand in the ith direction, and R_i represents the change in position due to collisions of the ligand with solvent particles. No electrostatic forces are included in this version of the model. Values of R_i are randomly selected from a set of Gaussian random numbers to have

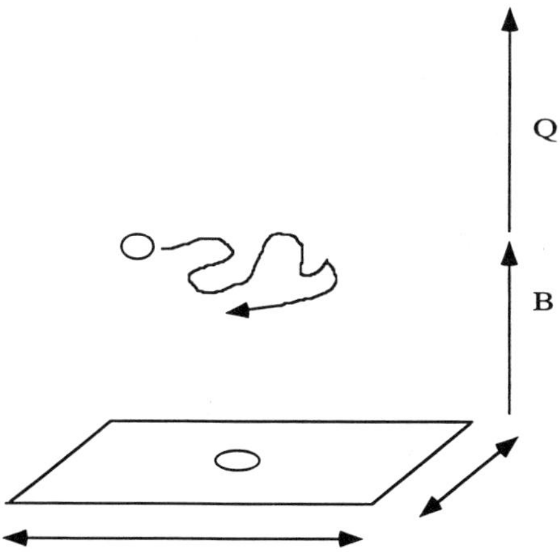

FIG. 15. Geometry of Brownian dynamic simulations. A ligand's trajectory is initiated at height B above the membrane surface. The trajectory continues until either ligand and receptor are ≤ 20 Å apart, or trajectory path escapes beyond the truncation distance Q.

a mean of zero and a variance of $2D_i \Delta t$, where D_i, is the ligand diffusion coefficient (ith direction). Hydrodynamic forces between the surface of the ligand and the membrane surface affect the ligand's diffusive motion and are reflected in the ligand diffusion coefficient. The ligand diffusion coefficient is

$$D_i = \frac{K_{\mathrm{B}}T}{6\pi\eta_{\mathrm{s}} s \Lambda_\iota}, \tag{57}$$

where

$$\Lambda_1 = \Lambda_2 = 1.0 - \left(\frac{9}{16} * \lambda\right) + \left(\frac{1}{8} * \lambda^3\right) - \left(\frac{45}{256} * \lambda^4\right) - \left(\frac{1}{16} * \lambda^5\right), \tag{57a}$$

$$\Lambda_3 = 1.0 - \left(\frac{9}{8} * \lambda\right) + \left(\frac{1}{2} * \lambda^3\right), \tag{57b}$$

$$\lambda = \frac{s}{x_3}, \tag{57c}$$

and x_i represents the position in the ith direction, K_{B} is Boltzman's constant, T is the absolute temperature, η_s is the viscosity of the extracellular medium, and s is the radius of the ligand molecule (Happel and Brenner, 1973). Directions 1 and 2 are parallel to the membrane face, while direction 3 is perpendicular. For gap distances between the membrane and the ligand of less than 90 Å, tabulated "exact" bipolar coordinate solutions to the Stokes equation can be linearly interpolated to obtain the corresponding diffusion coefficient (Cox and Brenner, 1967; Goldman *et al.*, 1967; Happel and Brenner, 1973). For the results given here, random numbers were generated using the Marsaglia–Zaman random-number generator (Marsagla *et al.*, 1990).

For each individual simulation, a ligand trajectory was initiated at a point equidistant from neighboring receptors and at a random height less than 100 Å above the membrane surface. Details of the secretion process at the cell surface are not well understood, and the proximity of newly secreted ligands to surface receptors is not known. One possible mechanism might be that of a uniform surface secretion. Secretion may occur from any point on the surface and in a random, continuous manner, similar to that of membrane turnover. Alternatively, ligand may be secreted from specific locations in a "spouting" or "plume" of molecules from concentrated exocytic vesicles. By choosing to initiate molecules equidistant from neighboring receptors at a height $\leq$ 100 Å above the surface, Forsten and Lauffenburger essentially placed molecules at their farthest possible point from the homogeneously distributed receptors and assumed that secreted particles may actually be exocytosed with bulk fluid convection such that their initial point of pure diffusion does not occur at the membrane surface. In order to determine if initial position biased the capture probability, the capture probability for particles released randomly over the receptor's unit space with initiation occurring at the cell surface was also calculated. In this way capture probabilities for alternative mechanisms were compared. The difference in probabilities was found to be $\leq 5\%$, except at very low receptor densities where the probability approached zero.

Three thousand separate trajectories were simulated for each receptor density and at each truncation height. In contrast to molecular dynamics, in BDS the solvent is treated as a viscous continuum and, hence, time steps on the order of 0.1 ps are appropriate. Diffusion-limited binding or instantaneous reaction upon ligand–receptor collision was assumed. Computationally, this condition was considered met when the center of the ligand particle and the center of the receptor were less than 20 Å apart. Trajectories were truncated when the ligand's height above the membrane surpassed Q, the truncation distance. Sample trajectories of both a successful capture and an escape are shown in Figs. 16a and 16b.

At each receptor density R and truncation height Q, a probability of capture P is obtained from

$$P(Q, R) = \frac{n_{\text{capture}}}{n_{\text{capture}} + n_{\text{escape}}}, \tag{58}$$

where n_{capture} and n_{escape} are the numbers of molecules which were captured or escaped. A plot of the results for 5×10^5 receptors/cell is shown in Fig. 17a. At low receptor densities, a small fraction of initiated trajectoreis were neither captured nor escaped beyond the truncation distance within the allotted length of time. These trajectories were not included in the probability calculation.

The overall probability of autocrine capture desired is given by the probability of capture at infinite truncation distance, or

$$P_\infty(R) = \lim_{Q \to \infty} P(Q, R). \tag{59}$$

Plotting the probability of capture, $P(Q, R)$, at a given receptor density and truncation height versus e^{-Q} reveals a roughly linear relationship,

$$P_\infty(R) = P(Q, R) - C^* e^{-Q}, \tag{60}$$

and allows us to calculate $P_\infty(R)$. An example plot is shown in Fig. 17b for one particular receptor density. Calculations were based on simulation

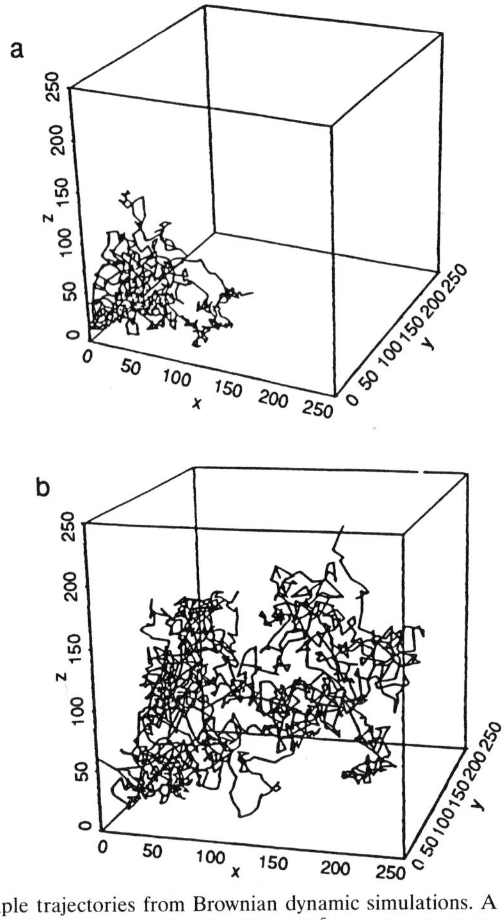

FIG. 16. Sample trajectories from Brownian dynamic simulations. A unit receptor's area is shown for a cell with a receptor density of 5×10^5 receptors/cell. Box length units are in angstroms; every 100th step is shown. (a) A successfully captured ligand trajectory is pictured. (b) A trajectory which escapes beyond the given truncation height of 250 Å is shown.

data obtained at truncation heights of 250 Å, 500 Å, and 1,000 Å. Additional simulation points at 750 Å, 400 Å, and 150 Å are shown to further demonstrate the near-linear relationship.

Results of simulations for several different receptor densities are summarized in Fig. 18. As expected, increasing receptor density leads to an increase in the probability of autocrine ligand capture. A cell with fewer than 10^4 receptors has a negligible probability of capturing its own secreted ligand. However, with an increase in receptor number of two

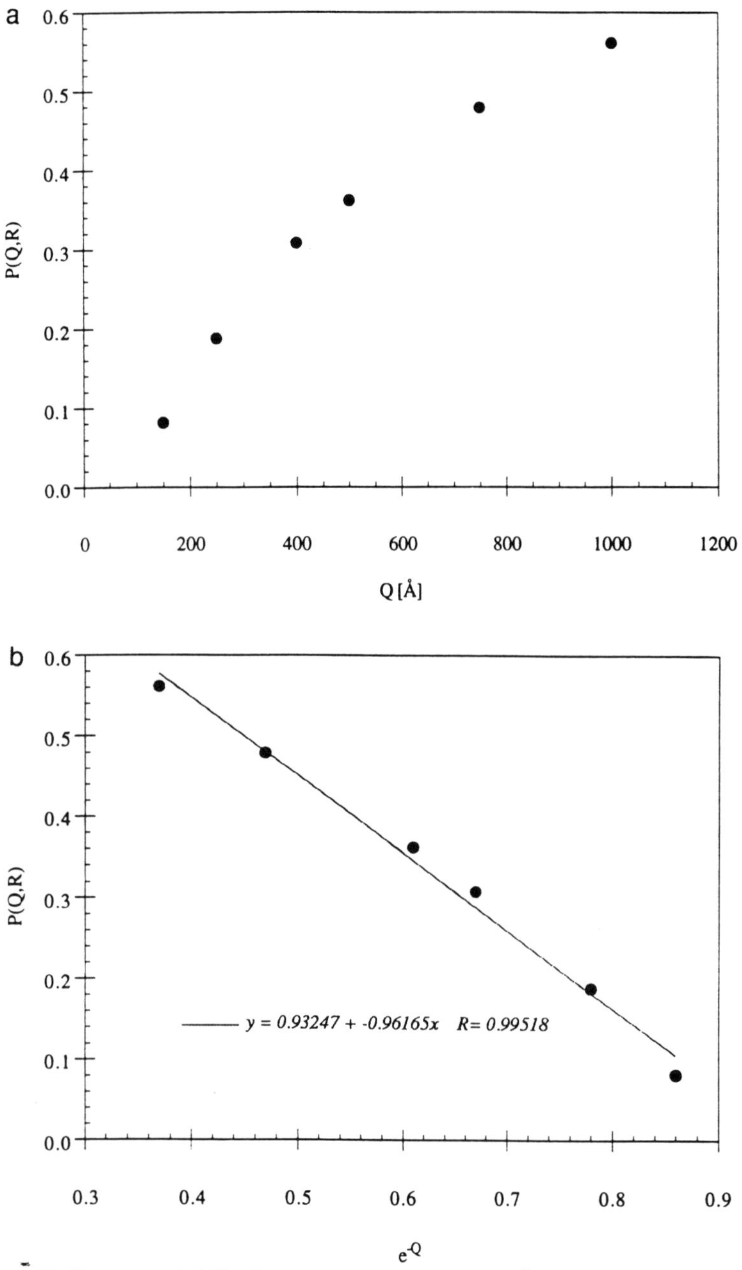

FIG. 17. Capture probability for receptor density of 5×10^5 receptors/cell. (a) Probability of autocrine ligand capture is shown for various truncation distances Q. (b) The probability of capture at infinite dilution can be calculated by plotting the capture probability versus e^{-Q}. A linear fit to the data provides the y-intercept $P_\infty(R)$.

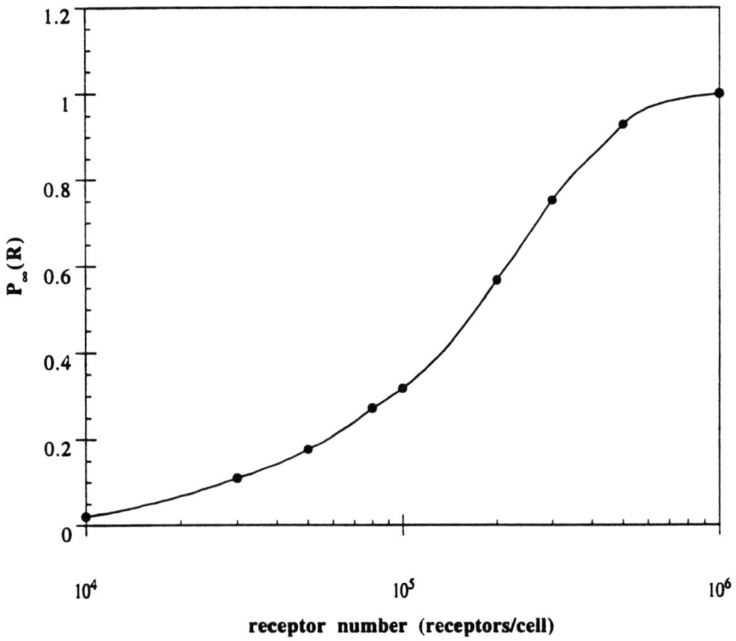

FIG. 18. Probability of autocrine ligand capture. The capture probability is plotted as a function of the receptor density. Typical growth factor receptor densities are 10^4 to 10^6 receptors/cell.

orders of magnitude, the probability of escape from the cell's microenvironment becomes essentially zero.

A qualitatively similar receptor density dependence was shown analytically by Berg and Purcell (1977) in their seminal paper addressing the diffusion of ligand to the cell surface and its probability of capture (Fig. 19a). They focused on the transport of exogenous ligand from a distant source and the subsequent binding that occurs within the cell's microenvironment. Solving the steady-state diffusion equation for ligand diffusing toward a spherical cell, they examined the cooperative effect competing receptors would have on the overall flux of molecules to the cell. Meandering of ligand molecules in the vicinity of the cell, once they have arrived at the cell surface, significantly increases the chance of capture over that expected solely on the basis of surface area coverage by the receptors. Note, however, that our analysis in this section has a rather different focus. We are interested in secreted ligand's immediate transport and transient search within the local microenvironment of the cell. Rather than a steady-state analysis in which a constant source of ligand exists at

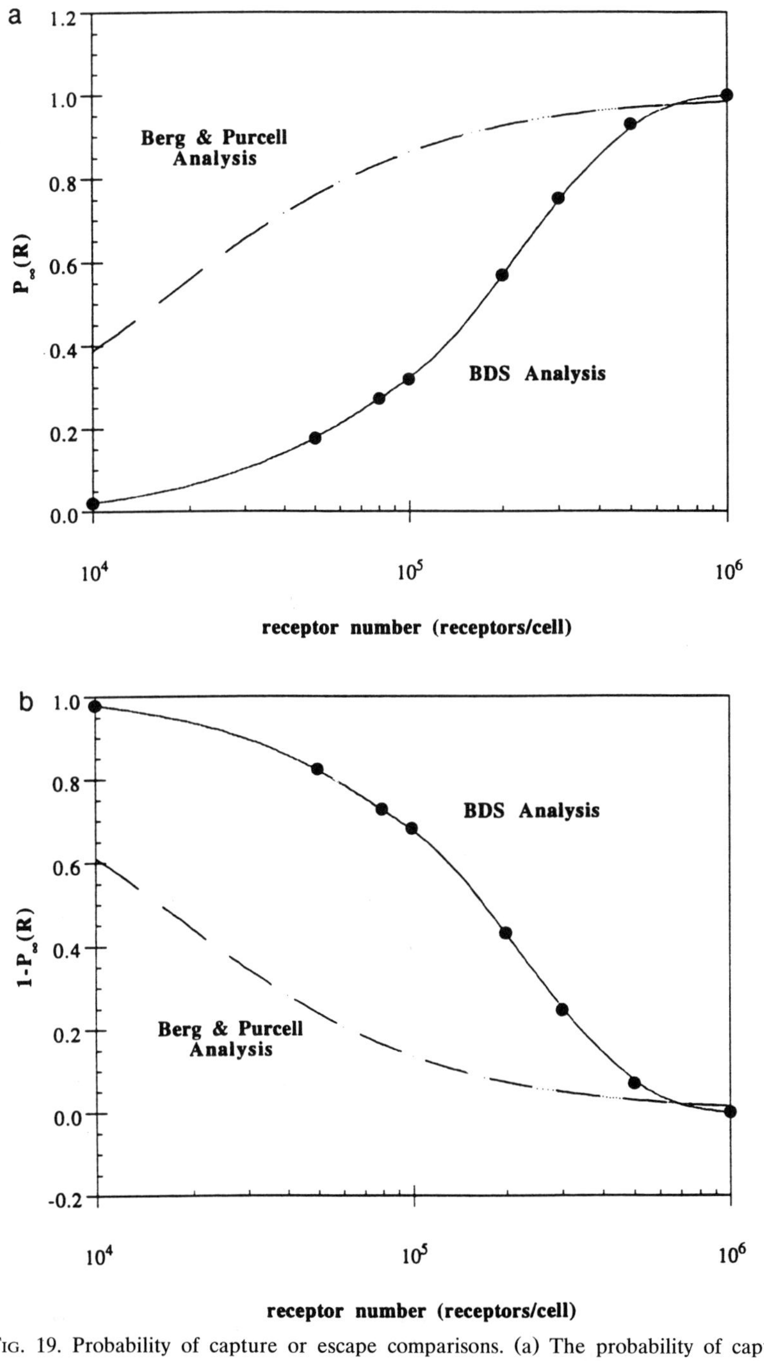

FIG. 19. Probability of capture or escape comparisons. (a) The probability of capture versus the receptor density as calculated using BDS techniques or the Berg and Purcell (1977) analysis is shown. (b) The escape probability as calculated using BDS techniques or the exogenous ligand Berg and Purcell type analysis is shown.

an infinite distance from the surface, we are examining here the retention of particles secreted within the cell's microenvironment. The significant hurdle that must be overcome by ligand diffusing a great distance to reach the cell surface does not exist for the autocrine ligand. The probability of capture for an autocrine ligand calculated in this section is a measure of the first-pass transient capture by the receptors. Consequently, while quite appropriate for the bulk ligand binding, the expression derived by Berg and Purcell would significantly overestimate the level of capture by the autocrine cell at low receptor coverage. The overall probability derived for their steady-state exocrine ligand model conceptually weights the transport to the microenvironment such that once relatively close to the surface, binding is probably inevitable. Autocrine ligands do not go through any type of extensive transport filtering, so the events within the cell microenvironment are critical.

For example, at a receptor density of 10^4 receptors/cell, the BDS analysis indicates about a 2% probability of any ligand being captured by the cell receptors, while a 40% chance would be predicted from the Berg–Purcell analysis (Fig. 19a). Alternatively, a more meaningful comparison might be that of comparing the escape probability derived in an analogous manner to the Berg–Purcell analysis (DeLisi, 1980) to the escape probability for an autocrine ligand derived via BDS. The escape probability of an autocrine ligand is significantly higher than that derived from the steady-state analysis (Fig. 19b). Again, conceptually this reflects both the first-pass capture within the autocrine system and the large distance which must be overcome by the endocrine-type ligand in order to be in a position to bind.

The primary result of the Forsten and Lauffenburger (1994a) analysis described here is a determination of the increase in the probability of autocrine ligand capture as a function of increasing receptor density (Fig. 18). McGeady *et al.* (1989) found that receptor density may play a privotal role in autocrine transformation. A retroviral vector with the gene for TGF-α was introduced into both a rat fibroblast cell line and a mouse mammary epithelial cell line. The fibroblast cell line expresses about 10^4 TGF-α receptors per cell, while the epithelial cells express about an order of magnitude more receptors. Autocrine ligand production resulted in transformation of the epithelial cells and not the fibroblasts. Although other factors may have contributed to these results, in light of the BDS analysis, it appears likely that the cells expressing only 10^4 may not have been capturing autocrine ligand and, hence, were not significantly different than their non-secreting progenitors. Autocrine transformation is likely a function not only of the ligand secretion rate, but also of the level of receptor expression.

Ligand secretion measurements have been used as a type of litmus test for classifying systems as autocrine. Recent experimental work with stimulated T cells and their autocrine ligand, IL-2, have verified that intrinsic capture can interfere with experimental measurements (Claret *et al.*, 1992). In the presence of blocking antibody, researchers found an average increase in measurable secreted ligand of a factor of over 300. Unfortunately, receptor densities were not presented. In light of the theoretical work presented in this section, it is not surprising that such a dramatic increase in measurable ligand would be obtainable. In the absence of blocking antibody, presumably all secreted ligand could be captured by the secreting cell. Once self-binding has been eliminated via antibody blockage, a true estimate of the secretion rate may be ascertained. The actual cell secretion rate can be predicted as the measured secretion rate divided by the capture probability. This has real implications for the understanding of both ligand–receptor activation and inhibitor inactivation. Thorough characterization and classification of receptor-mediated cell functions in response to autocrine ligands may, therefore, demand a quantitative understanding of the receptor number and regulatory dynamics.

Finally, the autocrine ligand capture probability found as described in this section has been used to analyze the role of low-affinity receptors on autocrine cells also possessing high-affinity receptors for the same ligand (Forsten and Lauffenburger, 1994b). There are many examples of such dual receptor systems, and their role in autocrine stimulation has not been fully explored (Lein *et al.*, 1991; Miyajima *et al.*, 1992; Smith, 1988c; Yahon *et al.*, 1991). Focusing on the IL-2 system, they used mathematical modeling to compare three potential functions for low-affinity receptors. First, the low-affinity receptors may function as ligand reservoirs, holding ligand close to the cell surface to enhance later binding by high-affinity receptors. Second, the low-affinity receptors may function as reservoirs for receptor subunits, for high-affinity receptors in this system are composed of subunits found also in the low-affinity receptors. Third, the low-affinity receptors may function as surface carrier/presentor molecules, transporting ligand to the high-affinity receptors. Using high-affinity complex levels as an indicator of low-affinity receptor's effect, it was found that with both the ligand and receptor reservoir mechanisms there was an inhibitory effect on complex levels due to binding competition. With the carrier mechanism, the binding competition actually led to an increase in high-affinity complexes, and this was especially true at low cell densities. Conflicting data has been reported on whether the low-affinity IL-2 receptor is necessary for cellular response and whether its presence actually enhances or reduces cell responsiveness (Collins *et al.*, 1990;

Jankovic *et al.*, 1990; Kumer *et al.*, 1987; Kuziel *et al.*, 1993; Tsudo *et al.*, 1989). Use of mathematical approaches such as this may help sort through this complicated question.

B. Receptor Coupling to G-Proteins for Signal Transduction

The simple binding of ligand to a cell surface receptor in itself is not sufficient to produce, for example, cell migration or secretion; the receptor must somehow convey to the cell interior the information that a binding event has occurred. In most cases, there is incomplete knowledge concerning the intracellular signal transduction events transforming receptor-mediated signals into cell behavioral responses. Tremendous efforts are currently underway in many laboratories to identify and characterize the intracellular mediators and kinetic pathways that lie between receptor binding and cell responses. As a result, a significant amount of information has been obtained during the past decade on the very early signal transduction processes which occur immediately after receptor/ligand binding (see Chapters 8 and 9 of Gennis, 1989, for a general background). These early signals are more closely connected to short time-scale responses, such as the secretion or release of certain cell products (e.g., cyclic AMP, histamine, antibodies), than to long time-scale behaviors of, for example, cell migration and proliferation.

There are three main modes of signal transduction for cell surface receptors bound with ligand: Receptors can act as ion channels; receptors can perform as enzymes (e.g., tyrosine kinases); and receptors can interact with GTP-binding proteins (G-proteins) to generate other signaling molecules. In this section we will focus on the third pathway, which involves the coupling of bound receptors and G-proteins in the two-dimensional lipid bilyaer. Receptors using this mode of transduction are many and diverse, but typically regulate physiological responses occurring on the time scale of minutes; examples include the chemotactic peptide receptor and the α- and β-adrenergic receptors. In a recent review, Birnbaumer *et al.* (1990) list approximately 80 identified receptors that interact with G-proteins.

A schematic of the interaction of G-proteins with receptors is shown in Fig. 20. The inactive form of the G-protein consists of α, β, and γ subunits with a molecule of GDP bound to the α subunit. The interaction of this inactive G-protein with a bound receptor promotes the release of GDP from the α subunit and the binding of GTP at the same site. The G-protein is then released from the receptor and dissociated into separate $\beta\gamma$ and α-GTP entities; α-GTP is an active form of the G-protein. The bound receptors thus serve to catalyze the formation of active G-protein.

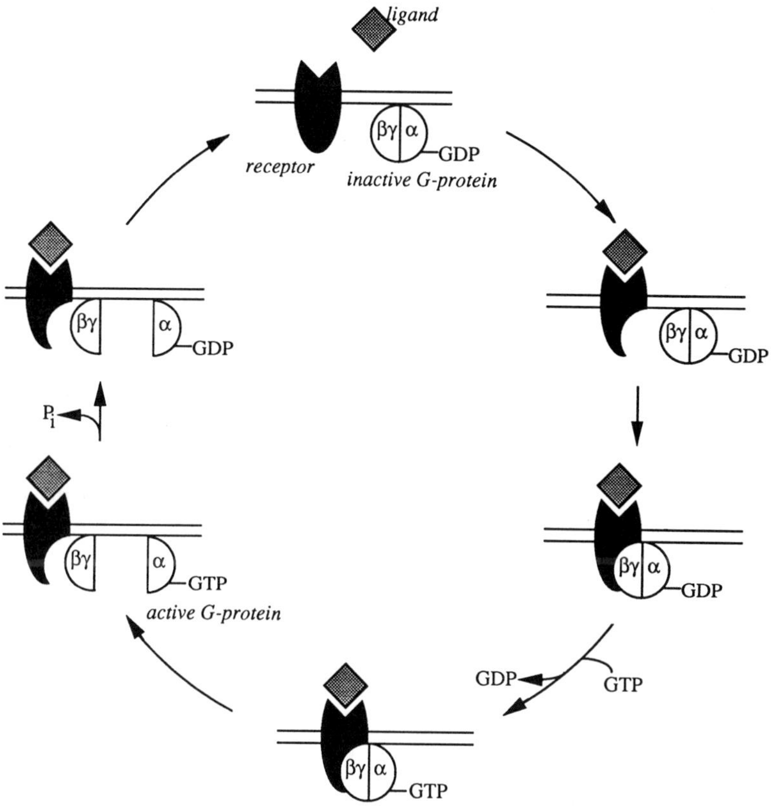

FIG. 20. Activation of G-proteins by bound receptors. The inactive form of the G-protein couples to bound receptors. After GDP is replaced by GTP, the α subunit with attached GTP dissociates from the $\beta\gamma$ subunit and acts on targets within the cell. Hydrolysis of GTP by the α subunit allows reformation of the inactive G-protein.

Active G-proteins are returned to their inactive state upon hydrolysis of GTP by the GTPase activity found in the α subunit itself, and the α-GDP and $\beta\gamma$ subunits may then recombine. We further note that the separate $\beta\gamma$ subunit may also play an active role in signal transduction, though this role is not well understood at present (Birnbaumer, 1992).

The active form of the G-protein, α-GTP, can modulate the activity of a true signal-generating enzyme or effector. For example (Fig. 21), α-GTP can activate the enzyme phosphatidylinositol-specific phospholipase C (PLC). PLC acts to break down the membrane phospholipid phosphatidylinositol-4,5-bisphosphate (PIP_2) to form two "second messengers": inositol 1,4,5-trisphosphate (IP_3) and 1,2-diacylglycerol (DG). IP_3 diffuses into the cytoplasm, where it binds to an intracellular receptor and causes

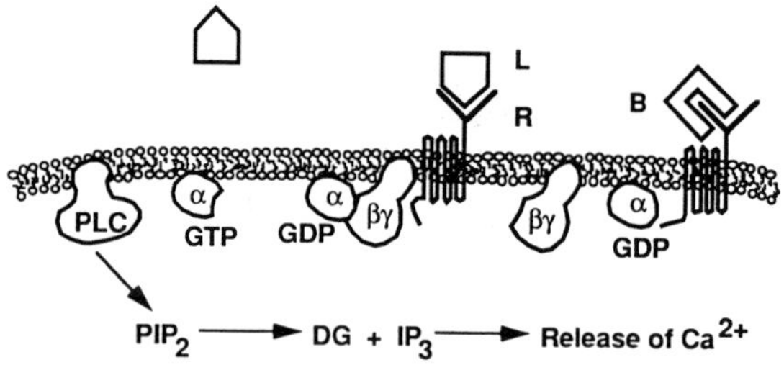

FIG. 21. Signal transduction pathway. Ligand (L) binds to a receptor (R) on the cell membrane, forming a receptor/ligand complex. The receptor/ligand complex associates with a G protein ($\beta\gamma\alpha$-GDP) in the cell membrane. Following exchange of GTP for GDP on the G protein, the receptor and G protein dissociate, and the trimeric G protein separates into two parts: the $\beta\gamma$ subunit and the active α-GTP subunit. α-GTP stimulates the activity of a phospholipase C (PLC), which converts phosphatidylinositol 4,5-bisphosphate (PIP_2) into diacylglycerol (DG) and inositol 1,4,5-trisphosphate (IP_3). IP_3 is soluble in the cytosol and binds to receptors on an internal calcium store, causing the release of calcium into the cytosol. Also shown is a receptor antagonist or blocker (B) which is able to bind to a receptor without activating the signaling pathway.

release of the second messenger calcium from various internal stores (Berridge, 1993; Burgoyne and Cheek, 1991). Calcium is a seemingly ubiquitous regulator of a diverse range of cell functions and can bind to a variety of proteins, particularly calmodulin (Heizmann and Hunziker, 1991). Calcium–calmodulin complexes modulate the activity of many intracellular enzymes, including various protein kinases (which phosphorylate proteins), as well as glycogen synthase and microtubule-associated proteins. DG diffuses within the membrane and activates the membrane-associated enzyme known as protein kinase C (pKC); this enzyme phosphorylates protein substrates on serine and threonine residues and thus modifies their activity. Nishizuka (1986) provides a listing of the numerous membrane and cytoplasmic proteins likely serving as pKC substrates, including a variety of cell surface receptors (e.g., EGF, insulin, transferrin, IL-2, and β-adrenergic receptors). Cytoplasmic proteins, including the cytoskeleton contractile protein myosin and the cytoskeleton/adhesion receptor-binding protein vinculin (both apparently involved in cell migration) and membrane transport proteins for glucose, Na^+, and H^+ (likely involved in cell metabolism for growth) also may serve as pKC substrates.

As described earlier, the interaction between bound receptors and G-proteins occurs on the two-dimensional cell membrane surface. The transient encounter between a ligand-occupied receptor and a G-protein last only a few milliseconds (Taylor, 1990). In order to compare this time with the likely time *between* encounters, the time for a receptor/ligand complex to diffusion to a G-protein can be estimated from $t = b^2/(4D)$, where t is the time between encounters of a receptor and any G-protein, D is the sum of the diffusion coefficients of the receptor and G-protein, and b is one-half the mean distance between G-proteins. If G-proteins are assumed to be uniformly distributed, b can be estimated from Eq. (46) with X equal to the number of G-proteins in the membrane. Sample calculations show that in the experimental system we have investigated, that of α_1-adrenergic receptors on BC_3H1 cells, the time between collisons of a single receptor with any G-protein is likely one to two orders of magnitude greater than the time required for activation of a G-protein already in contact with a receptor/ligand complex. Thus, the time required for diffusional encounter between receptors and G-proteins appears to be a limiting factor in the activation of G-proteins. Direct measurements of the effect of receptor and G-protein diffusion on signal transduction have not been made. However, the role of receptor and G-protein lateral diffusion in signal transduction is supported by experiments in which alteration of plasma membrane fluidity affects enzyme activation (Hanski *et al.*, 1979; Moscona-Amir *et al.*, 1989; Gorospe and Conn, 1987; Gantzos and Neubig, 1988, Bakardjieva *et al.*, 1979). Thus, we have chosen to describe the formation of active G-proteins (α-GTP) as diffusion-limited.

One might describe the rate of production of α-GTP by a term $k_c CG$, where C is the number of bound receptors per cell, G is the number of G-proteins available for activation (GDP-$\alpha\beta\gamma$), and k_c is the coupling rate constant described in Section IV, C. If the coupling is diffusion-limited, then k_c is simply equal to k_+. A simple deterministic model for the early events in signal transduction could then be written by following the appearance of bound receptors with Eq. (6) and the production of α-GTP with the equation

$$\frac{d(\alpha\text{-GTP})}{dt} = k_c CG - k_h(\alpha\text{-GTP}), \qquad (61)$$

where k_h is the rate constant for the hydrolysis of GTP to GDP and thus the inactivation of α-GTP. No information about the spatial location of molecules is available in this approach. Such a model predicts that cells with similar time courses of receptor/ligand binding will produce similar time courses of α-GTP production and, presumably, similar generation of second messengers such as calcium.

In fact, however, it has been found by Mahama and Linderman (1994b) that cells which are predicted to have similar numbers of bound receptors may not have similar calcium responses when receptor antagonists or blockers, molecules which bind to receptors and prevent ligand binding,

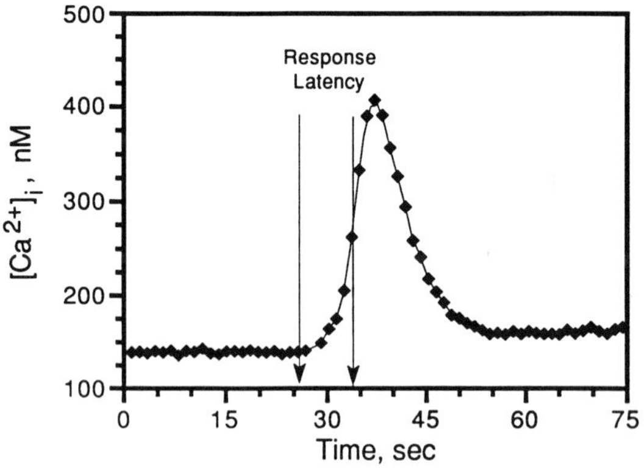

FIG. 22. Single-cell calcium response. Shown is the concentration of intracellular free calcium in a single cell as a function of time. The cell is stimulated with 10 μM PhE at a time indicated by the first arrow. The second arrow represents the time of maximum rate of calcium increase as determined by a nonlinear fit of the data. The time lag between the addition of PhE and the time of maximum rate of calcium increase is defined as the calcium response latency. The experimental methods used to derive the data of this figure and Fig. 23 are described in detail in Mahama and Linderman (1993a, b).

are used. In Fig. 22, the calcium response of a BC_3H1 cell stimulated with the ligand phenylephrine (PhE), which binds to α_1-adrenergic receptors, is shown. For this experimental system, receptor/ligand binding is rapid. Even for PhE concentrations as low as 0.1 μM, 95% of equilibrium receptor occupation is reached in less than 0.1 seconds. In comparison to receptor/ligand binding, calcium mobilization in these cells is slow, occurring 3–25 seconds after PhE stimulation. Thus, for simplicity, both the fraction of cells which mobilize calcium and the speed of calcium mobilization (defined as the time between ligand addition and the maximum rate of increase in intracellular free calcium concentration) are plotted as a function of the *equilibrium* receptor occupation by agonist in Fig. 23. In some of these experiments, the receptor blocker prazosin (Pz) was used; dissociation of prazosin during the time course of an experiment should be minimal because of its small dissociation rate constant. Note that for cases of equal receptor occupation by agonist, cells with inactivated or blocked receptors showed diminished calcium mobilization following ligand addition as compared to cells without inactivated receptors. Such a result is not anticipated from the simple model suggested earlier in this section [Eqs. (6) and (61)].

A clear difference between the experiments with and without receptor blocker is in the number of receptors actually available for ligand binding. Stickle and Barber (1989) have studied a similar experimental system, the binding of epinephrine to β-adrenergic receptors and the resulting activa-

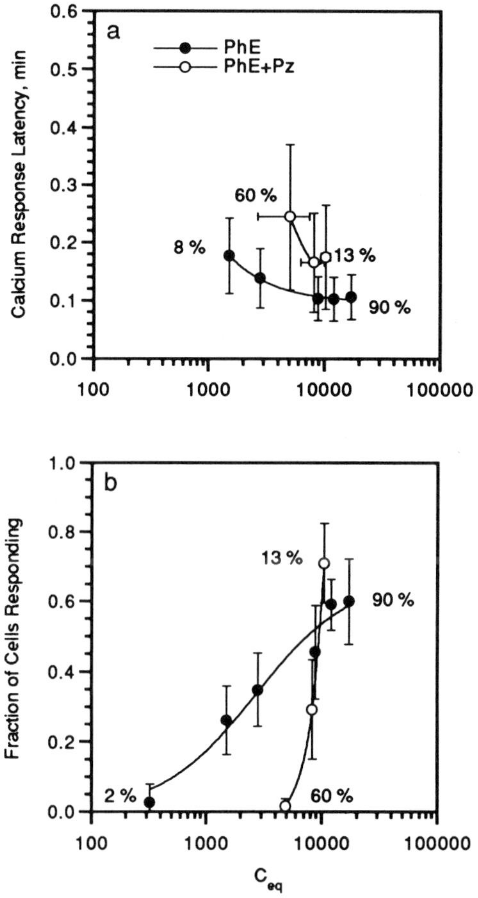

FIG. 23. Fraction of cells responding and calcium response latency. Both the fraction of cells responding and the calcium response latency depend on the equilibrium receptor occupation by phenylephrine (PhE), C_{eq}, which can be calculated from Eq. (7). Data without prazosin (Pz) pretreatment are shown as solid circles. Equilibrium receptor occupation for these data ranges from 2 to 90%. Open circles represent data for cells pretreated with prazosin to block cell receptors. For the three cases shown, prazosin treatment inactivates between 13 and 60% of the receptors. (a) The calcium response latency reaches a minimum at high equilibrium receptor occupation. For equal equilibrium receptor occupation, pretreatment with receptor blocker slows the calcium response. (b) The fraction of cells responding increases to a maximum at high equilibrium receptor occupation. As the fraction of receptors blocked by prazosin increases, the fraction of cells responding drops sharply.

tion of adenylate cyclase, and suggest that the receptor/ligand binding frequency, or rapid movement via diffusion of ligand among receptors, is important for enzyme activation at low ligand concentrations. This may partly explain the effect of receptor inactivation on calcium mobilization shown in the experiments of Fig. 23.

To examine the role of inactivated receptors, or reduced ability of ligand to move among receptors, Mahama and Linderman (1994b, c) have studied the two-dimensional diffusion and collision of receptors and G-proteins in the cell membrane using a dynamic simulation model. Receptor/ligand binding on the cell surface is described simply by

$$R + L \underset{k_r}{\overset{k_f}{\rightleftarrows}} C.$$

In simulations, conversion of receptors between ligand-occupied and unoccupied states was allowed to occur with a probability proportional to $k_f L$ and k_r, respectively.

Inactive G protein, $\beta\gamma\alpha$-GDP, is represented in the model formulation as G. As reasoned earlier, the activation of G-protein in the cell membrane was assumed to be diffusion-limited. Collision between a receptor/ligand complex and a G-protein results in the formation of a ternary receptor/ligand/G-protein complex. GTP binds to the α subunit within milliseconds, resulting in the dissociation of the ternary complex. Because the ternary complex is short-lived, G-protein activation is approximated by

$$G + C \longrightarrow C + \alpha\text{-GTP} + \beta\gamma.$$

The active α-GTP subunit has a limited lifetime, as its intrinsic GTPase activity results in hydrolysis of GTP to GDP:

$$\alpha\text{-GTP} \xrightarrow{k_h} \alpha\text{-GDP}.$$

Conversion of α-GTP to α-GDP in the simulations occurs with a probability proportional to the α-GTP inactivation rate constant, k_h. The inactive α-GDP subunit may combine with a $\beta\gamma$ subunit to reform the complete G-protein:

$$\alpha\text{-GDP} + \beta\gamma \longrightarrow G.$$

This reaction was assumed to be diffusion-limited and occurred upon collision of the two subunits. All reaction rate constants mentioned here, as well as other parameters used in the simulations, are summarized in Table II.

All simulations were run on a 1,000 × 1,000–grid mesh with a grid spacing of 7 nm, approximately a protein radius. Periodic boundary

TABLE II
PARAMETERS USED IN SIMULATIONS OF α-GTP PRODUCTION

Parameter	Meaning	Value	Ref.
K_D	Equilibrium receptor/ligand dissociation constant	5.8×10^{-6} M	*a*
k_f	Receptor/ligand association rate constant	$1 \times 10^{7}\ M^{-1}\ s^{-1}$	*b*
k_r	Receptor/ligand dissociation rate constant	$58\ s^{-1}$	
k_h	GTPase activity	$2\ s^{-1}$	*c*
R_T	Total number of α_1-adrenergic receptors	19,000 $cell^{-1}$	*d*
G_T	Total number of G-proteins	100,000 $cell^{-1}$	*e*
A	Cell surface area	2200 μm^2	
D	Diffusion coefficient	$1 \times 10^{-10}\ cm^2\ s^{-1}$	*f*

[a] Mauger *et al.* (1982); Amitai *et al.* (1984); Guellaen *et al.* (1978); Abel and Minneman (1986).

[b] Measurement of k_f and k_r have not been reported for the PhE/α_1-adrenergic system. Values used here are similar to those for epinephrine binding to β-adrenergic receptors (Richard Neubig, personal communication).

[c] Thompsen and Neubig (1989).

[d] Mauger *et al.* (1982); Hughes *et al.* (1982); Stickle and Barber (1989).

[e] Bokoch *et al.* (1988).

[f] Gennis (1989).

conditions were used. The simulations were initialized by placing receptors and G-proteins randomly on the simulation mesh. For simulations with inactive receptors, a fraction of the receptors placed on the mesh was randomly selected and permanently reidentified as antagonist-blocked receptors. All membrane species were allowed to move randomly and independently with the same mobility or diffusion coefficient. If a random move resulted in the collision of two nonreacting species, e.g., a receptor colliding with a receptor, the move was rejected. For collisions between reacting species such as $\beta\gamma$ and α-GDP subunits, the reaction was assumed to be diffusion-limited, and thus reaction occurred for every collision. The results shown are the average of 20 simulations converted to a single cell basis according to the cell surface area.

These dynamic simulations of receptors and G-proteins in the cell membrane were used to determine whether or not receptor inactivation significantly affects G-protein activation, and thus, presumably, calcium mobilization. Parameters for three test cases are listed in Table III. All test cases have equal numbers of G-protein and equal equilibrium receptor occupation. In test case 1, no receptors are blocked. In test cases 2 and 3, 59.5% and 74.4% of the receptors are blocked prior to ligand stimulation.

Simulation predictions for the time-course of G-protein activation for the three test cases are shown in Fig. 24. Test case 1, with no receptor

TABLE III
TEST CASES USED IN SIMULATIONS OF α-GTP PRODUCTION[a]

Parameters	Case 1: $f_B = 0.0$	Case 2: $f_B = 0.595$	Case 3: $f_B = 0.744$
Ligand concentration, L	2 μM	10 μM	10 mM
Total receptors per cell, R_T	19,000	19,000	19,000
Total G-protein per cell, G_T	100,000	100,000	100,000
Equilibrium number of receptor/ligand complexes, C_{eq}	~ 4900	~ 4900	~ 4900
Inactive receptors	0	~ 11,300	~ 14,100
Free receptors at equilibrium	~ 14,100	~ 2800	~ 0

[a]Cases compared have equal equilibrium receptor occupation. Case 1 has no blocked or inactivated receptors. Cases 2 and 3 have 59.5% and 74.4% of receptors blocked prior to ligand stimulation, respectively.

inactivation, leads to activation of approximately 20% more α-GTP than test case 2 and 40% more than test case 3 in the first three seconds.

The encounter rate constant k_c between receptor/ligand complexes and G-protein, calculated from simulation results, is shown for the three test cases in Fig. 25. The encounter rate constant for test case 1 remains approximately constant over the course of ligand stimulation. For cases 2 and 3, the encounter rate constants are initially lower than for test case 1. In addition, the encounter rate constants for cases 2 and 3 drop off quickly within the first two seconds of ligand stimulation to lower, approximately constant rates.

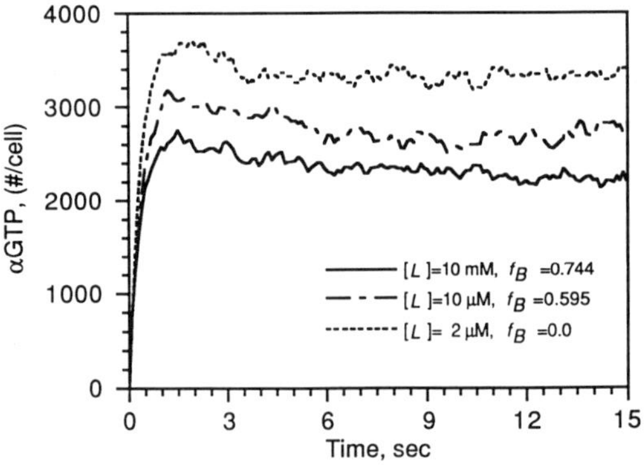

FIG. 24. Predictions of α-GTP production. For the three test cases with equal equilibrium receptor occupation, the simulations predict that inactivation of receptors inhibits G protein activation. In the first 3 seconds following ligand stimulation, test case 1 with $f_B = 0.0$ produces approximately 20% more α-GTP than test case 2 with $f_B = 59.5\%$, and 40% more α-GTP than test case 3 with $f_B = 74.4\%$.

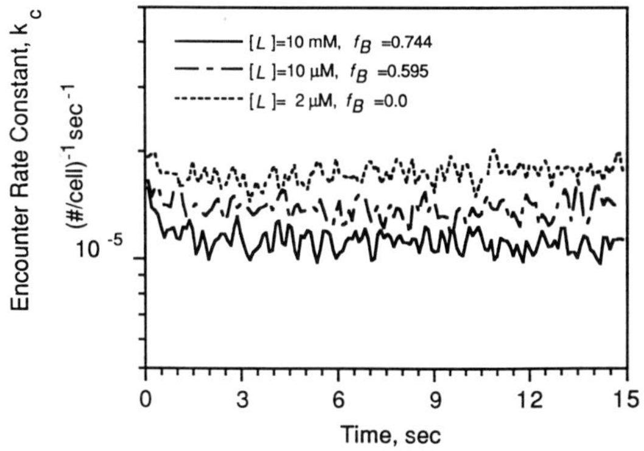

FIG. 25. Receptor/ligand complex and G protein encounter rate constant. For the three test cases with equal equilibrium receptor occupation, the simulations predict that inactivation of receptors reduces the rate of encounter between G protein and receptor/ligand complexes.

The differences in receptor/ligand complex and G-protein encounter rate constants between cases with and without receptor inactivation can be attributed to differences in the distribution of receptor/ligand complexes on the cell surface. To illustrate this difference, snapshots of receptor/ligand complexes and α-GTP from two simulations are shown in Fig. 26. The snapshots are from simulations of test cases 1 and 3. More α-GTP is produced in case 1 (Fig. 26a) than 3 (Fig. 26b), and the α-GTP is more evenly distributed over the cell membrane in case 1. For test case 3, α-GTP is segregated in patches in the membrane and all α-GTP is located very near a receptor/ligand complex. For test case 1, some α-GTP subunits are found more distant from receptor/ligand complexes than would be possible by diffusion of receptor/ligand complexes and G-proteins alone; ligand movement among receptors by diffusion above the cell surface has occurred.

In test case 1, then, the system is relatively "well-mixed," and Eq. (61) with a constant value of k_c is a reasonable model. In test cases 2 and 3, the system is not "well-mixed," and the spatial location of molecules, obtainable from this type of simulation, plays a role in the formation of α-GTP. Even when k_c is relatively constant, however, it may be poorly estimated by Eq. (50b) (Mahama and Linderman, 1994c).

For test case 1, no receptors are blocked, and the cells are stimulated with a low ligand concentration. Ligand binds to receptors on the cell surface, and by two-dimensional diffusion, receptor/ligand complexes collide with several G-proteins in their vicinity to produce α-GTP. Ligand may dissociate and bind to other receptors in the cell membrane, produc-

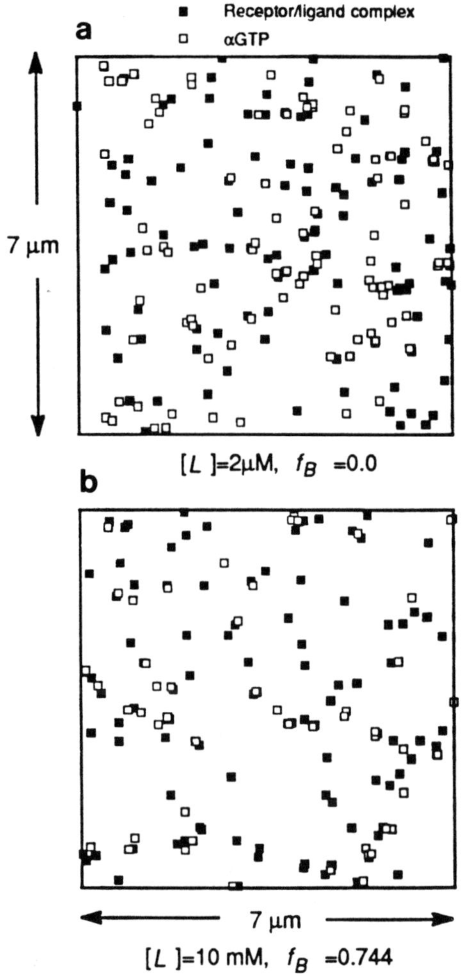

FIG. 26. Snapshots of receptor/ligand complexes and α-GTP. The simulation snapshots are for test cases 1 and 3 with equal equilibrium receptor occupation, and are taken at $t = 3$ seconds. For (a), movement of ligand among free receptors and diffusion are important in activation of G protein. For (b), ligand movement among receptors is insignificant in G protein activation because the number of free receptors is nearly zero; G protein activation occurs almost exclusively by 2-D diffusion. Because of the movement of ligand among receptors, α-GTP formation is greater and more evenly distributed in (a) than (b). Also, α-GTP is seen at greater distances from receptor/ligand complexes in (a) because of the effect of ligand movement. For easy visualization, symbols are not drawn to scale.

ing complexes over the entire cell surface. This movement of ligand among free receptors allows thorough access of receptor/ligand complexes to G-protein. Approximately 25% of the receptors are occupied at equilibrium, so a receptor is more likely to be unoccupied than occupied. Thus, for this case, movement or switching of ligand among receptors as well as receptor mobility is important for G-protein activation.

For test cases 2 and 3, a large fraction of the receptors is inactivated by the receptor blocker, so much higher concentrations of ligand are needed to produce the same equilibrium receptor occupation as in test case 1. Ligand again binds to receptors on the cell surface, and receptor/ligand complexes activate G-proteins in their vicinity by two-dimensional diffusion and collision. However, because the ligand concentration is higher, each receptor has a higher probability of rebinding ligand than in test case 1. At equilibrium, more than 63% and 99% of the available receptors are occupied by ligand in test cases 2 and 3, respectively. Therefore, a receptor is more likely to be ligand-occupied than unoccupied. With fewer free receptors in these cases, switching of ligand among receptors plays a less significant role in G-protein activation than in test case 1. For this reason, the receptor/ligand complexes tend to activate most of the G-proteins in their vicinity by two-dimensional diffusion, causing a local depletion of inactive G-protein. As this occurs, the encounter rate constant between G-proteins and complexes decreases to a steady-state value lower than that for test case 1.

Most importantly, the results of these dynamic simulations offer an explanation for the effect of receptor blockers (Fig. 23). The model predicts that for the same equilibrium dissociation constant, K_D, the association/dissociation rate constants of receptor/ligand binding may determine whether or not receptor blockers affect calcium mobilization. The behavior extremes occur when association/dissociation rates are fast and slow relative to the rate of two-dimensional diffusion.

For the case in which receptor/ligand binding is slow compared to two-dimensional diffusion, movement of ligand among free receptors will not play a significant role in G-protein activation at any ligand concentration. Activation of G-protein occurs mainly by two-dimensional diffusion, and activation by ligand movement is insignificant. In this situation, then, receptor inactivation will have little effect on G-protein activation. A model of calcium mobilization, based in part on Eqs. (6) and (61), will make reasonable predictions for cases with and without receptor blockers.

For the other extreme in which receptor/ligand binding kinetics are fast compared to two-dimensional diffusion, switching of ligand among free receptors may be a major contributor to G-protein activation. At low ligand concentrations, movement of ligand among receptors on the cell surface provides an increased encounter frequency between complexes and G-protein. The contribution of ligand movement to G-protein activation decreases as ligand concentration increases because the fraction of unoccupied receptors decreases. In this situation, then, receptor inactivation significantly reduces G-protein activation by reducing the component of G-protein activation produced by ligand movement among receptors. A model, based in part on Eqs. (6) and (61), will overestimate G-protein activation and thus calcium mobilization for fast receptor/ligand binding kinetics in the presence of receptor blocker because the reduction in ligand movement among free receptors caused by receptor inactivation is not considered; all G-proteins are assumed accessible.

The experimental system which motivated these computations, that of phenylephrine binding to α_1-adrenergic receptors, falls closest to this second extreme, the case in which receptor/ligand binding kinetics are rapid compared to two-dimensional diffusion. This suggests that use of the receptor blocker prazosin may significantly reduce G-protein activation by restricting ligand movement. Thus, the diminished cell responsiveness observed with receptor blocker may be partially accounted for through reduced G-protein activation, and thus lower PLC activation and calcium release. The movement of ligand among receptors is especially important for low levels of receptor occupation; this is where the greatest disparity in the calcium responses with and without receptor blocker is seen.

Receptor antagonists, or blockers, are a common target of pharmacologic agents, and more recently research has turned to the design of agents to inhibit receptor-catalyzed G-protein activation (e.g., Dalman and Neubig, 1991). Our findings suggest that a quantitative characterization of the effects of these agents may require analyses such as that presented here.

VI. Conclusions

In much previous work, receptor-mediated events such as binding and trafficking (see Fig. 3) have been treated as essentially chemical phenomena (reviewed in Lauffenburger and Linderman, 1993). That is, the rate constants representing the various kinetic events were considered to be characteristics of the particular molecular components involved. Although this is true to a large degree, receptor-mediated phenomena are not governed totally by purely intrinsic chemical properties. Merely physical features of the systems can sometimes significantly influence observed process rates. We have examined here two such physical aspects: diffusion and probabilistic effects. Diffusion effects will play a role in ligand binding to surface receptors when the receptor concentration is relatively large or when the binding rates are very fast. In two-dimensional molecular interactions taking place on a membrane, diffusion can be expected generally to play a crucial role. Probabilistic effects must be anticipated when receptor-mediated cell behavior is sensitive to changes in small numbers of molecules. Hence, the rates of receptor binding, trafficking, and signaling events can depend on quantities such as diffusion coefficients and receptor number. Although these quantities certainly reflect some characteristics of the molecular components involved, they are much less intimately related to molecular structure that might be altered dramatically by small changes in protein sequence.

Analysis of receptor/ligand interactions is made much more complicated by explicit consideration of these physical features. Without such considerations, we are often able to model receptor phenomena with first-order ordinary differential equations based on straightforward mass-action kinetic species balances. When diffusion and probabilistic effects are taken into account, the models can easily give rise to partial differential equations, second-order ordinary differential equations, extremely large sets of first-order ordinary differential equations, and/or probabilistic differential equations.

As an alternative to the formulation and analytical solution of such equations, we have successfully used simulations to investigate the movement of ligands prior to receptor/ligand binding and the movement of bound receptors and G-proteins leading to G-protein activation. Given the dramatically increasing power of computational facilities available to researchers, we anticipate widespread application of direct simulation methods to model situations of great complexity. Such simulations may prove to be increasingly important as investigators attempt to integrate the influence of these receptor and ligand properties through the various levels involved in behavioral responses: binding, trafficking, signaling, interaction with other cell components, and gene regulation.

At the heart of all future modeling work, though, must be model validation through experiment. To us, this is perhaps the most exciting aspect of this approach. Given the growing capabilities of molecular biologists to alter molecular structures of receptors, ligand, and effectors, there is no excuse for avoiding the direct testing of models with intentional modification of system parameter values. The coming years should be a golden age for molecular-based modeling of cell receptor phenomena, because models can be formulated and tested using manipulation of key molecular species in terms of their important quantitataive properties.

Acknowledgments

J. J. L. and D. A. L. express appreciation for grant funding from the following for helping support work related to this article: National Science Foundation, National Institutes of Health, Whitaker Foundation, Procter & Gamble, and University of Illinois National Center for Supercomputing Applications.

Notation

Symbol	Definition	Typical Units
a	cell radius	μm
A	cell surface area	μm^2
b	radius of a cell region	μm
C	constant	
C	receptor/ligand complex number	#/cell
C_{eq}	equilibrium receptor/ligand complex number	#/cell
C_0	initial receptor/ligand complex number	#/cell
D	diffusion coefficient	cm^2/s
D_{cell}	cell diffusion coefficient	cm^2/s
D_i	component of diffusion coefficient in i-direction	cm^2/s
D_R	receptor diffusion coefficient	cm^2/s
f_B	fraction of receptors blocked	
G	number of G-protein molecules	#/cell
G_T	total number of G-protein molecules	#/cell
$G(s,t)$	generating function	
h	membrane thickness	nm
k_c	coupling or encounter rate constant	$(\#/\text{cell})^{-1}\ s^{-1}$ or cm^2/s^a
k_f	rate constant for association of receptor/ligand complexes (per receptor)	cm^3/s^b
$(k_f)_{cell}$	association rate constant per cell	cm^3/s^b
k_h	rate constant for GTP hydrolysis	s^{-1}
k_{off}	intrinsic dissociation rate constant	s^{-1}
k_{on}	intrinsic association rate constant per receptor	$cm^3/s^{b,c}$
$(k_{on})_{cell}$	intrinsic association rate constant per cell	cm^3/s^b
k_r	rate constant for receptor/ligand complex dissociation	s^{-1}

k_u	uncoupling rate constant	s^{-1}
k_+	transport rate constant per receptor	$cm^3/s^{b,c}$
$(k_+)_{cell}$	transport rate constant per cell	cm^3/s^b
K_A	equilibrium association constant	M^{-1}
K_B	Boltzmann's constant ($= 1.38 \times 10^{-16}$ g-cm^2/s^2-K)	
K_D	equilibrium dissociation constant	M
l	characteristic system dimension	cm
L	ligand concentration	M
L_0	initial concentration of ligand	M
n	cell concentration	#/volume
$n_{capture}$	number of molecules captured	#
n_{escape}	number of molecules escaping	#
n_R	free receptor concentration on the cell surface	$\#/cm^2$
n_{Rb}	free receptor concentration at a distance b	$\#/cm^2$
N_{Av}	Avogadro's number ($= 6.02 \times 10^{23}$ #/mole)	
P	probability of capture at a finite truncation distance	
P_∞	probability of capture at an infinite truncation distance	
P_j	probability that there are j complexes	
Q	truncation height	nm
r	radial position	cm
R_i	change in position, direction i	cm
R	free receptor number	#/cell
R_T	total surface receptor number	#/cell
s	dummy variable	
s	encounter radius or molecule radius	nm
s'	reactive site radius	nm
S_i	new coordinate of ligand in i-direction	
S_i^0	previous coordinate of ligand in i-direction	
t	time	s
t_{sample}	time period	s
T	absolute temperature	K
u	dimensionless receptor/ligand complex number	
u_{eq}	dimensionless equilibrium receptor/ligand complex number	
u_0	initial dimensionless receptor/ligand complex number	
V	sampling volume	cm^3
x_i	position (ith coordinate)	

X	number of species X	#/cell
α-GTP	number of α-GTP molecules	#/cell
γ	capture probability for a receptor	
γ_{cell}	capture probability for a cell	
γ_E	Euler's constant (= 0.5772)	
δ	standard deviation in a quantity	
Δt	time interval	s
η_m	membrane viscosity	g/cm-s
η_s	solution viscosity	g/cm-s
θ	dimensionless ratio of membrane to solution viscosities	
θ_R	angle circumscribing reactive portion of receptor	radians
λ_0	dimensionless ligand concentration	
ρ	ρ_{cell} or ρ_{rec}	
ρ_{cell}	ratio of rate constants for binding to cell surface receptors	
ρ_{rec}	ratio of rate constants for binding to solution receptors	
σ_c^2	variance in C	#/cell
$(\sigma_c^2)_{eq}$	variance in C_{eq}	#/cell
τ	dimensionless time	
$\tau_{1/2}$	dimensionless half-time	
ϕ	fractional surface coverage of a cell with receptors	
$\langle \cdot \rangle$	expected or mean value of a quantity	

[a] More accurately, $(\#/cm^2)^{-1}\ s^{-1}$.
[b] More accurately, $(\#/cm^3)^{-1}\ s^{-1}$. Commonly converted to $M^{-1}\ s^{-1}$.
[c] For two-dimensional reactions the units are typically cm^2/s, or, more accurately, $(\#/cm^2)^{-1}\ s^{-1}$.

References

Abel, P. W., and Minneman, K. P., Alpha-1 adrenergic receptor binding and contraction of rat caudal artery. *J. Pharmacol. Exp. Ther.* **239**, 678 (1986).

Adam, G., and Delbruck, M., Reduction of dimensionality in biological diffusion processes. In "Structural Chemistry and Molecular Biology," (A. Rich and A. Davidson, eds.), p. 198. Freeman, San Francisco, 1968.

Akiyama, S. K., and Yamada, K. M., The interaction of plasma fibronectin with fibroblastic cells in suspension. *J. Biol. Chem.* **260**, 4492 (1985).

Amitai, G., Brown, R. D., and Taylor, P., The relationship between α_1-adrenergic receptor occupation and the mobilization of intracellular calcium. *J. Biol. Chem.* **259**, 12519 (1984).

Axelrod, D., Koppel, D. E., Schlessinger, J., Elson, E., and Webb, W. W., Mobility measurement by analysis of fluorescence photobleaching recovery kinetics. *Biophy. J.* **16**, 1055 (1976).

Baird, B., Erickson, J., Goldstein, B., Kane, P., Menon, A. K., Robertson, D., and Holowka, D., Progress toward understanding the molecular details and consequences of IgE-receptor crosslinking. *In* "Theoretical Immunology" (A. S. Perelson, ed.), Part One, p. 41. Addison-Wesley, Redwood City, CA, 1988.

Bajzer, Z., Myers, A. C., and Vuk-Pavlovic, S., Binding, internalization, and intracellular processing of proteins interacting with recycling receptors: A kinetic analysis. *J. Biol. Chem.* **264**, 13623 (1989).

Bakardjieva, A., Galla, H. J., and Helmreich, E. J. M., Modulation of the β-receptor adenylate cyclase interactions in cultured change liver cells by phospholipid enrichment. *Biochem.* **18**, 3016 (1979).

Barak, L. S., and Webb, W. W., Diffusion of low density lipoprotein-receptor complex on human, fibroblasts. *J. Cell Biol.* **95**, 846 (1982).

Berg, H. C., and Purcell, E. M., Physics of chemoreception. *Biophys. J.* **20**, 193 (1977).

Berg, O., and von Hippel, P. H., Diffusion-controlled macromolecular interactions. *Annu. Rev. Biophys. Biophy. Chem.* **14**, 131 (1985).

Berridge, M. J., Inositol trisphosphate and calcium signalling. *Nature (London)* **361**, 315 (1993).

Bharuca-Reid, A. T., "Elements of the Theory of Markov Processes and their Application." McGraw-Hill, New York, 1960.

Birnbaumer, L., Receptor-to-effector signaling through G proteins: Roles for $\beta\gamma$ dimers as well as α subunits. *Cell (Cambridge, Mass.)* **71**, 1069 (1992).

Birnbaumer, L., Abramowitz, J., and Brown, A. M., Receptor-effector coupling by G proteins. *Biochim. Biophys. Acta* **1031**, 163 (1990).

Bokoch, G. M., Bickford, K., and Bohl, B. P., Subcellular localization and quantitation of the major neutrophil pertussis toxin substrate, G_n. *J. Cell Biol.* **106**, 1927 (1988).

Brown, M. S., and Goldstein, J. L., Analysis of a mutant strain of human fibroblasts with a defect in internalization of receptor-bound low density lipoprotein. *Cell (Cambridge, Mass.)* **9**, 663 (1976).

Bruckert, F., Chabre, M., and Vuong, T. M., Kinetic analysis of the activation of transducing by photoexcited rhodopsin: Influence of the lateral diffusion of transducing and competition of guanosine diphosphate and guanosine triphosphate for the nucleotide site. *Biophys. J.* **63**, 616 (1992).

Brunn, P. O., Absorption by bacterial cells: Interaction between receptor sites and the effect of fluid motion. *J. Biomech. Eng.* **103**, 32 (1981).

Burgoyne, R. D., and Cheek, T. R., Locating intracellular calcium stores. *Trends Biol. Sci.* **16**, 319 (1991).

Bussell, S. J., Koch, D. L., and Hammer, D. A., The resistivity and mobility functions for a model system of two equal-sized proteins in a lipid bilayer. *J. Fluid Mech.* **243**, 679 (1992).

Bussell, S. J., Koch, D. L., and Hammer, D. A., The effect of hydrodynamic interactions on the diffusion of integral membrane proteins: Diffusion in plasma membranes. Submitted for publication (1994a).

Bussell, S. J., Hammer, D. A., and Koch, D. L., The effect of hydrodynamic interactions on the tracer and gradient diffusion of integral membrane proteins in lipid bilayers. *J. Fluid. Mech.* **258**, 167 (1994b).

Cantrell, D. A., Collins, M. K. L., and Crumpton, M. J., Autocrine regulation of T-lymphocyte proliferation: Differential induction of IL-2 and IL-2 receptor. *Immunology* **65**, 343 (1988).

Ciechanover, A., Schwartz, A. L., Dautry-Varsat, A., and Lodish, H. F., Kinetics of internalization and recycling of transferrin and the transferrin receptor in a human hepatoma cell line: Effect of lysosomtropic agents. *J. Biol. Chem.* **258**, 9681 (1983).

Claret, E., Renversez, J.-C., Zheng, X., Bonnefoiz, T., and Sotto, J.-J., Valid estimation of IL2 secretion by PHA-stimulated T-cell clones absolutely requires the use of anti-CD25 monoclonal antibodies to prevent IL2 consumption. *Immunol. Lett.* **33**, 179 (1992).

Collins, M. K. L., Malde, P., Miyajima, A., Arai, K.-I., Smith, K. A., and Mulligan, R. C., Evidence that the level of the p55 component of the interleukin (IL) 2 receptor can control IL 2 responsiveness in a murine IL 3-dependent cell. *Eur. J. Immunol.* **20**, 573 (1990).

Cox, R. G., and Brenner, H., The slow motion of a sphere through a viscous fluid towards a plane surface. II. Small gap widths, including inertial effects. *Chem. Eng. Sci.* **22**, 1753 (1967).

Cozens-Roberts, C., Lauffenburger, D. A., and Quinn, J. Q., Receptor-mediated cell attachment and detachment kinetics: I. Probabilistic model and analysis. *Biophys. J.* **58**, 841, (1990*a*).

Cozens-Roberts, C., Quinn, J. A., and Lauffenburger, D. A., Receptor-mediated cell attachment and detachment kinetics: II. Experimental model studies with the radial-flow detachment assay. *Biophys. J.* **58**, 857 (1990*b*).

Cuttitta, F., Carney, D. N., Mulshine, J., Moody, T. W., Fedorko, J., Fischler, A., and Minna, J. D., Bombesin-like peptides can function as autocrine growth factors in human small-cell lung cancer. *Nature (London)* **316**, 823 (1985).

Dalman, H. M., and Neubig, R. R., Two peptides from the α_{2A}-adrenergic receptor alter receptor G protein coupling by distinct mechanisms. *J. Biol. Chem.* **266**, 11025 (1991).

DeLisi, C., The biophysics of ligand-receptor interactions. *Q. Rev. Biophys.* **13**, 201 (1980).

DeLisi, C., and Wiegel, F. W., Effect of nonspecific forces and finite receptor number on rate constants of ligand-cell bound-receptor interactions. *Proc. Natl. Acad. Sci. U.S.A.* **78**, 5569 (1981).

Dickinson, R. B., and Tranquillo, R. T., A stochastic model for adhesion-mediated cell random motility and haptotaxis. *J. Math. Biol.* **31**, 563 (1993).

Doraiswamy, L. K., and Kulkarni, B. D., "The Analysis of Chemically Reacting Systems: A Stochastic Approach." Gordon & Breach, New York, 1987.

Earle, W. R., Sanford, K. K., Evans, V. J., Waltz, H. K., and Shannon, J. J. E., The Influence of inoculum size on proliferation in tissue culture. *J. Natl. Cancer Inst. (U.S.)* **12**, 133 (1951).

Echavarria-Heras, H., Convective flow effects in receptor-mediated endocytosis. *Math. Biosci.* **89**, 9 (1988).

Edidin, M., Zagyansky, Y., and Lardner, T. J., Measurement of membrane protein lateral diffusion in single cells. *Science* **191**, 466 (1976).

Erickson, J., Goldstein, B., Holowka, D., and Baird, B., The effect of receptor density on the forward rate constant for binding of ligands to cell surface receptors. *Biophys. J.* **52**, 657 (1987).

Ermak, D. L., and McCammon, J. A., Brownian dynamics with hydrodynamic interactions. *J. Chem. Phys.* **69**, 1352 (1978).

Faber, D. S., Young, W. S., Legendre, P., and Korn, H. Intrinsic quantal variability due to stochastic properties of receptor-transmitter interactions. *Science* **258**, 1494 (1992).

Forsten, K. E., and Lauffenburger, D. A., Autocrine ligand binding to cell receptors Mathematical analysis of competition by solution "decoys." *Biophys. J.* **61**, 1 (1992a).

Forsten, K. E., and Lauffenburger, D. A., Interrupting autocrine ligand-receptor binding: Comparison between receptor blockers and ligand decoys. *Biophy. J.* **63**, 857 (1992b).

Forsten, K. E., and Lauffenburger, D. A., Probability of autocrine ligand capture by cell-surface receptors: Implications for ligand secretion measurements. *J. Comp. Biol.* **1**, 15 (1994*a*).

Forsten, K. E., and Lauffenburger, D. A., The role of low-affinity interleukin-2 receptors in autocrine ligand binding: Alternative mechanisms for enhanced binding effect. *Mol. Immunol.* **31**, 739 (1994b).

Gantzos, R. D., and Neubig, R. R., Temperature effects on α_2-adrenergic receptor-G_i interactions. *Biochem. Pharmacol.* **37**, 2815 (1988).

Gardiner, C. W., "Handbook of Stochastic Methods for Physics, Chemistry, and the Natural Sciences." Springer-Verlag, New York, 1983.

Gennis, R. B., "Biomembranes: Molecular Structure and Function." Springer-Verlag, New York, 1989.

Goel, N. S., and Richter-Dyn, N., "Stochastic Models in Biology." Academic Press, New York, 1974.

Goldman, A. J., Cox, R. G., and Brenner, H., Slow viscous motion of a sphere parallel to a plane wall. I. Motion through a quiescent fluid. *Chem. Eng. Sci.* **22**, 637 (1967).

Goldstein, B., Diffusion limited effects of receptor clustering. *Comm. Theor. Biol.* **1**, 109 (1989).

Goldstein, B., and Wiegel, F. W., The effect of receptor clustering on diffusion-limited forward rate constants. *Biophys. J.* **43**, 121 (1983).

Goldstein, B., and Wiegel, F. W., The distribution of cell surface proteins on spreading cells. *Biophys. J.* **53**, 175 (1988).

Goldstein, B., Wofsy, C., and Bell, G., Interactions of low density lipoprotein receptors with coated pits on human fibroblasts: Estimate of the forward rate constant and comparison with the diffusion limit. *Proc. Natl. Acad. Sci. U.S.A.* **78**, 5695 (1981).

Goldstein, B., Wofsy, C., and Echavarria-Heras, H., Effect of membrane flow on the capture of receptors by coated pits. *Biophys. J.* **53**, 405 (1988).

Goldstein, B., Posner, R. G., Torney, D. C., Erickson, J., Holowka, D., and Baird, B., Competition between solution and cell surface receptors for ligand: Dissociation of hapten bound to surface antibody in the presence of solution antibody. *Biophys. J.* **56**, 955 (1989).

Gorospe, W. C., and Conn, P. M., Membrane fluidity regulates development of gonadotrope desensitization to GnRH. *Mol. Cell. Endocrinol.* **53**, 131 (1987).

Green, N. M., Avidin. *Adv. Protein Chem.* **29**, 85 (1975).

Guellaen, G., Yates-Aggerbeck, M., Vauquelin, G., Strosberg, D., and Hanoune, J., Characterization with [^{3}H]dihydroergocryptine of the α-adrenergic receptor of the hepatic plasma membrane. *J. Biol. Chem.* **253**, 114 (1978).

Hammer, D. A., and Apte, S. A., Simulation of cell rolling and adhesion on surfaces in shear flow: General results and analysis of selection-mediated neutrophil adhesion. *Biophys. J.* **63**, 35 (1992).

Hanski, E., Rimon, G., and Levitzki, A., Adenylate cyclase activation by the β-adrenergic receptors as a diffusion-controlled process. *Biochemistry* **18**, 846 (1979).

Happel, J., and Brenner, H., "Low Reynolds Number Hydrodynamics," 2 rev. ed. Noordhoff Int. Pub., Grøningen. Leyden; The Netherlands, 1973.

Heizmann, C. W., and Hunziker, W., Intracellular calcium-binding proteins: More sites than insights. *Trends Biol. Sci.* **16**, 98 (1991).

Hu, W., Meier, J., and Wang, D. I. C., A mechanistic analysis of the inoculum requirement for the cultivation of mammalian cells on microcarriers, *Biotechnol. Bioeng.* **27**, 585 (1985).

Hughes, R. J., Boyle, J. R., Brown, R. D., Taylor, R., and Insel, P. A., Characterization of coexisting alpha$_1$- and beta$_2$-adrenergic receptors on a cloned muscle cell line, BC3H-1. *Mol. Pharmacol.* **22**, 258 (1982).

Hulme, E. C., ed., "Receptor-Ligand Interactions: A Practical Approach." IRL Press, Oxford, 1992.

Imanishi, K., Yamaguchi, K., Kuranami, M., Kyo, E., Hozumi, T., and Abe, K., Inhibition of growth of human lung adenocarcinoma cell lines by anti-transforming growth factor—a monoclonal antibody. *J. Natl. Cancer Inst.* **81**, 220 (1989).

Jacobs, S., and Cuatrecasas, P., The mobile receptor hypothesis and "cooperativity" of hormone binding. *Biochim. Biophys. Acta* **433**, 482 (1976).

Jankovic, D. L., Rebollo, A., Kumar, A., Gibert, M., and Thèze, J., IL-2-dependent proliferation of murine T cells requires expression of both the p55 and p70 subunits of the IL-2 receptor. *J. Immunol.* **145**, 4136 (1990).

Jans, D. A., The mobile receptor hypothesis revisited: A mechanistic role for hormone lateral mobility in signal transduction. *Biochim. Biophys. Acta* **1113**, 271 (1992).

Kawano, M., Hirano, T., Matsuda, T., Taga, T., Horii, Y., Iwato, K., Asaoku, H., Tang, B., Tanabe, O., Tanaka, H., Kuramoto, A., and Kishimoto, T., Autocrine generation and requirement of BSF-2/IL-6 for human multiple myelomas. *Nature (London)* **332**, 83 (1988).

Keizer, J., Theory of rapid bimolecular reactions in solution and membranes. *Acc. Chem. Res.* **18**, 235 (1985).

Klein, R., Jing, S., Nanduri, V., O'Rourke, E., and Barbacid, M., The trk proto-oncogene encodes a receptor for nerve growth factor. *Cell (Cambridge, Mass.)* **65**, 189 (1991).

Kumer, A., Moreau, J.-L., Baran, D., and Thèze, J., Evidence for negative regulation of T cell growth by low affinity interleukin 2 receptors. *J. Immunol.* **138**, 1485 (1987).

Kuziel, W. A., Ju, G., Grdina, T. A., and Greene, W. C., Unexpected effects of the IL-2 receptor α subunit of high affinity IL-2 receptor assembly and function detected with a mutant IL-2 analog. *J. Immunol.* **150**, 3357 (1993).

Kwon, G., Lateral mobility of fluorescently labelled G protein subunits in intact cells Ph.D. Thesis, University of Michigan, Ann Arbor, 1992.

Kwon, G., and Neubig, R. R., Lateral mobility of alpha and beta-gamma subunits of G_0 in NG 108-15 cells. *Biophys. J.* **61**, A96 (1992).

Lauffenburger, D. A., and Cozens, C., Regulation of mammalian cell growth by autocrine growth factors: Analysis of consequences for inoculum cell density effects. *Biotechnol. Bioeng.* **33**, 1365 (1989).

Lauffenburger, D. A., and Linderman, J. J., "Receptors: Models for Binding, Trafficking, and Signaling." Oxford Univ. Press, New York, 1993.

Limbird, L. E., "Cell Surface Receptors: A Short Course on Theory and Methods." Martinus Nijhoff, Boston, 1986.

Lipkin, E. W., Teller, D. C., and de Haen, C., Kinetics of insulin binding to rat white fat cells at 15°C. *J. Biol. Chem.* **261**, 1702 (1986).

Maddox, J., Is molecular biology yet a science? *Nature (London)* **355**, 201 (1992).

Mahama, P. A., and Linderman, J. J., Calcium signaling in individual BC_3H1 muscle cells: Speed of calcium mobilization and heterogeneity. *Biotechnol. Prog.* **10**, 45 (1994a).

Mahama, P. A., and Linderman, J. J., Monte Carlo simulations of membrane signal transduction events: Effect of receptor blockers on G Protein activation. *Ann. Biomed. Eng.* (1994b) (in press).

Mahama, P. A., and Linderman, J. J., A Monte Carlo study of the dynamics of G-protein activation. *Biophys. J.* **67**, 1345 (1994c).

Marsagla, G., Zamen, A., and Tsang, W. W., Toward a universal random number generator. *Stat. Probab. Lett.* **9**, 35 (1990).

Mauger, J. P., Sladeczek, F., and Brockaert, J., Characteristics and metabolism of α_1 adrenergic receptors in a nonfusing muscle cell line. *J. Biol. Chem.* **257**, 875 (1982).

Mayo, K. H., Nuñez, M., Burke, C., Starbuck, C., Lauffenburger, D. A., and Savage, C. R., Jr., Epidermal growth factor receptor binding is not a simple one-step process. *J. Biol. Chem.* **264**, 17838 (1989).

McCammon, J. A., Computer-aided molecular design, *Science* **238**, 486 (1991).

McCammon, J. A., Northrup, S. H., and Allison, S. A., Diffusional dynamics of ligand-receptor association. *J. Phys. Chem.* **90**, 3901 (1986).

McGeady, M. L., Kerby, S., Shankar, V., Ciardiello, F., Salomon, D., and Seidman, M., Infection with a TGF-α retroviral vector transforms normal mouse mammary epithelial cells but not normal rat fibroblasts. *Oncogene* **4**, 1375 (1989).

McQuarrie, D. A., Kinetics of small systems. I. *J. Chem. Phys.* **38**, 433 (1963).

Mellman, I. S., and Unkeless, J. C., Purification of a functional mouse Fc receptor through the use of a monoclonal antibody. *J. Exp. Med.* **152**, 1048 (1980).

Menon, A. K., Holowka, D., Webb, W. W., and Baird, B., Clustering, mobility, and triggering activity of small oligomers of immunoglobulin E on rat basophilic leukemia cells. *J. Cell Biol.* **102**, 534 (1986).

Mitchison, T., and Kirschner, M., Dynamic instability of microtubule growth. *Nature (London)* **312**, 237 (1984).

Miyajima, A., Hara, T., and Kitamura, T., Common subunits of cytokine receptors and the functional redundancy of cytokines. *Trends Biol. Sic.* **17**, 378 (1992).

Moscona-Amir, E., Henis, Y. I., and Sokolovsky, M., Aging of rat heat myocytes disrupts muscarinic receptor coupling that leads to inhibition of cAMP accumulation and alters the pathway of muscarinic-stimulated phosphoinositide hydolysis. *Biochemistry* **28**, 7130 (1989).

Munson, P. J., and Rodbard, D., Ligand: A versatile computerized approach for characterization of ligand-binding systems. *Anal. Biochem.* **107**, 220 (1980).

Nishizuka, Y., Studies and perspectives of protein kinase C. *Science* **233**, 305 (1986).

Northrup, S. H., Diffusion-controlled ligand binding to multiple competing cell-bound receptors. *J. Phys. Chem.* **92**, 5847 (1988).

Northrup, S. H., Allison, S. A., and McCammon, J. A., Brownian dynamics simulation of diffusion-influenced bimolecular reactions. *J. Chem. Phys.* **80**, 1517 (1984).

Northrup, S. H., Cuvin, M. S., Allison, S. A., and McCammon, J. A., Optimization of Brownian dynamics methods for diffusion-influenced rate constant calculations. *J. Chem. Phys.* **84**, 2196 (1986).

Peters, R., and Cherry, R. J., Lateral and rotational diffusion of bacteriorhodopsin in lipid bilayers: Experimental test of the Saffman-Delbruck equations. *Proc. Natl. Acad. Sci. U.S.A.*, **79**, 4317 (1982).

Poo, M., Lam, J. W., and Orida, N., Electrophoresis and diffusion in the plane of the cell membrane. *Biophys. J.* **26**, 1 (1979).

Pruzansky, J. J., and Patterson, R., Binding constants of IgE receptors on human blood basophils for IgE. *Immunology* **58**, 257 (1986).

Rhee, H.-K., Aris, R., and Amundson, N. R., "First-Order Partial Differential Equations," Vol. 1. Prentice-Hall, Englewood Cliffs, NJ, 1986.

Rimon, G., Hanski, E., and Levitzki, A., Temperature dependence of β receptor, adenosine receptor, and sodium fluoride stimulated adenylate cyclase from turkey erythrocytes. *Biochemistry* **19**, 4451 (1980).

Robb, R. J., Munck, A., and Smith, K. A., T cell growth factor receptors. *J. Exp. Med* **154**, 1455 (1981).

Rodgers, W., and Glaser, M., Fluorescence microscopic imaging of membrane domains. *In* "Optical Microscopy: Emerging Methods and Applications," (B. Herman and J. J. Lemasters, eds.), p. 263 Academic Press, San Diego, 1993.

Ryan, T. A., Myers, J., Holowka, D., Baird, B., and Webb, W. W., Molecular crowding on the cell surface. *Science* **239**, 61 (1988).

Saffman, P. G., and Delbruck, M., Brownian motion in biological membranes. *Proc. Natl. Acad. Sci. U.S.A.* **72**, 3111 (1975).

Saxton, M. J., Lateral diffusion in a mixture of mobile and immobile particles: A Monte Carlo study. *Biophys. J.* **58**, 1303 (1990).

Scatchard, G., The attractions of proteins for small molecules and ions. *Ann. N.Y. Acad. Sci.* **51**, 660 (1949).

Sheetz, M. P., Glycoprotein motility and dynamic domains in fluid plasma membranes. *Annu. Rev. Biophys. Biomol. Struct.* **22**, 417 (1993).

Sheetz, M. P., and Elson, E. E., Measurement of membrane glycoprotein movement by single-particle tracking. *In* "Optical Microscopy: Emerging Methods and Applications" (B. Herman and J. J. Lemasters, eds.), p. 285. Academic Press, San Diego, 1993.

Shoup, D., and Szabo, A., Role of diffusion in ligand binding to macromolecules and cell-bound receptors. *Biophys. J.* **40**, 33 (1982).

Smith, K. A., Interleukin 2: A 10-year perspective. *In* "Interleukin 2" (K. A. Smith, ed.), p. 1. Academic Press, San Diego, 1988a.

Smith, K. A., Interleukin 2: Inception, impact, and implications. *Science* **240**, 1169 (1988b).

Smith, K. A., The interleukin 2 receptor. *Adv. Immunol.* **42**, 165 (1988c).

Smoluchowski, M. V., Versuch einer mathematische theorie der koagulationskinetic kolloider loesungen. *Z. Phys. Chem.* **92**, 129 (1917).

Sporn, M. B., and Roberts, A. B., Autocrine secretion—10 years later. *Ann. Intern. Med.* **117**, 408 (1992).

Sporn, M. B., and Todaro, G. J., Autocrine secretion and malignant transformation of cells. *N. Eng. J. Med.* **303**, 878 (1980).

Spudich, J. L., and Koshland, D. E., Jr., Non-genetic individuality: Chance in the single cell. *Nature (London)* **262**, 467 (1976).

Stickle, D., and Barber, R., Evidence for the role of epinephrine binding frequency in activation of adenylate cyclase. *Mol. Pharmacol.* **36**, 437 (1989).

Taylor, C. W., The role of G proteins in transmembrane signalling. *Biochem. J.* **272**, 1 (1990).

Thompsen, W. J., and Neubig, R. R., Rapid kinetics of α_2-adrenergic inhibition of adenylate cyclase. Evidence for a distal rate-limiting step. *Biochemistry* **28**, 8778 (1989).

Torney, D. C., and McConnell, H. M., Diffusion-limited reaction rate theory for two-dimensional systems. *Proc. R. Soc. London, Ser. A* **387**, 147 (1983).

Tranquillo, R. T., Theories and models of gradient perception. *In* "Biology of the Chemotactic Response" (J. P. Armitage and J. M. Lackie, eds.), p. 35. Cambridge Univ. Press, Cambridge, UK, 1990.

Tranquillo, R. T., and Lauffenburger, D. A., Analysis of leukocyte chemosensory movement. *Adv. Biosci.* **66**, 29 (1987a).

Tranquillo, R. T., and Lauffenburger, D. A., Stochastic model of leukocyte chemosensory movement. *J. Math. Biol.* **25**, 229 (1987b).

Tranquillo, R. T., Fisher, E. S., Farrell, B. E., and Lauffenburger, D. A., A stochastic model for chemosensory cell movement: Application to neutrophil and macrophage persistence and orientation. *Math. Biosci.* **90**, 287 (1988).

Tsudo, M., Kitamura, F., and Miyasaka, M., Characterization of the interleukin 2 receptor β chain using three distinct monoclonal antibodies. *Proc. Natl. Acad. Sci. U.S.A.* **86**, 1982 (1989).

Waters, C. M., Oberg, K. C., Carpenter, G., and Overholser, K. A., Rate constants for binding, dissociation, and internalization of EGF: Effect of receptor occupancy and ligand concentration. *Biochemistry* **29**, 3563 (1990).

Weisz, P. B., Diffusion and chemical transformation: An interdisciplinary excursion. *Science* **179**, 433 (1973).

Wey, C., and Cone, R. A., Lateral diffusion of rhodopsin in photoreceptor cells measured by fluorescence photobleaching and recovery. *Biophys. J.* **33**, 225 (1981).

Wier, M., and Edidin, M., Constraint of the translational diffusion of a membrane glycoprotein by its external domains. *Science* **242**, 412 (1988).

Wiley, H. S., Anomalous binding of epidermal growth factor to A431 cells is due to the effect of high receptor densities and a saturable endocytic system. *J. Cell Biol.* **107**, 801 (1988).

Yahon, A., Klagsbrun, M., Esko, J. D., Leder, P., and Ornitz, D. M., Cell surface, heparin-like molecules are required for binding of basic fibroblast growth factor to its high affinity receptor. *Cell (Cambridge, Mass.)* **64**, 841 (1991).

Zhang, F., Crise, B., Su, B., Rose, J. K., Bothwell, A., and Jacobson, K., Lateral diffusion of membrane-spanning glycosylphosphatidylinositol-linked proteins: Towards establishing rules governing the lateral mobility of membrane proteins. *J. Cell Biol.* **115**, 75 (1991).

Zigmond, S. H., Ability of polymorphonuclear leukocytes to orient in gradients of chemotactic factors. *J. Cell Biol.* **75**, 606 (1977).

Zigmond, S. H., Sullivan, S. J., and Lauffenburger, D. A., Kinetic analysis of chemotactic peptide receptor modulation. *J. Cell Biol.* **92**, 34 (1982).

Zwanzig, R., Diffusion-controlled ligand binding to spheres partially covered by receptors: An effective medium treatment. *Proc. Natl. Acad. Sci. U.S.A.* **87**, 5856 (1990).

TRANSPORT PHENOMENA IN TUMORS

Rakesh K. Jain

Department of Radiation Oncology
Harvard Medical School and Massachusetts General Hospital
Boston, Massachusetts 02114

ADVANCES IN CHEMICAL ENGINEERING, VOL. 19

I. Introduction

Cancer is the second leading cause of death in the United States and many Western nations. Roughly, cancerous diseases can be grouped into two categories—(i) hematologic (leukemias and lymphomas) and (ii) "solid-like," in which cancer cells form a solid "tissue-like" mass (e.g., carcinomas of lung, breast, colon). A more detailed classification of cancer is based on the cell or tissue of origin (Holland *et al.*, 1993; DeVita *et al.*, 1993). Although considerable progress has been made in the treatment of hematologic cancers in the past 20 years, solid tumors still remain the major cause of cancerous deaths (Beardsley, 1994). Depending upon the stage of the disease, a surgeon may remove the bulk of the primary tumor from a patient. Any residual tumor that might remain locally is often treated with radiation therapy. But such primary tumors may often spread, seeding metastases at distant sites in the body. For a tumor that has spread regionally or widely throughout the body, the most common treatment is systemic chemotherapy, i.e., treatment with a chemical that is distributed throughout the body via the blood stream. Other methods of systemic therapy include use of genetically engineered biological agents. Other methods for local treatment include hyperthermia, where the tumor's temperature is elevated to therapeutic levels, or photodynamic therapy, where a photosensitizer is first allowed to localize in the tumor and is then locally excited with laser light so that it causes toxicity to cancer cells.

In radiation therapy, which can be highly effective in certain localized cancers, the effectiveness of treatment partly depends on the presence of oxygen and may be enhanced by increasing the oxygen concentration in the hypoxic regions of the tumor. The concentration of oxygen in the tumor is governed by the delivery of oxygen via the blood and by subsequent consumption of this oxygen by cancer cells. To increase the sensitivity of cancer cells to radiation, certain compounds known as "radiation sensitizers" are currently in clinical trials. The effectiveness of these compounds in improving radiation response is dependent on their sufficient localization in a solid tumor. Similarly, in chemotherapy, immunotherapy, gene therapy, and photodynamic therapy, the effectiveness of treatment depends upon whether the relevant therapeutic agent has been delivered to all regions of the tumor in optimal quantities without harming the normal tissue. In hyperthermia, the therapeutic effectiveness is governed by the temperature achieved within solid tumors. Again, the achievable temperature is governed by physiological parameters such as

TABLE I
CANCER TREATMENT METHODS

Treatment	Therapeutically relevant agent
Radiotherapy	Oxygen, radiation sensitizers
Chemotherapy	Cytotoxic drugs
Biological therapy (immunotherapy and gene therapy)	Monoclonal antibodies, immunotoxins, cytokines, anti-sense compounds, gene carrying vectors, LAK cells, TIL cells
Photodynamic therapy	Photosensitizers, light
Hyperthermia	Heat, thermal sensitizers

tumor blood flow. The ability of various agents to kill cancer cells is also influenced by additional physiological variables such as the acid–base balance (pH) in the tumor.

Thus, transport phenomena and tumor physiology play a crucial role in the delivery of relevant agents (Table I) to tumors (Jain, 1993). Therefore, the objective of this article is to discuss applications of fundamental principles of mass and heat transfer in tumors with the overall goal of improving various methods of detection and treatment. It is to be emphasized from the outset that in no way is this article intended to be an exhaustive review of the literature on these subjects. Rather, it is intended to provide an introduction to cancer research for a newcomer with a background in physical sciences and engineering or for an investigator whose line of research requires knowledge of transport phenomena in normal and neoplastic tissues.

In the first part of this article (Section II), principles of cancer detection and treatment are discussed briefly. Emphasis is placed on methods relying on mass or heat transfer. A quantitative understanding of transport in tissues may be useful in improving these methods.

In the second part of this article (Section III), various tumor models, which can mimic several characteristics of human tumors, are summarized and compared. These models include single cells, multicell spheroids, and experimental solid tumors. The most obvious and observable characteristic of neoplastic diseases is uncontrolled growth, invasion, and metastasis. As a result, attempts to model growth kinetics of tumor are discussed briefly in this section.

In the third part of this article (Section IV), various physiological and transport parameters relevant to heat and mass transfer are compiled. These parameters include vascular morphology, blood flow, transvascular transport, interstitial transport, and thermal and metabolic properties. It must be pointed out here that mathematical models and equations that describe transport in normal and neoplastic tissues are identical. The differences—and they may be important—lie in the value of physiological and transport parameters.

In the fourth part of this article (Section V), various techniques to study mass transfer in tumors, both *in vitro* and *in vivo*, are discussed. Two theoretical approaches for describing mass transfer in normal and neoplastic tissue are discussed: lumped parameter compartmental models and distributed parameter models. In the lumped parameter approach, mass transport in the body is modeled by a set of interconnected well-mixed compartments that represent various body tissues. Using the available physiological, anatomical, and physicochemical information, and solving a set of mass transport equations, the model can be used to predict drug concentrations as a function of time in each body compartment. The distributed parameter approach incorporates parameters that characterize the diffusion, convection, and reactions that occur within the vascular, interstitial, and intracellular spaces. Also, parameters for the regional perfusion rates, regional vascular volumes, and regional vascular surface areas per unit volume are included. Distributed parameter models are thus able to provide a more detailed analysis of the mass-transfer process within solid tumors so as to account for the effects of necrosis and nonuniform blood flow on the distribution of drugs within a tumor.

In the fifth part of this article (Section VI), heat transfer in tumors is discussed with application in thermography and hyperthermia. Similar to mass transfer, two theoretical approaches—lumped and distributed parameter—to describing heat transfer in normal and neoplastic tissues are described and used to predict temperature distributions during normo- and hyperthermia. Various techniques to induce localized and whole-body hyperthermia are also summarized.

By providing a unified theoretical basis for the quantification of mass and heat transfer in tumors and then compiling recent experimental findings of various investigators, this article points out several gaps in our present knowledge and suggests some directions for future work.

II. Principles of Cancer Detection and Treatment

Various methods of cancer detection and treatment are discussed in oncology textbooks (for example, Holland *et al.*, 1993; DeVita *et al.*, 1993). In what follows, we will outline these methods with emphasis on approaches based on mass and heat transfer.

A. Cancer Diagnosis

The success of treatment largely depends on how early cancer is detected. A variety of methods are used for the detection of this disease, including physical and radiological examination. The most reliable method for identification and classification of the disease is the microscopic examination of the tissue/cells which are suspected to be malignant. The tissue (cells) are mostly obtained by surgical excision, but in some cases cells may shed from the surface of tissues into a body cavity (e.g., the "Pap" test to detect cancer of uterine cervix). Radiological methods of cancer detection include x-rays and computerized axial tomography (CAT), magnetic resonance imaging (MRI), positron emission tomography (PET), sonography, tracer techniques, and thermography. Since the precise knowledge of heat and mass transfer is useful for improving the application of the last two techniques, we will discuss these two methods briefly here.

1. Tracer Techniques

Tracers (usually radioisotopes) that tend to accumulate selectively in particular body tissues are useful in both detection and treatment of cancer. Normal thyroid tissue, for example, collects most of the body's iodine to use in the production of thyroid hormone. Since thyroid cancer cells that have spread to other parts of the body continue to collect iodine, it is possible to detect iodine-collecting deposits of cancer cells spread all over the body. (In a cancer patient, after the surgical removal of the thyroid gland, the patient is given hormones to eliminate activity in the thyroid tissue that has spread to other parts of the body. The patient then is given a "large" dose of radioactive iodine which destroys cancer cells that accumulate sufficient amounts of iodine.) Nonradioactive tracers used for detection include contrast agents for x-rays and MRI, and fluorescent agents such as porphyrins.

The advent of hybridoma technology and genetic engineering has led to the design and large-scale production of monoclonal antibodies (MABs) and other biological molecules with some degree of specificity for markers on cancer cells (referred to as the tumor-associated antigens). Once hailed as "magic bullets," these molecules have not lived up to initial expectations, primarily because of their inadequate uptake in solid tumors (Jain, 1989; Sands, 1992). A detailed analysis of mass transfer in tumors may provide insights into the poor localization and may offer some strategies for improved delivery of these macromolecules to tumors.

2. *Thermography*

The existence of some neoplastic tissues at a higher temperature than the surrounding normal tissues of the host has been exploited in thermography for the diagnosis of tumors. This difference in temperature is usually attributed to the higher rate of metabolic heat generation in tumors and to the lower perfusion rate of tumors (Jain *et al.*, 1979; Gullino *et al.*, 1982). Several extensive reviews on medical thermography have appeared in the last 20 years (e.g., Shitzer and Eberhart, 1985).

Despite recent developments in the instrumentation for thermography, including liquid crystals and microwave scanners, thermography remains an underdeveloped diagnostic modality for several reasons: (i) the lack of data on temperature distributions in tumors and surrounding tissues under "normal" conditions, (ii) the lack of precise knowledge of blood flow distribution and metabolism in tumors, (iii) the technical difficulties in instrumentation, and (iv) the unavailability of precise algorithms which can be used to extract physiological parameters from the thermal information. Some of these points will be discussed further in Section VI.

B. Cancer Treatment

Currently, there are six major methods available for cancer treatment: surgery, radiotherapy, chemotherapy, immunotherapy, hyperthermia, and photodynamic therapy. The first three are the most widely used, and the last three are under development. Surgery, radiotherapy, hyperthermia, and photodynamic therapy are primarily local, while chemotherapy and immunotherapy are primarily systemic methods. In most cases a combination of methods is used for cancer treatment. Except for surgery, the application of the remaining five methods can be improved considerably by developing quantitative understanding of mass and/or heat transfer in tumors and normal tissues. In what follows, we will discuss the problems and promises of each of these five techniques from the point of view of mass and heat transfer, and mention anti-angiogenic approaches.

1. *Radiotherapy*

The purpose of radiotherapy is to deliver a large radiation dose to the tumor and a minimal dose to the surrounding normal tissues. Depending upon the location and volume of the tumor, the radiation can be a photon source (e.g., x-ray tubes, cobalt teletherapy unit, linear accelerator, Betatrons) or a source for a high-energy particle (e.g., electrons, protons).

When the radiation is absorbed by cells, a few of the atoms and molecules of the cells are ionized. The ionization leads, either directly or via the formation of free radicals, to chemical reactions in the cells and ultimately to cellular damage. Despite the significant use of radiotherapy, the chemical and physical mechanisms of this damage are not completely understood (Hall, 1988).

The cellular damage depends primarily upon the dose of radiation. A low radiation dose can cause cancer; a high dose can kill cancer. When healthy tissue receives a low to moderate dose, cell genes may undergo mutations leading to cancer. At a higher dose, the cells may die because of irreparable damage.

The response of cells to radiotherapy also depends upon the rate of cell division, and the cell's physiological environment. Normal tissues that are characterized by a comparatively high rate of cell division (e.g., bone marrow, lymph nodes, gonads, intestinal mucous membrane, skin) have a high radiosensitivity. Among the most radiosensitive cancerous diseases are leukemia, malignant lymphoma (lymph-node cancer), Ewing's sarcoma (tumor of the skeleton), and myeloma. Even moderately radiosensitive tumors, e.g., cervical cancer in women, can often be treated successfully with radiotherapy alone.

The radiosensitivity of the cancer cells is also influenced by the physiological environment in which they are located during the time of irradiation. These environmental factors include radiosensitizers (i.e., agents which increase the radiosensitivity) and radioprotectors (i.e., agents which prevent cell damage). Poor oxygenation decreases the radiosensitivity. Under "normal" conditions some regions of a large tumor may be hypoxic because of poor vascularization and perfusion rate (chronic hypoxia) or because of transient fluctuations in blood flow (acute hypoxia), and therefore may be resistant to radiation. Attempts have been made to increase the oxygen tension in tumors by placing the patient in a hyperbaric oxygen atmosphere. However, poor convective mass transfer with blood flow makes it difficult to oxygenate the tissue in and near the poorly vascularized regions of the tumors. Radiosensitizers have also been used to increase the effectiveness of radiotherapy; however, poor perfusion may have limited their access to tumors, rendering radiotherapy ineffective in these cases. Therefore, a better understanding of diffusive and convective mass transfer in tumors may be helpful in improving the results of therapy.

2. *Chemotherapy*

Most cancer deaths are due to an inability to cure widespread disease. While localized cancer often can be removed by surgery or controlled by radiation, these methods can rarely cure cancers that have metastasized widely, nor can they cure cancers of the blood or blood-forming tissues, such as leukemia, which are widespread from the beginning. Chemotherapy (i.e., the use of anti-cancer drugs), therefore, seems a logical way to treat these cancers.

Since the 1940s, more than 50 drugs have been developed that are effective against some types of cancer. The problem with most of these agents is that they are highly toxic to several normal tissues. As soon as the drug is injected into the circulation, it is transported by blood to the tumors and normal organs. Therefore, organs such as the liver and kidney which have higher blood perfusion rates than most solid tumors (especially carcinomas) may have a high uptake of drug. Furthermore, normal tissues, such as bone marrow, that are equally or more sensitive to the drug than cancer cells can be dose-limiting. Thus, chemotherapy often leads to side effects such as nausea, vomiting, diarrhea, temporary loss of hair, and impaired production of blood cells. Of course, when the cancer cells are spread in blood (e.g., leukemia) or when the tumors have very high perfusion rates, these drugs may produce cures without significant side effects. In most cases, more than one drug is used in combination for cancer treatment. The drug combination is used partly to overcome the resistance cancer cells develop against some of these agents, and partly to reduce the toxicity which may result from the use of massive doses of one drug.

Each year, several hundred materials are tested for anticancer activity *in vitro* and, in some cases, in rodents. These agents include plant extracts, antibiotics, hormones, alkylating agents, and newly synthesized compounds related to known drugs. Those that appear promising are then tested in larger animals for evidence of toxicity. Almost one out of every 1,000 to 2,000 of these chemicals is considered promising and safe enough to be studied in patients. In the application of each drug, one faces the problem of scale-up from small animals to human subjects and searches for an optimal schedule and dose to minimize the concentration of drug in the normal cells and maximize in the neoplastic cells. The use of a physiologically based pharmacokinetic model may facilitate such scale-up and optimization (Section V,C).

3. *Immunotherapy*

This method of cancer treatment is based on using the body's natural defense, its immunological system, to control cancer. The immune response of the body can be either specific or nonspecific. The "specific" system consists of specialized groups of cells that recognize and reject some foreign substances or antigens, or directly interact with the antigen-bearing substrate and destroy it with lytic enzymes, toxic proteins, and chemicals. They produce specific counter-substances called antibodies that react with and inactivate the antigens. The "nonspecific" system consists of cells such as macrophages which recognize and engulf the foreign cells or particles.

One approach in immunotherapy is to use a vaccine made of cancer cells to stimulate production of antibodies against cancer. While this objective has been achieved in a few cancers in some animals, such a treatment for humans is still in the future. A number of human tumors were once thought to be antigenic and therefore potentially within the reach of immunotherapy. However, only Burkitt's lymphoma is considered a strong candidate. Agents such as BCG and *C. parvum* have received attention from the medical community, but these agents are nonspecific stimulators of hosts' immune response and have not shown any success in cancer treatment when used alone. Recent advances in biotechnology and immunology have led to the ready availability of monoclonal antibodies and various biological response modifiers (e.g., interleukins, cytokines), as well as the ability to isolate, activate, expand, and/or transfect subpopulations of immune cells with the appropriate genes. The availability of these agents and techniques has led to a resurgence of interest in immunotherapy. A quantitative understanding of the biodistribution and disposition of the biological response modifiers and effector cells, and subsequent chemical reactions leading to cancer cell death, may be useful in improving this method of cancer treatment.

4. Hyperthermia

Heat in various forms has been exploited by mankind for therapeutic purposes since ancient times (Licht, 1965). The Egyptians (~ 3000 B.C.) were the first to use cautery against tumors and various non-malignant diseases. The Hindus (~ 2000 B.C.) used cautery to control surface lesions during the Aryan civilization. The importance of therapeutic heat in the Greek civilization is reflected in the aphorism, "Fire will succeed when all other methods fail," credited to the well-known Greek physician Hippocrates (460–357 B.C.). He recommended cautery (with red-hot iron) for small tumors and many other diseases. The application of cautery using heated metals or lenses remained popular among the medical community until the early to mid-20th century, when more sophisticated methods for elevating local tissue temperatures (e.g., diathermy and ultrasound) became available and when it was realized that heat may be lethal to some tumors at moderately elevated temperatures (40–42°C).

In 1866 in Germany, Busch reported a cure for a histologically verified sarcoma of the face after an attack of erysipelas which induced fever. Busch suggested the possibility of heat being selectively lethal to neoplastic cells. About 25 years later, Coley (1893) administered bacterial toxins in cancer patients in New York which resulted in fever and led to regression of advanced and inoperable cancers. While Coley's toxins led to sustained response in some patients for up to 50 years, because of the uncertainty in preparations and biological activity of the mixed bacterial toxins (MBT) used by Coley, the method was later abandoned, as it proved disastrous for the patients.

In 1967 Cavaliere and his co-workers in Rome heated human tumors in the extremities by local perfusion with warm blood and showed that heat alone can lead to total regression of melanomas and sarcomas and increase in survival of patients. In 1969, Stehlin in the USA showed that heat and an anti-cancer drug (Melphalan) together not only led to regression of the primary tumor, but also reduced the incidence of metastases from these tumors. Limited but encouraging work of these two groups, coupled with the discouraging results by surgery, radiotherapy, and chemotherapy, led to a new resurgence of interest in hyperthermia worldwide for the next 20 years. However, despite a large effort to treat cancer by hyperthermia, the long-term survival results in patients taken collectively from different centers have been less than impressive. The reasons why the full potential of hyperthermia, used either alone or in conjunction with other currently available methods for human cancer treatment, has not been realized are as follows: (i) The technical difficulties of heating tumors adequately; (ii) the lack of precise knowledge and control of temperature distributions within tumors and the surrounding normal tissues during local or whole-body hyperthermia; (iii) the lack of data on the susceptibility of human tumors to various thermal doses, as determined by the temperature and duration of heating; (iv) poor understanding of the physiological, biochemical, and immunological responses of normal and neoplastic tissues at elevated temperatures; and (v) the paucity of data on optimal sequencing of hyperthermia with other modalities of cancer treatment to minimize the damage to normal tissues while maximizing it to neoplastic tissue.

5. Photodynamic Therapy (PDT)

This is a relatively new treatment modality in which a photosensitizing agent is first injected into a patient. Once the agent is localized in the tumor in adequate quantities, the tumor is illuminated with light of appropriate wavelength so that the photosensitizer is activated. In the presence of oxygen, cytotoxicity results from the generation of free radicals and singlet oxygen. While an elegant concept, PDT is currently limited by (i) the lack of suitable sensitizers, (ii) heterogeneous localization of photosensitizers in tumors, (iii) lack of penetration of light throughout a large lesion, (iv) phototoxicity to normal tissues, and (v) inability to treat widespread metastatic disease (Pass, 1993). Development of novel photosensitizers, and better understanding and control of transport of photosensitizers and light, should alleviate some of these problems.

6. *Antiangiogenic Therapy*

The realization that solid tumors cannot grow beyond a critical size ($\sim$ 1 mm) without recruiting new blood vessels, and that they cannot metastasize via blood without blood vessels, led to the concept in the early 1970s that any agent that interferes with angiogenesis (i.e., formation of blood vessels) should be able to control tumor growth (Folkman, 1971). In the past 20 years, various molecules involved in stimulating and suppressing angiogenesis have been discovered (Folkman, 1993). Some of these agents are currently under clinical trials. If successful, this approach would augment the currently used methods of cancer treatment. Furthermore, if a molecule or a set of molecules specific for tumor vasculature is discovered, then the transport limitations posed by the tumor vessel wall and the interstitium would not be a problem.

III. Tumor Models and Their Growth Characteristics

In order to understand the nature of human tumors, we need tumor models which have many of their characteristics. In this section, I will describe three such models briefly and discuss their advantages and disadvantages. Since a key characteristic of cancerous diseases is uncontrolled growth, we will discuss their growth kinetics briefly. [For a comprehensive review of various experimental and theoretical studies on growth kinetics of tumor, the reader is referred to two excellent monographs by Steel (1977) and Swan (1977), respectively.]

A. Tumor Models

Knowledge about heat and mass transfer in tumors has been obtained using primarily three types of biological systems:

1. Single cells from humans and animals can be grown in culture (*in vitro*) or inside the body (*in vivo*), for example, in the peritoneal cavity.

Studies using single cells allow precise control of the extracellular environment and, therefore, can provide useful information on the cellular uptake of drugs and cell cycle kinetics during various types of treatment. Such detailed information cannot be obtained directly from whole-tissue (e.g., solid-tumor) studies because of the heterogeneous nature of tumor blood flow and vascular structure, and a variety of host factors. However, caution must be exercised in extrapolating the information obtained from single cells to the solid tumor *in vivo*.

2. Multicell spheroids provide an *in vitro* model for tumors which is intermediate in complexity between solid tumors and single cell cultures. Spheroids are three-dimensional, spherical clusters of a variety of animal and human cells about 0.1–1 mm in diameter. Spheroids can be grown in suspension culture, in quiescent liquid, or in semi-solid medium.

Cells in a spheroid receive nutrients by diffusion from the growth medium towards its core. As spheroids grow, they reach a critical size at which cells in their center begin to die because of diffusion limitation of oxygen and/or glucose. With continued increase in the size of the spheroid, the size of the central necrotic core also increases. Like solid tumors, spheroids provide a heterogeneous array of cells in three-dimensional contact, in various nutritional states, with spontaneous development of hypoxic and necrotic zones, redistribution of cells in various phases of cell cycle, and diffusion gradients of nutrients and waste products. It is believed that in the early stages of *in vivo* development, a tumor exists as a small nodule of tissue less than a millimeter in diameter. Similar to spheroids, this small tumor has no blood vessels and therefore mostly depends upon diffusion from nearby host vessels to supply nutrients and remove wastes.

Multicell spheroids have been used to study the transport of molecules and cells. They have been used for *in vivo* studies by injecting spheroids into the peritoneal cavities of experimental animals. This approach has been used to study tumor cell response to drugs and also to study immune response to tumors. As a result of lack of vasculature, caution must be exercised in using spheroid information to plan treatment in animals and patients (Sutherland, 1988).

3. Solid tumors can arise in animals and humans spontaneously. They can also be induced chemically, virally, by irradiation, or by transfecting or deleting genes. The spontaneous or induced tumors, in turn, can be transplanted into another animal. Although arguments have been presented both for and against the use of transplanted tumors, they remain of prime importance in modern-day investigations in experimental cancer

research. The problems involved in the use of spontaneous and induced tumors include the long time needed in their production, and their biological individuality and more pronounced internal heterogeneity. The advantages of using transplanted tumors include relative ease of obtaining reasonably reproducible samples of neoplastic tissue, growing at a fairly predictable rate and available in large quantities. As a result, the use of transplanted tumors in the screening and testing of various anti-cancer agents has provided an opportunity and wealth of information that could never have been accumulated in a comparable period of time utilizing spontaneous tumors. Needless to say, there are a variety of problems that can be explored only with the spontaneous tumor system, especially those related to the development of cancer (i.e., the role of genetics, viruses, and specific immune responses). The ready availability of genetically engineered animals, in which the desired gene has been deleted or modified, should overcome some of these problems (Capecci, 1994).

The most common method of transplanting tumors is by subcutaneous (usually near the abdominal wall or the thigh) inoculation. Other sites of tumor implantation include muscle (usually the leg), peritoneal cavity, kidney, liver, adrenal, spleen, ovaries, uterus, and intestine. In order to observe the tumor while it is growing, several investigators have transplanted tumors in transparent windows or chambers placed on the rabbit ear, hamster cheek pouch or dorsal skin of rodents (Fig. 1).

One important factor in the transplantation of normal and neoplastic tissue is the compatibility between the graft and the host. Depending upon the tumor, the following types of transplants are possible: Autogenic—one in which an individual is grafted with its own tissue. Syngenic or isogenic—graft between genetically identical individuals, i.e., within inbred strains, between identical twins. Allogenic—graft between genetically different individuals of the same species, i.e., between two different strains of rats. Xenogenic—graft between species. Depending upon its success in growing, a tissue may be referred to as histocompatible with the host (Lieblet and Lieblet, 1967; Begg, 1961). The ready availability of immunodeficient rodents (e.g., nude mice, nude rats, severe combined immunodeficient mice) has made it possible to grow human tumor xenografts. Of course, these xenografts have blood vessels of the host. Nevertheless, these models have been quite useful for testing agents against human cancers (Kallman, 1987).

Since solid tumors are the primary cause of cancerous deaths, in this article we will focus our attention on these tumors. Results obtained from single cells and multicell spheroids will also be discussed to compare the information obtained from all three systems.

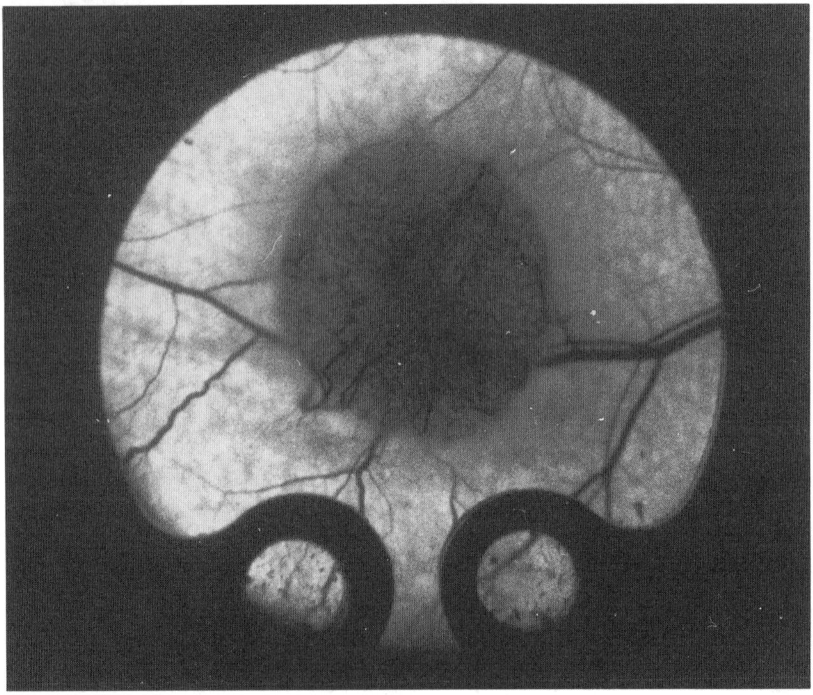

FIG. 1. Microcirculation of a human colon carcinoma grown in the dorsal skin chamber in a severe-combined immunodeficient mouse. (Adapted from Leunig *et al.*, 1992b.) Note that angiogenesis leads to formation of numerous blood vessels. Such a transparent preparation can permit noninvasive, continuous measurement of transport processes in normal and tumor tissues (Jain, 1985b). Parameters we can measure include hemodynamic (e.g., blood flow, vasomotion); metabolic (e.g., pH, pO_2, Ca^{2+}); transport (e.g., permeability, diffusion, binding), and cell–cell interactions (e.g., adhesion, deformability).

B. Growth Kinetics of Tumors

Numerous mathematical models have been proposed or adapted for describing the growth of normal and neoplastic tissues. One school of thought uses the model to "fit" various overall properties of the tissue (weight, diameter, etc.) as a function of time or some other measurable quantity. The second school has seen fit to develop models based on underlying biological mechanisms of tissue growth and subsequently tested the various models on available data. The second approach seeks to understand, as opposed to "fit," the characteristics of tissue growth.

1. *Empirical Models*

The observation that the specific growth rate of many normal tissues and tumors decays approximately exponentially with time led to the extensive use of the Gompertz equation (Gompertz, 1825):

$$W = W_0 \exp\left[\frac{a}{b}(1 - e^{-bt})\right].$$

Here, W_0 is the initial weight of tissue, and constants a and b are determined by fitting the equation with data. At early time intervals, this equation reduces to the well-known exponential growth rate:

$$W = W_0 \exp(at), \qquad t \to 0,$$

and at long time intervals, the tissue size tends to its asymptote:

$$W = W_0 \exp\left(\frac{a}{b}\right), \qquad t \to \infty.$$

This function has been used by a large number of investigators to simulate the growth of normal and neoplastic tissue over a 1,000-fold range (Steel, 1977). The limitation of this model is that it exhibits retardation in growth from the onset of growth to the asymptotic phase, and consequently does not simulate the growth adequately in the early time periods. One possible remedy for this discrepancy is to split the growth curve into two phases—the early phase, characterized by exponential growth, and the later phase by the Gompterzian growth (Steel, 1977).

2. *Physiologically Based Models*

Physiologically based models that incorporate the availability of nutrients for growth through the vasculature have been limited. Assuming that the critical nutrient is oxygen diffusing into a spherical tumor from its periphery, Burton (1966) derived a criterion for the onset of necrosis in tumors. This model is adequate to describe the growth of a tumor spheroid, but is unable to describe the growth of tumors in which the vessels penetrate the tumor. Greenspan (1972, 1974) and Wette *et al.* (1974a, b) extended Burton's analysis by considering both the nutrients and waste products of metabolism as parameters of growth. Deakin (1975) extended Burton's model by assuming that oxygen consumption per unit tissue volume in a tumor is not constant (zeroth-order), but follows a saturable (Michaelis–Menten) kinetics.

Tannock (1968) used the diffusion equation for a cylindrical geometry to calculate the radius of viable tissue around a capillary on the basis of four critical agents—oxygen, carbon dioxide, glucose, and lactate. Tannock's work provided the first clear-cut example of the relationship of growth with the vascular structure of a tumor. However, cords (tissue cylinder around a capillary) of this type are not common in tumors, and therefore, the results of Tannock cannot be extrapolated to a tumor mass with irregular topology of blood vessels. Assuming that the growth rate of tumors depends on the *total* functional area of capillaries, Summers (1965) developed an approximate formulation for tumor growth. However, Summers's model did not account for the heterogeneous distribution of blood flow rate in tumors, and variations in the diameter of vessels in a vascular bed. It is of interest to mention here that under appropriate limiting conditions, both Burton's and Summers's models yield the well-known cube-root growth law of tumors, which was put forward by Mayneord in 1932. Such a growth curve (in which the cube root of tumor volume varies linearly with time) has been used by some investigators (Steel, 1977). Of course, cube-root growth is observed only for a limited period in growth.

The mathematical models discussed heretofore ignore mechanisms of growth regulation at the cellular level and of angiogenesis. The first important step in this direction was taken by Weiss and co-workers (Weiss and Kavanau, 1957). Assuming that a tissue consists of generative and differentiated mass, Weiss developed a theory of growth based on a negative feedback mechanism of self-regulation, which can account not only for the sigmoid time course of growth, but also for compensatory growth after injury, as well as for growth stimulation by organ extracts (now referred to as growth factors). The analysis of Shymko and Glass (1976) considers diffusion of nutrients and growth-stimulating and -inhibiting factors to explain growth in tissues. As our knowledge of oncogenes and growth factors increases, future efforts must be directed to test specific biological hypotheses using mathematical models. Such models may also be used to examine the role of necrosis and apoptosis (programmed cell death) in tumor growth and regression.

Mathematical models that correlate neovascularization with growth of tissue are limited in number. Liotta *et al.* (1977) developed a mathematical model which describes the spatial and temporal growth of vessels and cancer cells in a transplanted tumor by two coupled partial differential equations with nonlinear birth and death rate terms. While these authors made no attempt to fit their data quantitatively, their model simulates the density of tumor cells and endothelial cells qualitatively and predicts the onset of necrosis in tumors.

We developed a distributed parameter model that describes the spatial and temporal growth of granulation tissue during wound-healing (Zawicki *et al.*, 1981). The growth process was modeled by a set of three partial differential equations simulating the interaction among three coexisting cell populations: dead tissue, granulation tissue, and endothelial cells. The functional forms for the birth and death rate of these species were based on our understanding of the biological mechanisms of growth process. The mathematical model not only described our data adequately, but also exhibited two striking properties of observable growth kinetics: (i) provisional matrix formed by the dead tissue debris or some chemical exuded from the debris is required to trigger revascularization, and (ii) vessel density overshoots in most cases before reaching the steady-state (or equilibrium) value (Zawicki *et al.*, 1981). The need to develop a model to describe the growth of vessels and cancer cells in tumors based on molecular mechanisms is urgent.

Most of the mathematical models to date have ignored the role of interstitial matrix in growth. Recent studies have shown the interstitial matrix not only forms the scaffold to support the cancer cells and blood vessels, but also can "direct" their growth. Furthermore, it can contribute to stresses generated as a result of growth. To this end, our current efforts are directed towards including residual stresses and the viscoelastic nature of tissue in growth models of solid tumors (McElwain and Ponzo, 1977; Skalak *et al.*, 1982; Fung, 1990; Chaplain and Sleeman, 1993).

3. Models for Metastatic Process

One key factor that characterizes most neoplastic diseases is the capacity of the tumor mass for local destructive invasion and for distant spread, also referred to as metastasis. Cancer cells can metastasize via blood and/or lymph vessels. Hematogeneous (i.e., blood-borne) metastases develop from a solid tumor in the following stages: (i) neovascularization of tumor, which provides a route for cancer cells to leave the tumor; (ii) penetration of tumor cells into the blood vessel walls to become exposed to blood flow; (iii) dislodging of tumor cells from the vessel wall by flowing blood and entry into the circulatory system; (iv) arrest of circulating cells or cell clumps in the blood vessels of the target organ; and (v) penetration of arrested cells into the target tissue and eventual formation of metastatic foci (Jain and Ward-Hartley, 1987).

Saidel *et al.* (1975) developed a lumped parameter, deterministic model to describe these five steps in the metastatic process. This model describes their data on pulmonary metastatic formation from a fibrosarcoma implanted in mice and simulates the effects of various perturbations (e.g., external tumor massage, primary tumor amputations) on metastatic process. These authors also developed a stochastic model of metastasis formation to account for the random variation in sizes of cell clumps and metastatic foci (Saidel *et al.*, 1977; Liotta *et al.*, 1974, 1977). Future efforts of this nature must include the molecular mechanisms underlying cell–cell interactions (Hammer and Apte, 1992; Dickinson *et al.*, 1993; Lauffenberger and Linderman, 1993; McIntire, 1994).

IV. Physiological and Transport Parameters

Transport of mass and heat in normal and neoplastic tissues is determined primarily by convection and diffusion. A blood-borne molecule or cell that enters the vasculature reaches cancer cells via (i) distribution through the vascular compartment; (ii) convection and diffusion across the microvascular wall; (iii) convection and diffusion through the interstitial compartment; and (iv) transport across cell membrane. Movement of molecules through the vasculature is governed by the vascular morphology (i.e., the number, length, diameter, and geometrical arrangement of various blood vessels) and the blood flow rate. Transport across vessel wall, through interstitial space and across cell membrane depends on the physical properties of the molecules (e.g., size, charge, configuration), physiological properties of these barriers (e.g., transport pathways) and driving force (e.g., concentration and pressure gradients). Furthermore, movement of a molecule through a barrier may be altered by specific or nonspecific binding to tissue components.

Convection of heat via blood depends primarily on the local blood flow in the tissue and the vascular morphology of the tissue. Thermal diffusion is determined by thermal conductivity in the steady state, and thermal diffusivity in the unsteady state. In addition to these transport parameters, we need to know the volumes and geometry of normal tissues and tumor. In general, tumor volume changes as a function of time more rapidly than normal tissue volume. In special applications, such as hyperthermia induced by electromagnetic waves or radiofrequency currents, we need electromagnetic properties of tissues—the electrical conductivity and the relative dielectric constant. In the case of ultrasonic heating, we need to specify the acoustic properties of the tissue—velocity of sound and attenuation (or absorption) coefficient.

It must be reiterated here that mathematical analyses of transport in normal and neoplastic tissues are identical. The only difference lies in the physiological, geometric, and transport parameters. In what follows, we will discuss parameters which will be used in Sections V and VI for model development. We will place emphasis on parameters measured for tumors, and point to appropriate references for normal tissues.

A. Vascular Morphology

The tumor vasculature consists of (i) vessels recruited from the preexisting network of the host vasculature and (ii) vessels resulting from the angiogenic response of host vessels to cancer cells (Gullino, 1975; Folkman, 1993; Jain, 1988). Although the tumor vasculature originates from the host vasculature, its organization may be completely different, depending on the tumor type, its growth rate, and its location. The architecture may be different not only among various tumor types, but also between a spontaneous tumor and its transplants (for review, see Jain, 1988).

Macroscopically, the tumor vasculature can be envisioned in terms of two idealized categories: peripheral and central. In tumors with peripheral vascularization, the centers are usually poorly perfused (Fig. 2). In those with central vascularization, one would expect the opposite; hence, the delivery of blood-borne substances should follow the same pattern. In reality a tumor may consist of many territories, each exhibiting one or the other of these two types of idealized vascular patterns.

Microscopically, the tumor vasculature is highly heterogeneous and may not conform to the typical normal vascular organization (i.e., artery to arteriole to capillaries to postcapillary venule to vein). A key difference between normal and tumor vessels is that the latter are dilated, saccular, and tortuous, and may contain tumor cells within the endothelial lining of the vessel wall (Jain, 1988). In addition, unlike a normal tissue with a fixed route between arterial and venous sides, a tumor may have blood flowing from one venule to another via a network of vessels, or directly via a shunt. The branching patterns of blood vessels in a tumor are significantly different from those in a normal tissue, with many trifurcations, self-loops and sprouts (Less *et al.*, 1991, 1994). Furthermore, because of the peculiar nature of the vasculature, the organization of vessels may be different from one location to another and from one time to the next. As a result one would expect different routes for blood flow in the well-perfused zone, semi-necrotic zone, and necrotic zone (Fig. 2).

The vascular space in tumors varies from 1% to 20% depending upon the tumor type, its weight, and the method of measurement (Jain, 1988). Some studies show that the fractional vascular volume of tumors remains fairly constant during growth (suggesting an increase in the number of blood vessels with sluggish flow), while others show that the fractional vascular volume decreases as a tumor grows [in agreement with the observation that tumor perfusion rate (flow rate per unit tissue volume) decreases as a tumor grows] (Jain, 1988). Possible reasons for this discrepancy include errors associated with different measurement techniques, as well as the presence of arteriovenous shunts and blood vessels with

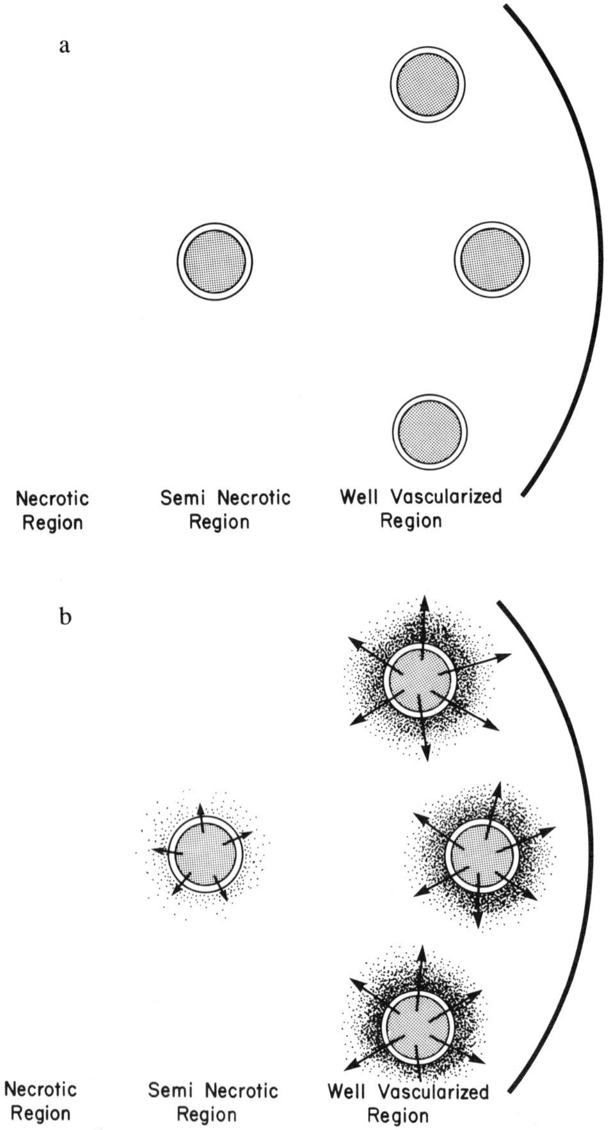

FIG. 2. Physiological barriers that a blood-borne molecule encounters before it reaches a cancer cell in a solid tumor. (a) Schematic of a heterogeneously perfused tumor showing well-vascularized periphery; a semi-necrotic, intermediate zone; and an avascularized, necrotic central region. Note that immediately after i.v. injection, the molecules are delivered to perfused regions only. (b) Low interstitial pressure in the periphery permits adequate extravasation of fluid and macromolecules.

c

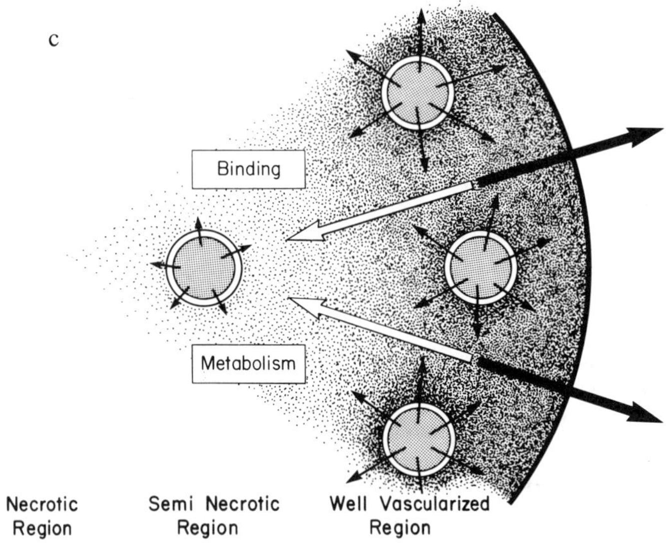

FIG. 2 *Continued.* (c) These macromolecules move toward the center by the slow process of diffusion (⇒). In addition, interstitial fluid oozing from tumor carries macromolecules with it by convection (→) into the normal tissue. Note that the interstitial movement may be further retarded by binding. Products of metabolism may be cleared rapidly by blood. (Reproduced with permission from Jain, 1989.) These transport processes have been mathematically modeled by Jain and Baxter (1988) and Baxter and Jain (1989, 1990, 1991a, b).

stagnant blood in them. Whether the fractional vascular volume decreases or not, a reduction in vascular surface area would lead to a reduction in the transvascular exchange of molecules. In addition, an increase in the intercapillary distance would require the molecules to traverse longer distances in the interstitium to reach all regions of a tumor.

B. Blood Flow Rate

Most investigators have measured the local blood flow rate of tumors based on uptake or clearance of a tracer from a single or a limited number of regions of the tumor (Vaupel *et al.*, 1989; Vaupel and Jain, 1991; Eskey *et al.*, 1994). Because of the noticeable spatial and temporal heterogeneity in tumor blood supply, these values may not be representative of the whole tumor. A limited number of studies in which the blood flow rate of the whole tumor has been measured show that the *average* perfusion rate of carcinomas is less than that of the host tissue or the tissue of origin. Sarcomas and lymphomas have higher *average* blood flow rates per unit tumor volume than carcinomas (Jain and Ward-Hartley, 1984). The data on blood flow in human tumors are limited and inconclusive because of methodological problems (Vaupel and Jain, 1991). In general, as tumors grow larger they may develop necrotic foci and, as a result, the average flow rate per unit volume decreases with tumor size (Jain and Ward-Hartley, 1984). Note that, even in these large necrotic tumors, therapeutic agents would be delivered in the well-perfused regions.

Blood flow in tumor vessels has been found to be intermittent (Endrich *et al.*, 1979a, b; Eskey *et al.*, 1992). There are random periods of flow reduction and stasis followed by resumption of flow, sometimes in the opposite direction. Tumor microcirculation is characterized by increased geometric and viscous resistance (Sevick and Jain, 1989a, b, 1991b; Less *et al.*, 1994; Zlotecki *et al.*, 1993, 1994). Quantitative studies on the macroscopic spatial heterogeneities in the tumor perfusion rate as a function of tumor growth (size) are limited. Based on perfusion rates, four regions can be recognized in a tumor: (a) an avascular, necrotic region; (b) a semi-necrotic region; (c) a stabilized microcirculation region, and (d) an advancing front (Fig. 2). In general, blood flow rates in necrotic/semi-necrotic regions of tumors are low, while those in non-necrotic regions are variable and substantially higher than in surrounding/contralateral host normal tissues. As a result of these spatial and temporal heterogeneities in blood supply, coupled with variations in the vascular morphology at both macroscopic and microscopic levels, it is not surprising that the spatial distribution of therapeutic agents in tumors is heterogeneous and the average uptake may decrease with increasing tumor weight.

C. Transvascular Transport

Once a blood-borne molecule has reached an exchange vessel, its extravasation rate, J_S (g/s), is governed by diffusion and convection and, to some extent, by transcytosis (Fig. 3). Diffusion is proportional to the exchange vessel's surface area and the difference between the plasma and interstitial concentrations. Convection is proportional to the rate of fluid leakage from the vessel. Fluid leakage, in turn, is proportional to surface area and the difference between the vascular and interstitial hydrostatic pressures minus the difference between the vascular and interstitial oncotic (i.e., osmotic pressure exerted by proteins) pressures. The proportionality constant which relates transluminal diffusive flux to concentration gradients is referred to as the vascular permeability, P (cm/s), and the constant which relates fluid leakage to pressure gradients is referred to as the hydraulic conductivity, L_p (cm/mm Hg-s). The effectiveness of the

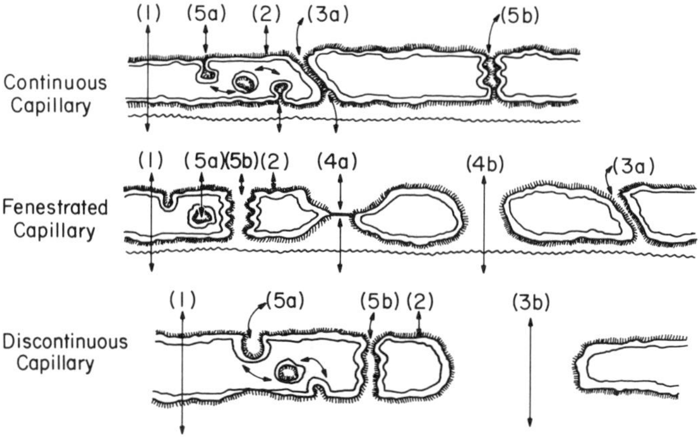

FIG. 3. Transvascular exchange. Transport pathways in normal capillary endothelium. (1) endothelial cell; (2) lateral membrane diffusion; (3) interendothelial junctions—(a) narrow, (b) wide; (4) endothelial fenestrae—(a) closed, (b) open; (5) vesicular transport—(a) transcytosis, (b) transendothelial channels. Note that water and lipophilic solutes share pathways (1), (3), and (4). Lipophilic solutes may use pathway (2) as well. Hydrophilic solutes and macromolecules use pathways (3) and (4). Macromolecules may also follow pathway (5). Note that in tumors these pathways have a "leakier" structure. [From Jain (1987a), with permission.]

transluminal oncotic pressure difference in producing fluid movement across a vessel wall is characterized by the osmotic reflection coefficient, σ; σ is close to 1 for a macromolecule and close to zero for a small molecule (Jain, 1987a; Deen, 1987). Thus, transport of molecules across normal or tumor vessels is governed by three transport parameters, P, L_p, and σ; the surface area for exchange; and the transvascular concentration and pressure gradients.

Ultrastructural studies of animal and human tumors have shown that tumor vessels have wide interendothelial junctions, a large number of fenestrae and transendothelial channels formed by vesicles, and discontinuous or absent basement membrane (Jain, 1987a; Dvorak *et al.*, 1988) (Fig. 3). These characteristics of tumor vessels suggest that they should have relatively high L_p and P (Sevick and Jain, 1991a; Gerlowski and Jain, 1986; Yuan *et al.*, 1993, 1994) (Fig. 4). If tumor vessels are indeed "leakier" to fluid and macromolecules compared to several normal tissues, what leads to their poor extravasation? As discussed next in Section D, tumors contain regions of high interstitial pressure, which lowers the fluid extravasation. Since the transvascular transport of macromolecules under normal conditions occurs primarily by convection (Jain, 1987a), a decrease in fluid extravasation would lead to a decrease in extravasation of macro-

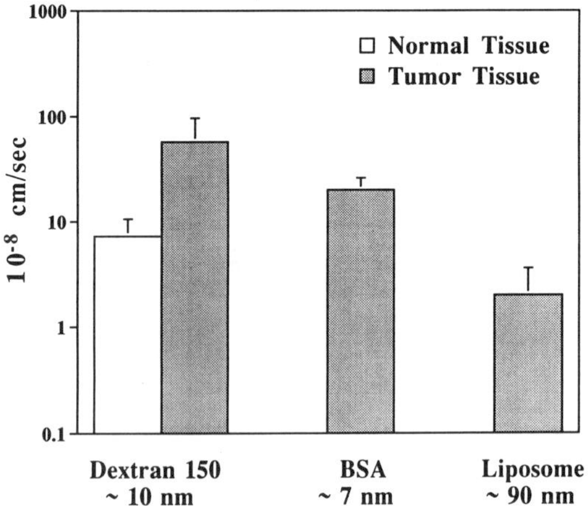

FIG. 4. Molecular-weight dependence of effective vascular permeability. Vascular permeability to 150,000 MW dextran (D150) is about one order of magnitude higher in tumor vessels than in the host tissue (data from Gerlowski and Jain, 1986). Even though albumin has a lower molecular weight (~ 70,000), because of its globular configuration, it has a lower permeability than D150 (Yuan *et al.*, 1993). Liposomes with diameters between 80 and 100 nm have even lower permeability in the tumor (Yuan *et al.*, 1994).

molecules (Jain and Baxter, 1988). Furthermore, the average vascular surface area per unit tumor volume decreases with tumor growth; hence one would expect reduced transvascular exchange in large tumors compared to smaller ones (Baxter and Jain, 1990).

D. Transvascular Pressure Gradients

Since the initial work of Young *et al.* (1950), several investigators have shown that interstitial fluid pressure, P_i, in animal tumors is significantly higher than in normal tissues (for a review, see Jain, 1987b). Recently, we have quantified interstitial hypertension in human melanomas, cervical carcinomas, head and neck tumors, and primary and metastatic breast and colorectal cancers (Boucher *et al.*, 1991; Roh *et al.*, 1991; Gutmann *et al.*, 1992; Less *et al.*, 1992) (Table II). Further, as the tumor grows, P_i rises in some tumors (Fig. 5), presumably because of the proliferation of tumor cells in a confined space, high vascular permeability, and the absence of functioning lymphatic vessels (Boucher *et al.*, 1990; Boucher and Jain, 1992). This increase in P_i is often associated with a reduction in tumor blood flow and the development of necrosis in a growing tumor (Jain, 1987b). Recent investigations of intratumor pressure gradients show that

TABLE II
INTERSTITIAL PRESSURE IN HUMAN TUMORS[a]

Tumor types	N	Mean	S.D.	Range
Head and neck carcinomas	27	19.0	17.3	1.5–79.0
Cervical carcinomas	26	22.8	20.5	6.0–94.0
Lung carcinomas	26	10.0	7.5	1.0–27.0
Metastatic melanomas	12	14.3	12.5	2.0–41.0
Breast carcinomas	8	15.0	9.0	4.0–33.0
Colorectal liver metastasis	8	21.0	12.0	6.0–45.0
Renal cell carcinoma	1	38.0	—	—
Normal skin	5	0.4	1.7	−1.0–3.0
Normal breast	8	0.0	1.0	−0.5–3.0

[a]Pressure values are in mm Hg.

the interstitial pressure is elevated throughout the tumor, and it drops precipitously to normal physiological value in the tumor periphery (Fig. 6a) (Boucher *et al.*, 1990). This pressure profile is in agreement with the predictions of our mathematical model (Jain and Baxter, 1988; Baxter and Jain, 1989). Direct measurements in two-dimensional tumors, and in the superficial layer of three-dimensional tumors, have shown that on the arterial side vascular pressure does not differ significantly between non-tumor and tumor vessels, whereas venous pressures may be lower in tumor vessels compared to those in normal vessels (for a review, see Jain, 1988). Our recent measurements show that the microvascular pressures in tumors may be as high as P_i, and may be a key source of interstitial hypertension (Boucher and Jain, 1992) (Fig. 6b).

In normal tissues vascular and interstitial oncotic pressures (π_v and π_i) are approximately 20–25 and 5–15 mm Hg, respectively (Baxter and Jain, 1989). Although there are no direct measurements of π_i in tumors, based on high vascular permeability and high interstitial diffusion coefficient in tumors, one would expect higher concentration of endogenous plasma proteins in the tumor interstitium than in normal interstitium. This hypothesis is supported by the data in the literature (Sylvén and Bois, 1960). As a result, π_i in tumors may be higher than that in normal tissues.

As shown in Fig. 6a, P_i in tumors is lower in the periphery; therefore, the filtration of fluid from vessels, J_F, would be close to normal. However, as one moves towards the center of the tumor, the increase in P_i would reduce the transvascular pressure gradient and thus the extravasation of fluid, J_F. As stated earlier, convective transport of a macromolecule is proportional to J_F; therefore, the rate of extravasation of a blood-borne macromolecule would be negligible in the center of a tumor (Baxter and

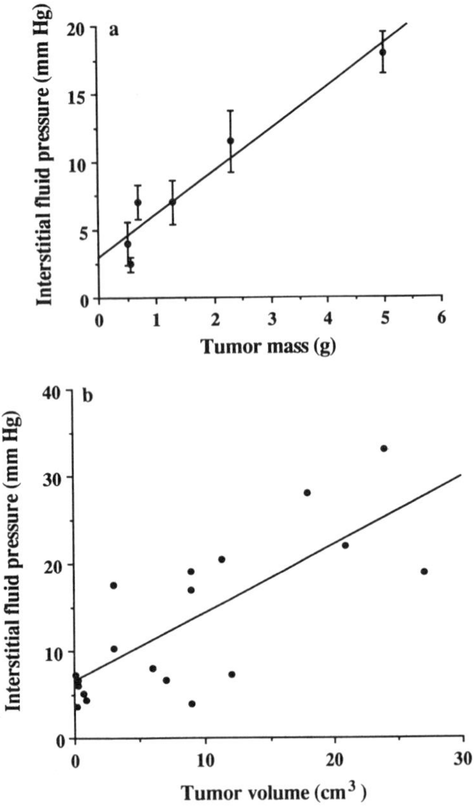

FIG. 5. Tumor size dependence of interstitial pressure. (a) In Walker 256 mammary carcinoma grown as tissue-isolated tumor, the mean central pressure ($\pm$SD) is linearly related to the tumor weight [pressure = 3.05 $\times$ weight (g) $\pm$ 3.02 mm Hg]. However, not all tumor types exhibited such correlation. In some tumors the interstitial pressure increased initially with tumor growth and reached a maximum value (Lee *et al.*, 1992). (b) We have also measured interstitial pressure in various human tumors (see text). In head and neck tumors in patients, pressure rises with tumor size (Gutmann *et al.*, 1992). We have found that several agents (e.g., nicotinamide, pentoxyfylline, dexamethesone, hemodilution, heat, radiation) can lower the interstitial fluid pressure in tumors (Lee *et al.*, 1992, 1994a, b; Leunig *et al.*, 1992a, 1994a; Kristjansen *et al.*, 1993; Roh *et al.*, 1991; Zlotecki *et al.*, 1993, 1994). We are exploring the possible use of high pressure in tumor localization during needle biopsy.

Jain, 1989). Since transvascular transport by diffusion is slow for a macromolecule to begin with, macromolecular extravasation would be very small in the high interstitial pressure regions of a tumor. Since high-pressure regions usually coincide with regions of poor perfusion rate and lower vessel surface area, leakage of blood-borne macromolecules from vessels would be further restricted (Baxter and Jain, 1990).

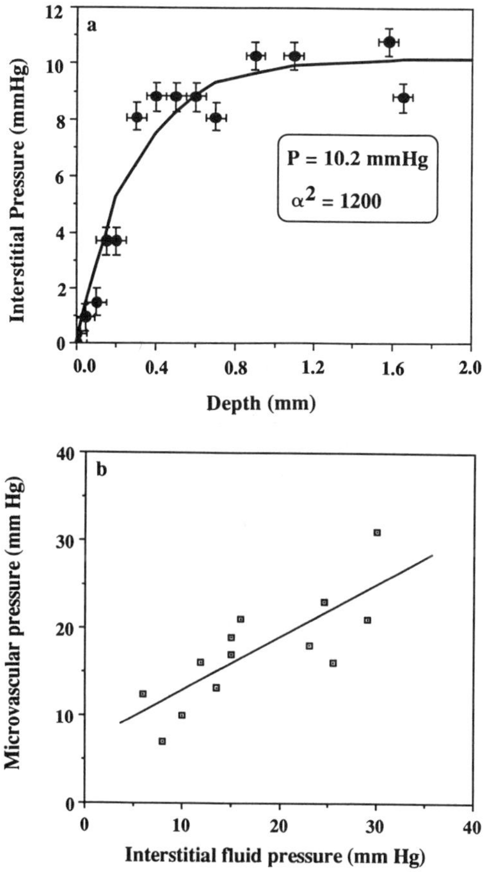

FIG. 6. (a) Interstitial pressure gradients in the mammary adenocarcinoma R3230AC as a function of radial position. The circles (●) represent data points (Boucher *et al.*, 1990), and the solid line represents the theoretical profile based on our previously developed mathematical model (Jain and Baxter, 1988; Baxter and Jain, 1989). Note that the pressure is nearly uniform in most of the tumor, but drops precipitously to normal tissue values in the periphery. Elevated pressure in the central region retards the extravasation of fluid and macromolecules. In addition, the pressure drop from the center to the periphery leads to an experimentally verifiable, radially outward fluid flow. (Reproduced from Boucher *et al.*, 1990, with permission.) (b) Microvascular pressure (MVP) in the peripheral vessels of the mammary adenocarcinoma R3230AC is comparable to the central interstitial fluid pressure (IFP) (adapted from Boucher and Jain, 1992). These results suggest that osmotic pressure difference across vessel walls is small in this tumor.

E. Interstitial Transport

Once a macromolecule has extravasated, its movement occurs by diffusion and convection through the interstitial space (Chary and Jain, 1989). Diffusion is proportional to the concentration gradient in the interstitium, and convection is proportional to the interstitial fluid velocity. The latter, in turn, is proportional to the pressure gradient in the interstitium. The proportionality constant which relates diffusive flux to the concentration gradient is referred to as the interstitial diffusion coefficient, D (cm^2/s), and the constant which relates interstitial velocity to the pressure gradient is referred to as the interstitial hydraulic conductivity, K (cm^2/mm Hg-s) (for a review, see Jain, 1987b). Values of transport coefficients D and K are determined by the structure and composition of the interstitial compartment, as well as the physicochemical properties of the solute molecule. Larger values of these parameters lead to less hindered movement of fluid and macromolecules through the interstitium. Similarly, large values of interstitial pressure and concentration gradients lead to large convective and diffusive fluxes.

Despite the importance of interstitial transport parameters, it has been difficult to obtain accurate measurements of these values. Accumulation of molecules in tumor or normal tissue can be detected, but it is difficult to distinguish the roles of diffusion, convection, and binding, as well as transvascular transport. One experimental method that has been used successfully to quantitate interstitial diffusion, convection, and binding is fluorescence recovery after photobleaching (FRAP), in conjunction with tumors grown in transparent windows (Chary and Jain, 1987, 1989; Jain *et al.*, 1990; Kaufman and Jain, 1990, 1991, 1992a, b; Berk *et al.*, 1993).

The interstitial space in tumors, in general, is very large compared to that in host normal tissues (for a review, see Jain, 1987b). An order of magnitude higher values of D and K in tumors compared to several normal tissues should favor movement of macromolecules in the tumor interstitium (Gerlowski and Jain, 1986; Nugent and Jain, 1984a, b; Clauss and Jain, 1990; Swabb *et al.*, 1974) (Fig. 7). Why, then, do the exogenously injected macromolecules not distribute uniformly in tumors? As discussed later, there are two reasons for this apparent paradox.

The time constant, τ_D, for a molecule with diffusion coefficient D, to diffuse across distance l is approximately $l^2/4D$. For diffusion of IgG (MW ~ 155,000) in tumors, τ_D is of the order of 1 h for 100 μm distance, ~ 2 days for 1 mm distance, and ~ 7–8 months for 1 cm distance (Jain and Baxter, 1988; Clauss and Jain, 1990). Now consider a hypothetical tumor which is uniformly perfused, has nearly zero P_i, and has exchange vessels ~ 200 μm apart. In such a tumor, IgG would reach uniform

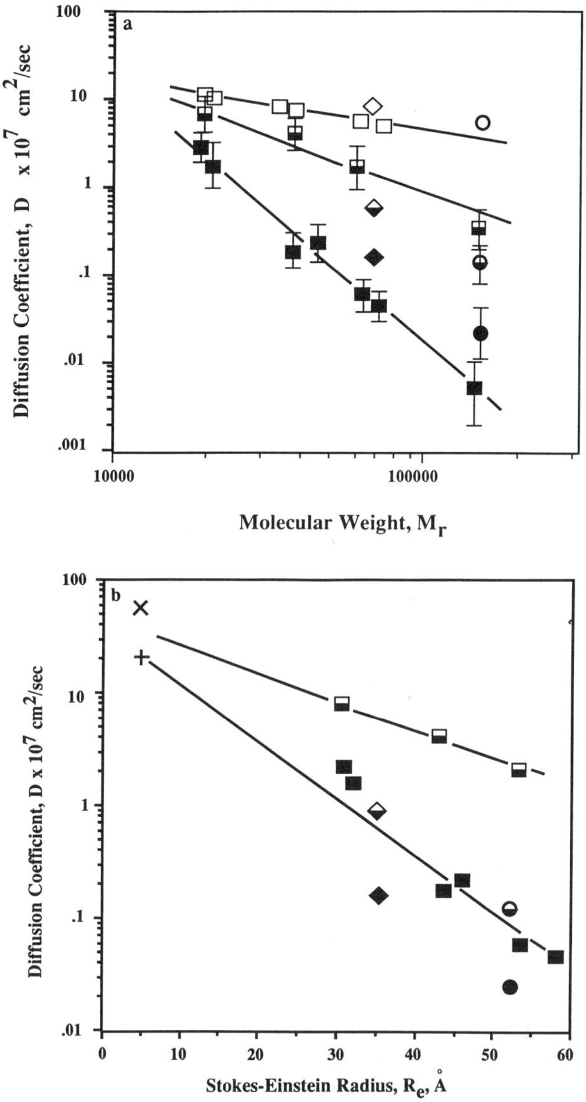

FIG. 7. Molecular weight dependence of diffusivity. (a) The effective diffusion coefficient, D, has been plotted as a function of molecular weight for dextrans (Nugent and Jain, 1984a, b; Gerlowski and Jain, 1986), albumin (Nugent and Jain, 1984a, b), and IgG (Clauss and Jain, 1990) in water, normal tissue, and tumor tissue. Symbols: □, dextran, aqueous; ◇, bovine serum albumin, aqueous; ○, rabbit IgG, tumor; ■, dextran, normal tissue; ◆, bovine serum albumin; normal tissue; ●, rabbit IgG, normal tissue. The half-filled symbols refer to the tumor data. (b) The effective diffusion coefficient plotted versus the Stokes-Einstein radius. Symbols as in (a) plus: ×, sodium fluorescein, tumor; +, sodium fluorescein, normal tissue. (From Clauss and Jain, 1990, with permission.) Currently, we are measuring diffusion coefficient of molecules and particles larger than 50 Å in radius.

concentration in ~ 1 h post-injection, provided the plasma concentration remains constant. In a normal tissue with the value of D lower by an order of magnitude, it will take ~ 10 h to reach ~ 16% concentration.

Now consider a more realistic situation, where the tumor vessels are ~ 200 μm apart and uniformly perfused, but P_i has increased in the center so that fluid extravasation, and hence convective transport of macromolecules across vessels, has stopped. In such a case the only way macromolecules extravasate in the center is by the slow process of diffusion across vessel walls. Also, they can reach the center from the periphery (where P_i is near zero) by interstitial diffusion. As stated earlier, if the distance between the center and periphery is ~ 1 mm, it would take days for them to get there, and if it is ~ 1 cm, it would take months (Clauss and Jain, 1990). If, owing to cellular proliferation, the central vessels have collapsed completely, then there is no delivery of macromolecules by blood flow to the necrotic center (Jain, 1988; Baxter and Jain, 1990). In such a case there are no molecules available for extravasation by diffusion across the vessel wall, and consequently the central concentration would be even lower (Baxter and Jain, 1990). However, once the molecules have arrived there, the central region may serve as a reservoir for slow release later when the periphery has been cleared by plasma.

So far the interstitial movement of molecules which do not bind to any extravascular sites or undergo metabolism has been discussed. It is well known that the binding reaction lowers the apparent diffusion rate of molecules (Astarita, 1967). Therefore, although higher affinity of antibody to antigen significantly increases the antibody's concentration proximal to the vessel, it retards their movement to distal locations in the interstitium unless the antigens are saturated (Baxter and Jain, 1991a, b; Dedrick and Flessner, 1989; Fujimori *et al.*, 1989; Kaufman and Jain, 1990, 1991, 1992a, b; Sung *et al.*, 1993). The metabolism of antibodies in normal and tumor tissues is poorly understood. However, the products of metabolism are usually smaller in molecular weight, and hence may diffuse and be cleared relatively rapidly.

As discussed earlier, P_i is high in the center of tumors and low in the surrounding normal tissue. Therefore, one would expect interstitial fluid motion from the tumor's periphery into the surrounding normal tissue. Using a tissue-isolated tumor preparation, Butler *et al.* (1975) measured this fluid loss to be 0.14–0.22 mL/h-gram of tissue in four different rat mammary carcinomas. In various animal and human (xenograft) tumors studied to date, 6–14% of plasma entering the tumor has been found to leave from the tumor's periphery (Jain, 1988). This fluid leakage leads to a radially outward interstitial fluid velocity of 0.1–0.2 μm/s at the periphery of a 1 cm "tissue-isolated" tumor (Jain 1987a). [Because of the resistance offered by the surrounding normal tissue, the radially outward velocity is expected to be an order of magnitude lower in a tumor grown in the subcutaneous tissue or muscle (Baxter and Jain, 1989)]. A macromolecule at the tumor periphery has to overcome this outward convection to penetrate into the tumor by diffusion. The relative contribution of this mechanism to heterogeneous distribution of antibodies in tumors is, however, smaller than the contribution of heterogeneous extravasation due to elevated pressure and necrosis (Baxter and Jain, 1989, 1990, 1991a, b). Using fluorescence recovery after photobleaching, we have recently measured interstitial convective velocities around normal and tumor vessels (Chary and Jain, 1987, 1989; Jain *et al.*, 1990) (Fig. 8).

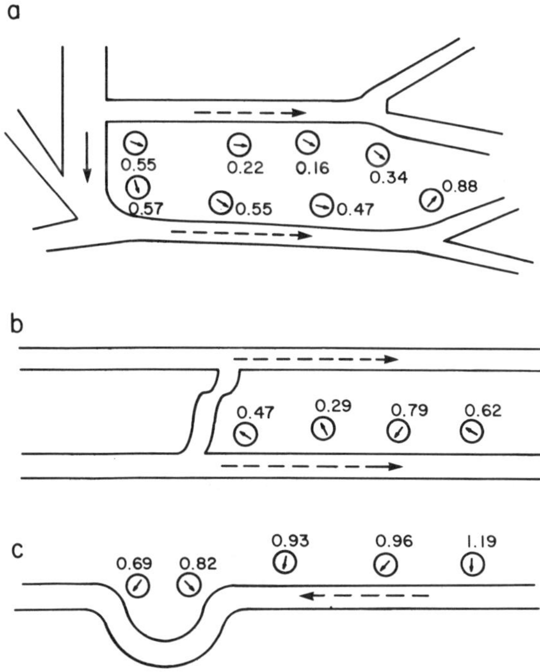

FIG. 8. Interstitial velocity profiles. Representative regions in the microcirculation. Circles represent locations of fluorescence photobleaching experiments. The arrows inside the circles represent the direction of the interstitial fluid velocity at these locations. The nearby values show magnitudes of the velocity in $\mu m/s$. (a) An area where interstitial flow parallels blood flow in the vessels. (b) Interstitial flow is opposite prevailing blood flow. (c) Fluid is absorbed from the interstitium into a postcapillary venule. (From Chary and Jain, 1989, with permission.) The photobleaching technique has provided the first and to date the only measurements in the literature of interstitial convective velocities. We have now further improved this technique to permit measurements of binding parameters (Kaufman and Jain, 1990, 1991, 1992a, b) and of transport parameters in light-scattering media (Berk *et al.*, 1993).

F. Cellular Transport

Transport of molecules across the cell membrane occurs by passive and facilitated diffusion and active transport (Stein, 1986; Finkelstein, 1987). Passive transport is governed by a mass-transfer coefficient, surface area for exchange, transmembrane concentration difference, and a partition coefficient. The partition coefficient can be modified by charge, pH, temperature, and presence of other drugs. Facilitated transport may be most simply described by Michaelis–Menten kinetics. Depending upon the carrier system, symmetric or asymmetric models may be used.

In most studies, the intracellular space has been assumed to be well mixed. Several investigators have shown that a simple diffusion equation coupled with appropriate reaction terms is adequate to describe intracellular transport (Kushmerick and Podolsky, 1969; Lauffenburger and Linderman, 1993).

Values of transport and kinetic parameters have been obtained primarily using *in vitro* approaches. The need to make these measurements *in vivo* and to compare them with *in vitro* values is urgent. Such comparisons may, in part, explain why certain agents that work in Petri dishes do not work as well *in vivo*.

G. Thermal Properties

A comprehensive tabulation of the thermal properties of tissues can be found in Shitzer and Eberhart (1985). Using a non-invasive probe technique, Jain *et al.* (1979a) measured the thermal conductivity (~ 3 mW/cm-K) and thermal diffusivity ($\sim 10^{-3}$ cm^2/s) of a tumor of mammary origin, Walker 256 carcinoma. In this study, tumors weighing between 2 and 11 g and with blood perfusion rates between 1 and 6 h^{-1} were used. While the effective thermal conductivity of these tumors decreased as they grew larger, no definite correlation was found between the true thermal conductivity of tumor and its weight. When the blood flow rate of a tumor was modified by increasing or decreasing the blood volume of the animal, its effective thermal conductivity (as measured by the temperature rise in the heating probe embedded in tumor) varied proportionally to the square root of the perfusion rate (Peclet number). This work shows that in order to obtain a biologically significant increase in the effective thermal conductivity, a substantial increase in the blood flow rate is needed. In these experiments, thermal conductivity measured *in vitro* was found to be within 10% of the *in vivo* value (Jain and Gullino, 1980). Various investigators have since measured thermal properties of tumors using invasive-probe techniques and have found the values close to that of normal tissues. In the absence of *in vivo* data on the thermal properties of tumors, an order of magnitude estimate can be obtained using the correlation of Cooper and Trezek (1971). This correlation relates the thermal properties of the tissue to its composition (water, protein, and fat).

The physical property which determines the absorption of ultrasonic (US) energy in a tissue is the attenuation (or absorption) coefficient, α, of the tissue. As a plane parallel beam penetrates into a homogeneous tissue, its intensity, I, decreases exponentially with distance, x, as a result of absorption:

$$I = I_0 \exp(-\alpha x).$$

Values of α as a function of the wave frequency have been obtained for the various normal tissues (Jain, 1985a). Note that the value of α is largest for bone, smallest for fat, and in between for muscle, suggesting a similar trend in the energy absorption by these tissues. Similar data are needed for various types of tumors.

Wavelength λ, and frequency, f, of sound are related to the speed of propagation, C, in the medium by the following equation:

$$\lambda f = C.$$

The velocity of sound in most tissues (except bone) is approximately equal to that in water, about 1,500 m/s. Air, on the other hand, does not allow the transmission of ultrasound from the source to the tissue. Therefore, ultrasound cannot be used to heat tissues which contain even minute amounts of air—for example, the chest cavity.

Similar to ultrasound, the strength of an electric field resulting from the absorption of plane parallel microwaves in a homogeneous tissue decreases exponentially (Bladel, 1964). The absorption coefficient, α, is related to the dielectric constant, ε, the electrical conductivity, σ (mho/cm) and wavelength in air, λ (cm). Both ε and σ are functions of the wave frequency and temperature. A number of investigators have measured ε and σ of various normal tissues. We have measured σ and ε of various mammary carcinomas and 9L-glioma at 37 and 43°C, and have compared the results with normal tissues (Peloso *et al.*, 1984). These data have been fitted by the following equations:

$$\log \varepsilon = a + b \log f + \frac{c}{\log f},$$

$$\log \frac{\sigma}{\omega \varepsilon_0} = d + e \log f.$$

The parameters incorporated in these two equations were estimated for various tumors at 37 and 43°C. Here, $\omega = 2\pi f$ and $e_0 = 1/(36\pi \times 10^{11})$ in farads/cm. For normal tissues, both ε and σ vary with the temperature according to the following relationships (Schwan, 1965):

$$\frac{\Delta\varepsilon}{\varepsilon} \approx -0.05\%/°\text{C} \quad \text{and} \quad \frac{\Delta\sigma}{\sigma} = 2\%/°\text{C}.$$

For neoplastic tissues, we found that the temperature coefficients are of the same order of magnitude (Peloso *et al.*, 1984). Whether dielectric properties of tumors are significantly different from that of the host tissues is not yet resolved (Smith *et al.*, 1986; Zywietz and Knöchel, 1986; Surowiec *et al.*, 1988; Foster and Cheever, 1992).

H. Metabolic Properties

The *in vivo* metabolic microenvironment (e.g., pH, pO_2) plays an important role in determining tumor response to certain therapies. These metabolic parameters reflect the availability of nutrients and removal of waste products, as well as the rate of metabolism (e.g., consumption of oxygen and glucose, and production of lactic acid and carbon dioxide) (Aisenberg, 1961). Since the pioneering studies of Gullino (1976), several investigators have measured the consumption of metabolites by tumors and related them to blood flow, energy level and growth characteristics of tumors (Vaupel *et al.*, 1989; Vaupel and Jain, 1991; Eskey *et al.*, 1993). Similarly, several investigators have shown that some regions of animal and human tumors may have low pO_2 and/or pH (Wike-Hooley *et al.*, 1984; Vaupel *et al.*, 1989; Jain *et al.*, 1984; Sevick and Jain, 1988; Vaupel and Jain, 1991). However, pH and pO_2 have not yet been related with the consumption and production of metabolites in a tumor to understand and quantify metabolic pathways in a tumor (Eskey *et al.*, 1993). With the advent of non-invasive microscopic methods (Torres-Filho *et al.*, 1994; Martin and Jain, 1993, 1994), it may be possible to resolve these issues in the near future.

I. Determinants of Cell Delivery

So far, we have discussed the delivery of molecules. In recent years, immunologically active cells (e.g., lymphokine-activated killer cells, tumor-infiltrating lymphocytes) have also been used as injected therapeutics (Rosenberg, 1990; Melder and Jain, 1993). In some cases, these cells have been transfected with an appropriate gene to produce the desired agent (e.g., cytokine, antibody, enzyme) at the site where these cells have accumulated. As with the delivery of molecules, heterogeneous blood supply is a major barrier to the delivery of cells to the tumor vasculature. Once these cells have arrived in the tumor vasculature via the blood stream, their retention in the tumor depends upon their adhesion to the vessel wall, and subsequent migration across the vessel wall (extravasation) and through the interstitium. If the tumor vasculature itself is the target of these cells, then they need not extravasate for a therapeutic effect (Sasaki *et al.*, 1991; Melder *et al.*, 1993). However, if cancer cells are the target of these effector cells or the target of their gene products, then these cells must extravasate and accumulate in the interstitial space.

The adhesion of these cells to the tumor vessel wall occurs when the force between the adhesion molecules on the surfaces of endothelium and effector cell is greater than the hydrodynamic force exerted by blood flow. The deformability of these cells also plays an important role in this process, since it can alter the surface area of contact (Sasaki *et al.*, 1989; Melder and Jain, 1992). Measurement of forces exerted by various adhesion molecules as well as cell deformability *in vitro* and *in vivo* is an active area of research in many laboratories, including our own (Ohkubo *et al.*, 1991; Munn *et al.*, 1994).

Extravasation and interstitial movement of these effector cells is more complicated, because unlike molecules, cells can exhibit active motility. In simple terms, they can move on their own by attaching to certain substrates in the vessel wall or the interstitial matrix, and by moving in a specific direction defined by chemical cues by a process called chemotaxis. Thus, their motion *in vivo* is governed by their deformability and adhesion properties, in addition to the physiological and immunological characteristics of the tissue. As a result of these physiological barriers, the number of effector cells localized in tumors is usually suboptimal. Increased understanding of various biophysical parameters should be helpful in optimizing delivery of therapeutic cells to tumors.

V. Mass Transfer in Tumors

After a drug is injected into the body and enters the blood stream, mass transfer takes place by the following processes: (a) flow through the vascular subcompartment of a tissue; (b) transport across the capillary walls into the interstitial space; (c) diffusion and convection within the interstitial space; (d) transport across the cell membrane into the intracellular space; and (e) diffusion within the intracellular space. For fluid and macromolecules, reabsorption by lymphatic vessels must also be considered. One important difference between normal and tumor tissues is that the lymphatic system may not be functional in the latter. In each of these subcomponents, the drug may metabolize or degrade into its subcompartments or bind to proteins or other components. In addition to this nonspecific binding, specific binding with an enzyme or other cellular element may occur, thereby explaining the therapeutic effectiveness of a particular drug.

Ideally, one would like to measure the mass transfer rates and concentrations in each compartment of a tissue as a function of both time and space and develop precise mathematical models on the basis of these data. Such models could then be used to predict spatial and temporal concentrations of various agents in a variety of normal and neoplastic tissues. Since the selective tumor cell kill depends on the concentration–time history of a drug, such information could be used in developing optimal dose schedule of anticancer agents. However, there are several practical problems in carrying out such detailed measurements directly, and in developing such detailed, dynamic, predictive mathematical models. Nevertheless, it is possible to obtain considerable useful information about mass transfer in tumors, using the experimental and theoretical approaches discussed in the next two sections.

A. Experimental Techniques

1. Single Cell Studies

a. In Vitro. The purpose of these studies is to measure cellular uptake of drugs and to determine parameters which characterize the passive and active transport across the membrane, and diffusion, binding and metabolism within the cell. In these experiments, dispersed normal or neoplastic cells are exposed to an artificial environment that simulates the physiological conditions. To measure the drug uptake from the extracellular fluid, the tissue culture medium is brought to a desired level of drug concentration, and intracellular drug concentration as a function of time is measured. To measure the efflux rate of drug, the cells which have accumulated drug are exposed to fresh medium, and intracellular drug concentration is measured periodically.

b. In Vivo. In these studies the suspended cells are grown *in vivo*, for example, in the peritoneal cavity of an animal. These studies involve injection of drug into an animal, and measurement of drug concentrations as a function of time in the cells and the extracellular fluid they are bathing in. Since the concentration of drug in the extracellular fluid is time-dependent, the analysis of *in vivo* data is more complex than that of the *in vitro* data (Weissbrod *et al.*, 1978).

2. *Multi-cell Spheroid Studies*

In these studies spheroids are exposed to the culture medium at a known drug concentration. If the culture medium is well stirred (in the case of suspension culture), the spheroids are exposed to a symmetric environment. If the culture medium is still and the spheroids rest on some surface, they are exposed to an asymmetric environment, resulting in an asymmetric concentration profile. The methods to measure concentration profiles include microelectrodes (which can be inserted into a spheroid up to various desired radial positions), autoradiography, and fractional disaggregation of various spheroid layers to measure cellular concentration in each layer. Each method has its own advantages and limitations.

3. *Solid Tumors—Standard Preparations*

In these studies, animals bearing spontaneous, induced or transplanted tumors are used.

a. In Vitro Studies. Once the tumor has reached a desired size, the tumor is removed from the animal and a slice of the tissue is exposed to a known drug concentration in a "diffusion-cell," and resulting concentration profiles are measured for later analysis. Care is taken to maintain the matrix structure of the tissue. Although the absence of blood flow (convection) and one-dimensional diffusion make the analysis of data relatively simple, caution must be exercised in using the parameter values obtained for *in vivo* simulation (Swabb *et al.*, 1974).

b. In Vivo Studies. Extrapolation to solid tumors of the results obtained from the techniques discussed heretofore has obvious limitations. Therefore, *in vivo* studies are most important for analyzing drug transport in solid tumors. These studies involve injection of drug into an animal, measurement of drug concentrations as a function of time in normal and tumor tissues by sequential sacrifice of animals, and estimation of the transport parameters using various mathematical models. The drug can be injected intravenously, intramuscularly, intraperitoneally, subcutaneously, or via other routes. Depending upon the drug, the concentration of drug can be measured using radioassay, chemical assay, bioassay or immunoassay, or a combination thereof. Depending upon the objective of the experiments, drug concentration can be measured as a function of spatial position in the tissue or averaged over the entire tissue mass. When high spatial resolution is not required, concentrations can be measured noninvasively using, for example, positron emission tomography.

4. Solid Tumors—Special Preparations

a. Tissue-Isolated Tumors—In Vivo Perfusion. Standard tumor preparations have multiple arteries and multiple veins, which make it difficult to study a tumor as an anatomical entity separated from the host. In 1961, Gullino developed a procedure to transplant a tumor, which can be treated as an organ, connected to the host's vasculature by a single artery and vein, and isolated from surrounding tissues such as the kidney (Gullino and Grantham, 1961). In 1973, Gullino and co-workers extended their technique to primary mammary tumors (spontaneous or induced) (Grantham *et al.*, 1973). Recently, we have adapted this preparation for human tumors in patients (Less *et al.*, 1994), and for human tumor xenografts in immunodeficient mice (Kristjansen *et al.*, 1994). The tissue-isolated tumor preparation permits one to collect the tumor efferent blood by placing a catheter in the tumor vein. By infusing equal amounts of blood into the animal via its jugular vein, it is possible to maintain the animal's blood pressure and volume in the physiological range. In addition, the blood flow to the tumor can be increased or decreased by inducing hyper- and hypovolemia in the animal, respectively. Therefore, such a preparation allows one to study directly the blood flow rate, transport, and metabolism of tumors (for a review, see Kristjansen *et al.*, 1994).

b. Tissue-Isolated Tumors—Ex Vivo Perfusion. The goal of these experiments is to develop a tumor preparation which can be perfused as an isolated organ *ex vivo*. A complete normal organ bearing a tumor or a segment of intestine "acting as supporting tissue" for the growth of tumor has been used by Folkman and co-workers (1962, 1963, 1966) for this purpose. However, a significant amount of residual normal tissue in these preparations precludes their use to study pathophysiology of tumors. On the other hand, the tissue isolated preparation developed by Gullino (1968), as described in the previous subsection, contains a negligible amount of host tissue. In Gullino's preparation, once the tissue-isolated tumor reaches an adequate size, the artery and vein of the pedicle are cannulated and the tumor is transferred into an *ex vivo* perfusion setup. Although physiologists routinely use isolated, perfused normal tissues/organs to study mass transfer, surprisingly, such a preparation has not been used to study mass transfer in tumors, presumably because of difficult surgical procedure. We have used this preparation to study determinants of tumor blood flow (Sevick and Jain, 1989a, b, 1991b; Less *et al.*, 1994), fluid transport (Sevick and Jain, 1991a), and metabolism (Eskey *et al.*, 1993), as well as residence time distribution of various tracers (Eskey *et al.*, 1994).

c. Tumors Incorporating a Micropore Chamber. The methods described so far can be used to measure the concentration of chemicals in the afferent and efferent blood of tumors or in the tissue as a whole. They do not provide continuous *in vivo* non-invasive sampling of the interstitial fluid. The interstitial compartment of a tissue provides a medium of exchange of chemicals among cells, and between cells and vessels, and therefore information about it can be useful.

In 1964, Gullino and Grantham developed a procedure to sample the tumor interstitial fluid (TIF) based on two observations—(i) tumors have the tendency to grow on and around extraneous material and to incorporate it into themselves, and (ii) tumors, perhaps because they lack a lymphatic system, ooze out the interstitial fluid in large amounts compared to the normal tissues. In this procedure, a cylindrical chamber with walls made of membrane (pore diameter less than 0.45 μm) is incorporated into a solid tumor. TIF flows into the chamber in about 24 h post-implant, and continues for as long as the chamber remains in the tumor. The fluid collected in the chamber either can be drained continuously via a catheter by siphon action (0.5–5 mL/day), or can be withdrawn periodically into a syringe placed in the catheter. Gullino and co-workers placed similar chambers in the subcutaneous space of the animals to collect the subcutaneous interstitial fluid (SIF), although at a considerably slower rate (Gullino, 1970).

So far this chamber technique has been used to monitor concentration of O_2, CO_2, glucose, lactic acid (Gullino, 1975, 1976), pH (Jain *et al.*, 1984), and a drug (methotrexate) (Jain *et al.*, 1979b) in TIF and SIF.

5. *Transparent Chamber Preparation*

The techniques discussed in the previous two sections provide useful "macroscopic" (i.e., tissue-level) information on mass transfer in normal and neoplastic tissues. These techniques, however, do not provide direct information on mass transfer at the "microscopic" (i.e., capillary or microcirculatory) level. Over the years various techniques have been developed to study the microvasculature and microcirculation in living animals. Some of the tissues that lend themselves to direct observation include cat, dog, rat, rabbit, and frog mesentery; cat, dog, and rabbit omentum; the hamster cheek pouch; the bat wing; the choriollantoic membrane of the chick embryo; the rat cremaster muscle and various other muscles in other species; cerebral, pancreatic, hepatic, and renal tissues, predominantly in the rat; and the human nailfold and retina. A review of these tissue preparations and the work done with them would necessitate an almost complete review of the field of microvascular research. Therefore, we will concentrate on one special preparation which has been used quite frequently in cancer research, namely, the transparent chamber technique.

The transparent chamber technique in its broadest sense covers all transparent devices which allow living tissue to be studied microscopically for more than a few hours. A large assortment of devices exist for numerous animals and various tissues (Baker and Nastuk, 1986). Internal organs that have been exteriorized by chamber techniques include a loop of small intestine with its attached mesentery in the rabbit and dog, the pancreas of the mouse, and the ovary and Fallopian tube in the rabbit. Body surfaces that have been replaced by transparent windows include the rabbit and monkey cranium, atrium, and stomach wall, and the dog and rabbit thorax. The original transparent chamber designed for the rabbit ear has since been modified and adapted to the lateral body-wall skin flap of rabbits, the ear of the dog, the hamster cheek pouch, the dorsal skin fold of the mouse and the rat, and even to the upper-arm skin fold in man.

Originally developed by Sandison in 1924 for rabbit ear, the chamber was adapted to the rat cranium by Forbes (1928) and to mice dorsal skin by Algire and Chalkley (1945). We have used these preparations to study vascular and interstitial transport of molecules and cells in mouse, rat, rabbit, and human tumors (Fig. 1). With the use of various optical and electronic devices and fluorescence microscopy, these chambers permit non-invasive, continuous, and quantitative measurement of a variety of physiological parameters. These parameters include angiogenesis and blood flow (Dudar and Jain, 1983, 1984; Ward-Hartley and Jain, 1987; Leunig *et al.*, 1992b, 1994b); metabolic microenvironment (Torres-Filho *et al.*, 1994; Martin and Jain, 1993, 1994); cell–cell interactions (Ohkubo *et al.*, 1991; Sasaki *et al.*, 1991); and vascular and interstitial transport (Nugent and Jain, 1984a, b; Gerlowski and Jain, 1985, 1986; Jain, 1985b; Chary and Jain, 1987, 1989; Clauss and Jain, 1990; Yuan *et al.*, 1993, 1994; Berk *et al.*, 1993). Of course, this technique has its limitations as well, including the ability to monitor only the superficial layer of the tumor.

B. Mathematical Models

Analogous to the experimental approaches discussed in the previous section, mathematical models have been developed to describe mass transfer at all three levels—cellular, multi-cellular (spheroid), and tissue levels. For each level two approaches have been used—the lumped parameter and distributed parameter models. In the former approach, the region of interest is considered to be a perfectly mixed reactor or compartment. As a result, the concentration of each region has no spatial dependence. In the latter approach, a more detailed analysis of the mass transfer process leads to information on the spatial and/or temporal changes in concentrations. Models for single cells and spheroids were reviewed in Section III,A and are part of the tissue-level models (Jain, 1984); hence, we will focus here only on tissue-level models.

1. Lumped Parameter Models

Lumped parameter models for tissues are also referred to as compartmental or pharmacokinetic models. These models can be divided into two categories—classical and physiological (or whole-body) compartmental analyses. In the classical approach, the body or a region of body is represented by one or more compartments, without relating the content or inputs or outputs associated with these compartments to available physiological and physicochemical information. These models are useful when it is sufficient to know and to be able to control the blood (plasma) concentration, and the details of any distribution in various tissues are not necessary (for details on classical pharmacokinetics, see Wagner, 1971).

In the whole-body pharmacokinetic model, mass transfer in the body is modeled by a set of interconnected lumped compartments that represent various organs of the body as shown in Fig. 9. The model predicts drug concentrations in each compartment using the available physiological, anatomical, and physicochemical information. With the use of these parameters, the physiologically based pharmacokinetic model provides a rational basis on which to extrapolate from one species to another, once the basic principles and primary mechanisms for distribution, metabolism, and excretion are understood (Gerlowski and Jain, 1983). Since only limited human data are available, the model is a valuable tool for carrying out this scale-up to from rodents to larger species and humans (Dedrick, 1973; Dedrick *et al.*, 1973a).

A physiologically based pharmacokinetic model capable of predicting the distribution of drugs in blood, organs, and other tissues of mammalian systems was originally developed by Bischoff, Dedrick, and their co-workers (Bischoff and Dedrick, 1968; Dedrick *et al.*, 1970; Bischoff *et al.*, 1970,

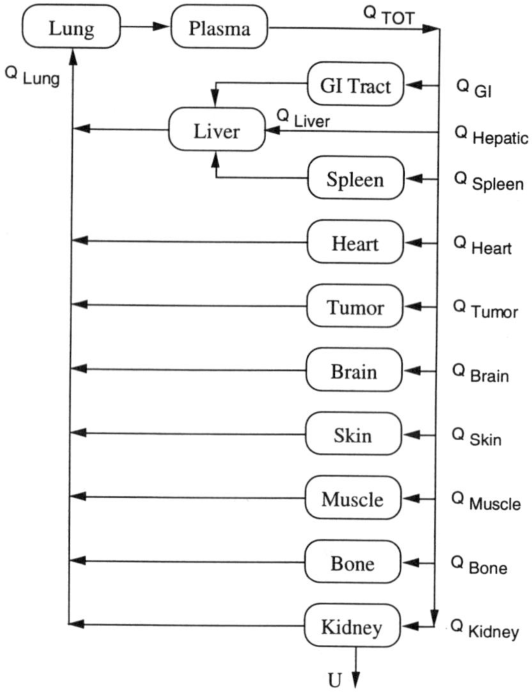

FIG. 9. Schematic of the physiologically based pharmacokinetic model for antibody distribution in mice and humans (reproduced with permission from Baxter *et al.*, 1994a).

1971). This approach has been successfully applied for the pharmacokinetics of more than 50 agents—anticancer and others (Dedrick *et al.*, 1973b, 1975; Gerlowski and Jain, 1983; Baxter *et al.*, 1994a).

In the most general case, the following unsteady-state material balance equations are written for the vascular, interstitial, and intracellular compartments, respectively:

$$V^{\mathrm{v}}\frac{dC^{\mathrm{v}}}{dt} = Q(C_{\mathrm{P}} - C^{\mathrm{v}}) - N^{\mathrm{vi}},$$

$$V^{\mathrm{i}}\frac{dC^{\mathrm{i}}}{dt} = N^{\mathrm{vi}} - N^{\mathrm{ic}},$$

$$V^{\mathrm{c}}\frac{dC^{\mathrm{c}}}{dt} = N^{\mathrm{ic}},$$

where V^{v}, V^{i}, V^{c} are the respective subcompartment volumes; C^{v}, C^{i}, C^{c} are the respective subcompartment drug concentrations; Q is the plasma flow rate for a particular compartment; C_P is the plasma drug concentration entering a particular compartment; N^{vi} is the rate of drug transport from the vascular to interstitial subcompartment; and N^{ic} is the rate of drug transport from the interstitial to intracellular subcompartment. Such equations can be written for each tissue or organ. In addition, the following unsteady-state mass balance equation is written for plasma:

$$V_P \frac{dC_P}{dt} = \sum_j (Q_j C_j^v) - Q_p C_P + g(t)$$

where V_p is the plasma compartment volume, C_p is the plasma drug concentration, and Q_j is the plasma flow rate of the jth compartment (which then enters the central plasma compartment). C_j^v is the vascular drug concentration in the jth compartment. Q_p is the total flow which enters the plasma compartment from the other compartments, and $g(t)$ is the injection function which models the intravenous injection of drug. Other modes of injection can be incorporated by modifying the injection function accordingly (Dedrick, 1988). Finally, unsteady-state mass balance equations are written for bile duct and gut lumen. Previous investigators have divided the bile duct and gut lumen into several subcompartments to simulate the time delays associated with bile clearance and reabsorption of drug by the intestine. In special tissues, such as the brain, a brain's cellular compartment may be added to account for the blood–brain barrier that restricts entry into brain cells of water-soluble, ionized materials, including most anticancer drugs (Gerlowski and Jain, 1983; Jain, 1984).

Metabolism of drug into its metabolites, which may be important for some drugs, can be accounted for in the model by writing a parallel set of equations for metabolites.

In writing the material balance equations for a compartment, several assumptions are made. The transport terms between each of the subcompartments are defined, the binding of drug in each subcompartment is quantified and incorporated into the equations, and additional terms are included where necessary to account for liver clearance, kidney clearance, and intestinal absorption. Each subcompartment, i.e., the vascular, the interstitial, and the intracellular, is considered to be a perfectly mixed continuous-stirred-tank reactor (CSTR). This means the concentration of each subcompartment has no spatial dependence.

The total concentration of drug in each subcompartment, j, can be divided into two compartments—free ($\overline{C}^j$) and bound ($\overline{\overline{C}}^j$):

$$C^j = \overline{C}^j + \overline{\overline{C}}^j.$$

The vascular subcompartment equation of liver includes two terms for plasma flow, corresponding to the systemic and enterohepatic circulations. The vascular subcompartment equations of the kidney and liver include additional terms to account for urine excretion and secretion into the common bile duct from the liver. Terms for intestinal reabsorption from the gut lumen and for fecal excretion are also included.

Using the available flow rates, volumes, transport parameters, binding relationships, metabolism information, and drug clearance rates for each organ, a set of differential equations is obtained. If the resulting equations are linear, analytical solutions can be obtained by standard methods. When nonlinear terms are present, numerical integration methods can be used to solve for drug concentration as a function of time in each subcompartment of an organ or tissue and in the plasma compartment.

It is not practical to write the material balance equations in their most general form, since detailed knowledge of the transport among the vascular, interstitial, and intracellular subcompartments is not always available. Therefore, based on the known transport properties of the agent, each organ is characterized by the process that may be limiting the transport. For example, if the rate of exchange of an agent across the vascular and cellular wall is rapid compared to the delivery of the drug to the organ via blood flow, then the organ may be considered as "flow-limited" for that particular drug. In such a case, we need not write mass balances for each of the three subcompartments. Instead, one equation can describe the uptake by that organ. Of course, when the vascular or cellular membrane are significant barriers, two equations are needed for such a "membrane-limited" case. Bischoff and Dedrick (1970) developed a criteria for classifying organs based on the values of dimensionless groups that are ratios of various transport rates. This way, we can reduce the numbers of equations to be solved simultaneously and the number of parameters that have to be specified. Of course, these assumptions must be reexamined as more data become available and our knowledge of the drug transport increases.

Until the mid-1980s, the application of physiologically based models was limited primarily to low molecular-weight agents (for a review, see Jain, 1984). With the advent of monoclonal antibodies and other macromolecules made by genetic engineering, this approach has now been applied to antibodies and their fragments (Covell *et al.*, 1986; Baxter *et al.*, 1994a). Instead of an exhaustive review of all agents studied to date, results for a low molecular-weight anticancer agent (methotrexate) and for macromolecules (antibodies) will be summarized to illustrate the use of this approach.

Distribution of methotrexate in various tissues and animal tumors for various doses and modes of injection has been experimentally obtained and modeled (Jain, 1984). Dedrick and co-workers have analyzed the time-dependent uptake of methotrexate in mice bearing Lewis lung carcinoma (Zaharko *et al.*, 1974) and spontaneous canine lymphosarcoma (Straw *et al.*, 1974; Lutz *et al.*, 1975). They reported maximum facilitated transport rates (V_{max}) ranging from 0.002 to 0.004 μg/mL and a Michaelis constant (K_m) equal to 0.2 μg/mL. They also quantified the extracellular methotrexate loosely bound to proteins or cell membranes. Yang *et al.* (1979) reported on methotrexate transport into the Lewis lung tumor in mice and found a permeability parameter (V_{max}/K_m) of about 0.01 min^{-1}, which is compared to 0.03 min^{-1} for the small intestine. They used this finding to account partially for the resistance of the Lewis lung tumor to methotrexate and for the relative toxicity to the small intestine. Such work focusing on the drug transport differences between resistant tumors and normal sensitive tissues is needed.

Jain *et al.* (1979b) studied the transport of methotrexate into Walker carcinoma 256 and hepatoma 5123 in rats after a pulse injection and continuous infusion of the drug. Transport in hepatoma 5123 was found to be flow-limited, and transport in Walker carcinoma 256 was found to be tissue-limited. Relative uptake by the tumors was reported to be almost eight-fold more with low as compared to higher doses.

Covell *et al.* (1986) were the first to develop a physiologically based pharmacokinetic model to describe the distribution of a nonspecific monoclonal antibody and its fragments (MW ~ 150,000; ~ 100,000; ~ 50,000, respectively) in mice. In addition to not incorporating a tumor or specific binding, a major limitation of their model was the use of the Patlak equation for the transcapillary solute flux, which is essentially a single-pore model (Patlak *et al.*, 1963). The one-pore model, while satisfactory for small solutes, requires physiologically unrealistic high values of permeability, lymph flow rate, and nonspecific binding (Baxter *et al.*, 1994a). Other investigators have treated the extravasation of macromolecules as a unidirectional process (Sung *et al.*, 1990, looked at the role of plasma kinetics, vascular permeability and extravascular binding on uptake of immunotoxins). In this case the solute escapes from the vascular space by convection, but may not return. Instead it is reabsorbed by nearby lymphatics. The lymphatic system is important for the return of fluid and proteins from the tissue spaces back to the bloodstream. Physiologically, not all fluid escaping from blood vessels becomes lymph. There may be recirculation of fluid caused by filtration from large pores and absorption via small pores, or from the arterial to venous ends of capillaries. This recirculation of fluid (and hence solute efflux by convection) may occur even under isogravimetric conditions (no *net* filtration). The two-pore model proposed by Rippe and Haraldsson (1987) for transcapillary exchange was used in our model to account for this recirculation. The reason for this recirculation is the difference in the osmotic pressure driving forces between large and small pores. Across both the large and small pores there exist two modes for extravasation of antibodies (active transport and vesicular transport notwithstanding): diffusion, with a flux proportional to the permeability–surface area product and the concentration difference; and convection, in which the fluid to be absorbed by the lymphatics carries along solute material. For the tumor compartment, although there is no functional lymphatic system, fluid is able to ooze from the tumor periphery, where it may be collected by lymphatic vessels in surrounding normal tissue. Figure 10 shows the comparison between our model and data for IgG distribution in plasma, tumor, bone, kidney, liver, lung, muscle, skin, heart, spleen, and GI tract of mice. Similar agreements between the model and data were obtained for the antibody fragments, and a nonspecific antibody using as few adjustable parameters as possible (Baxter *et al.*, 1994a). Sensitivity analysis showed that the lymph flow rate and transvascular fluid recirculation rates are important determinants of the antibody uptake, while specific binding is the key parameter for their retention.

An important conclusion of our transport studies in tumors (see the following section on the distributed parameter model) is that an ideal antibody should have a high specificity and low molecular weight. To this end, recent developments in recombinant DNA technology have already yielded smaller antibody fragments (e.g., single-chain antibody, antibody binding site, molecular recognition unit). In addition, two other approaches seem to satisfy the requirement of low molecular weight with increased specificity: the use of low molecular-weight chelates with bifunctional antibodies (BFA), and the use of low molecular-weight prodrug with enzyme-conjugated antibodies (ECA) (Yuan *et al.*, 1991; Baxter *et al.*, 1992). In these two-step approaches, BFA (or ECA) is injected into a patient, permitted to bind to antigenic sites in the tumor, and then cleared from the normal tissues. At an appropriate time later, a radionuclide attached to a low molecular-weight chelate (or a prodrug) is injected into the patient with the advantage of rapid delivery to the tumor and clearance from the body. The optimization of these two-step approaches may be facilitated by physiologically based pharmacokinetics. Such a model must consider transport of both large and small molecules simultaneously. To this end we have measured the biodistribution of BFA and a radiolabeled hapten in mice, and have developed a physiologically based model to describe these data (Baxter *et al.*, 1994a). We have used these models to scale up biodistributions to humans (Baxter *et al.*, 1994b; *cf*. Scale-up) and to calculate radiation dose delivered to normal and tumor tissues (Zhu *et al.*, 1994a, b). Similar models are now needed for other molecules made using genetic engineering to optimize their dose and schedule.

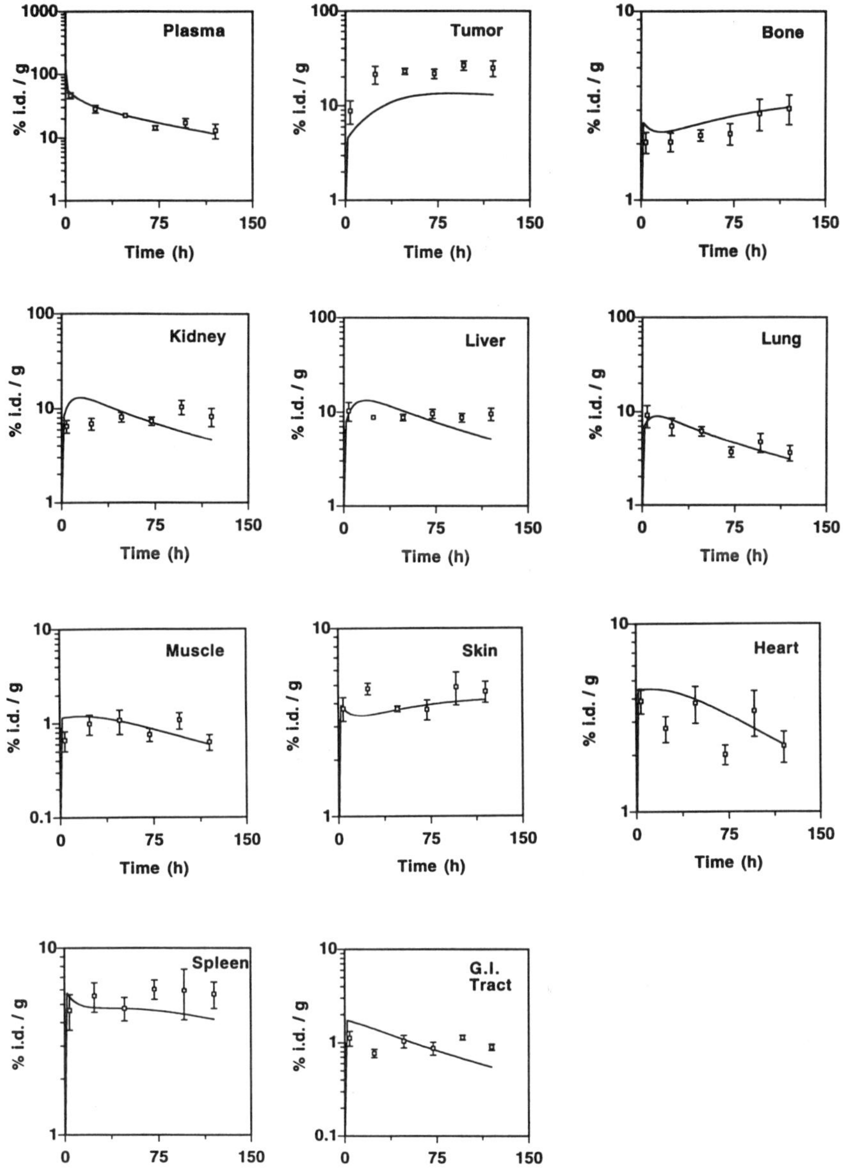

FIG. 10. Experimental data and model simulations for specific IgG_1 ZCE025 (10.9 μg, i.v.) distribution in plasma, bone, heart, kidney, liver, lung, muscle, skin, spleen, tumor, and GI tract in nude mice (reproduced with permission from Baxter *et al.*, 1994a). Similar agreement between model simulations and data was obtained for a nonspecific antibody and fragments of the specific antibody (Baxter *et al.*, 1994a).

2. Distributed Parameter Models

August Krogh's paper (1919) introducing the single-capillary model has been the basis of most distributed parameter analysis of transport in tissues. The basic functional unit of the Krogh model is a uniform cylindrical capillary surrounded by an isotropic tissue. A capillary bed can be viewed as an ensemble of Krogh cylinders interconnected with one another. Isolated Krogh cylinder analysis has been used to gain insight into the transport of nutrients (e.g., Tannock, 1970), antibodies alone (Fujimori *et al.*, 1989; Baxter and Jain, 1991b), and antibodies in combination with haptens or prodrugs (Baxter *et al.*, 1992, 1994a, b). These models have provided useful information regarding the parameters that control the microscopic profiles of various agents around individual blood vessels. Conversely, the experimentally measured concentration profiles in conjunction with these models have been used to estimate transport coefficients for tumor vessels and interstitium (Nugent and Jain, 1984a, b; Gerlowski and Jain, 1985, 1986; Clauss and Jain, 1990; Yuan *et al.*, 1993, 1994; Chary and Jain, 1987, 1989; Berk *et al.*, 1993).

Although useful, the simple Krogh cylinder model has two key limitations: It ignores the interaction among neighboring vessels, and more importantly, it cannot be used to provide three-dimensional concentration profiles in a tissue. Secomb *et al.* (1993) have addressed the first problem by using a Green's function based method to simulate pO_2 profiles in tumor vascular network. They used experimentally measured values for vessel diameter, length and branching patterns, and blood flow rates in individual vessels and compared calculated pO_2 values with their measured tissue pO_2 values. The value of oxygen consumption thus calculated was in the range reported for various tumors. Lack of vascular morphometry data and the tremendous computer time required currently preclude the application of such an approach to three-dimensional tumors.

For three-dimensional (spherical) tumors, most investigators have considered tumors to be avascular and have used models developed for spheroids (e.g., McFadden and Kwok, 1988; Van Osdol *et al.*, 1993). Theoretically, these models are analogous to the Krogh cylinder model, except for the boundary conditions and the use of spherical instead of radial coordinates. Therefore, they do not provide significant insights into the role of vasculature and transvascular flux.

Jain and Wei (1977) developed a distributed parameter model for the distribution of small solutes (methotrexate and sulfur mustard) in vascularized tumors. The model included regional variations in vascular volume, surface area, and perfusion, and described the radial distribution of methotrexate and sulfur mustard as a function of time. The model showed that the "necrotic region" of a tumor, hard to penetrate for a blood-borne drug, can serve as a reservoir for later release of drug when it has been washed from the tumor periphery. Flessner *et al.* (1992) looked at tissue concentration profiles both experimentally and mathematically for the bidirectional peritoneal transport of immunoglobulins in rats. The role of physiological pharmacokinetics on membrane transport was also investigated by Dedrick *et al.* (1978) and Lutz *et al.* (1980).

Nakagawa *et al.* (1987) developed a distributed parameter model for macromolecular transport in a brain tumor and surrounding tissue, but they did not consider the high interstitial pressure and the resulting nonuniform filtration of fluid from vessels. To this end, we developed a general theoretical framework for transvascular exchange and extravascular transport of fluid and macromolecules in tumors (Jain and Baxter, 1988). The model was first applied to a homogeneous, lymphatic tumor, with no extravascular binding (Baxter and Jain, 1989). For nonbinding molecules, the interstitial pressure was found to be a major contributing factor to the heterogeneous distribution of macromolecules within solid tumors. A steep pressure gradient was predicted at the periphery of the tumor, and verified by experiments (Boucher *et al.*, 1990; Boucher and Jain, 1992) (Fig. 6). The second paper in this series looked at the role of heterogeneous perfusion and lymphatics on the interstitial pressure distribution and concentration profiles of nonbinding macromolecules (Baxter and Jain, 1990). The third paper examined the role of specific binding and metabolism in macromolecular uptake and distribution (Baxter and Jain, 1991a). In this investigation the interstitial concentration profiles for IgG and its fragment, F(ab), were modeled with a convective-diffusion equation which includes extravascular binding and metabolism as well as transvascular exchange. The effects of molecular weight, binding affinity, antigen density, initial dose, plasma clearance, vascular permeability, metabolism, and necrosis were considered. An expression for optimal affinity was derived. The main conclusion was that an antibody with the highest possible binding affinity should be used except when (i) there are significant necrotic regions; (ii) the diffusive vascular permeability is very small; and (iii) a uniform concentration is required on a microscopic scale. The highest concentrations are achieved by continuous intravenous infusion, but the specificity ratio is highest for bolus injections. Antibody metabolism reduces both the total concentration and the specificity ratio, especially at later times. Additionally, specific binding reduces the amount of material sequestered in a necrotic core. Our model was compared with three previous models for antibody binding found in the literature. Unlike earlier models, this model combined nonuniform filtration, binding, and interstitial transport to determine macroscopic concentration profiles. In addition to supporting previous conclusions, our model offered some new strategies for therapy using two-step approaches. We are currently extending the model to two-step approaches.

C. Scale-up

Besides analyzing and integrating fundamental transport processes, the ultimate goal of the mathematical models is to improve detection and treatment in the clinic. In a typical clinical situation, only plasma and urine data are available. By no means could the precise uptake of a diagnostic or therapeutic agent by normal and neoplastic tissues be specifically inferred from the plasma data. The physiologically based pharmacokinetic models have been useful in scaling up the concentration levels of several low molecular-weight drugs from small animals (e.g., mice, rats) to humans (Dedrick, 1973). We have recently carried out such a scale-up for monoclonal antibodies in one-step and two-step approaches (Baxter *et al.*, 1994a, b; Zhu *et al.*, 1994a, b).

Prediction of drug uptake in humans requires specification of various physiological, biochemical, thermodynamic, and transport parameters. While the values of these parameters are available or can be measured for rodents, the data on human tissues are absent or limited. Intra- and inter-tumor variability adds another dimension to this complex problem of prediction for human tumors. In the scale-up studies done so far, wherever possible, investigators have used the human parameter values. When such values are not available, organ volumes are scaled up proportionally to body weight or other allometric relationships, while the rate processes (e.g., blood flow rate, transport coefficients) are scaled up as body weight to the three-fourth power (Dedrick, 1973; Pierson *et al.*, 1978; Jain *et al.*, 1981; Schmidt-Nielsen, 1990). Despite such simplifications, these models have provided an order of magnitude estimate of drug uptake by various human tissues. Continued success in this area is contingent upon further efforts of this nature to test and verify these models as more clinical data become available. Given the increasing financial constraints and ethical issues associated with human trials, the mathematical models described earlier can provide the pharmacokinetic rationale for the dose and route of administration of a new anticancer agent.

D. Summary and Recommendations

In this section, we have discussed the previous work of engineers and physical scientists, biologists, and clinicians on the characterization of mass transfer in tumors and normal tissues, and its application to cancer detection and treatment. Several important and not well understood problems have been pointed out at various places in the text in the hope of stimulating interest in this multidisciplinary area of research. Several areas that deserve further attention are listed here.

1. The strength of a model depends on the underlying assumptions and parameter values. The need for understanding fundamental physiological phenomena that govern transport, and for measuring the transport parameters for various agents, remains crucial.

2. *In vivo* microscopy of various microcirculatory preparations provides detailed information on mass transfer at the capillary level. Imaging methods such as PET, NMR, and CAT provide information on the organ level. Future experimental and modeling efforts need to bridge the gap between microscopic and macroscopic approaches.

3. There have been limited efforts in the past to combine cell-kill kinetics with drug concentration to stimulate tumor growth or regression in response to a given dose and schedule of an agent. Such an integrated approach can provide a quantitative basis for deciding clinically useful dose and schedule. Such models need to incorporate inherent and acquired drug resistance, and cell death by apoptosis and necrosis.

4. While the focus of modeling efforts to date has been on conventional agents, the approaches discussed here are equally useful for gene therapy, cellular therapy, etc. The need for measuring parameters for various genetically engineered molecules, cells, and particles and for quantifying their delivery is urgent to realize the fruits of molecular medicine. Mathematical models for cell delivery need to include details of cell adhesion and deformability.

VI. Heat Transfer in Tumors

The principal objective of this section is to present various theoretical frameworks which can be used to estimate heat transfer from an external or internal source to a tissue, and to predict resulting temperature distributions in the normal and neoplastic tissues of various mammals during normothermia and hyperthermia. Although not studied as extensively as mass transfer, this information is important for improving tumor detection by thermography and in designing heating protocols for hyperthermia treatment. Whereas the response of the normal and neoplastic tissues to thermal stress depends upon the absolute temperature obtained, the duration of that temperature, and the treatment history, there are many physical, physiological, biochemical, and immunological factors which must be considered in evaluating the effectiveness of hyperthermia in cancer treatment. Since these factors have been discussed in depth elsewhere (Jain, 1984, 1985a; Ward and Jain, 1988; Matsuda, 1992), this presentation will focus on the measurement and analysis of heat transfer and temperature distribution. Heat transfer in tissues has also been studied in the context of cryosurgery and laser surgery (Diller, 1992).

There are four major problems in analyzing heat transfer in normal and neoplastic tissues during hyperthermia:

1. The exact description of convective heat transfer in tissues is mathematically intractable. In most cases, therefore, a simplified scalar term is used to describe the heat dissipation by blood.
2. Actual geometries of tumors and normal tissues are usually unknown and/or complex. While finite element techniques can be used to solve the system equations for irregular geometries, most investigators have obtained numerical and analytical solutions for "simple" geometries.
3. The physiological parameters (i.e., blood flow and metabolic heat generation) and biophysical parameters (i.e., thermal, electrical, and acoustic properties) are not available for most tissues. In addition, these parameters vary during the course of the treatment.
4. Analytical expressions for the thermal energy absorbed in a tissue due to microwave, radiofrequency, and ultrasonic fields are not available for realistic geometries. Therefore, prediction of temperatures in the presence of these fields involves numerical solution of two problems—energy absorption and dissipation—each being complex by itself.

In light of these problems, two approaches have been used by investigators in this area of research: lumped and distributed parameter approaches. In this review, we will discuss both approaches. Wherever possible, relevant problems in the prediction of temperature distribution will be identified. Finally, some directions for future research in heat-transfer–related areas will be pointed out.

A. Lumped Parameter Approach

While the distributed parameter approach provides the detailed temporal and spatial distribution of temperature in a tissue, the solution of system equations is often tedious and requires precise knowledge of the tissue geometry, anisotropy, and orientation with respect to the surrounding tissues or heat source. Lumped parameter models overcome these problems at the cost of detailed information which may not be needed in some cases of interest. In what follows, we will discuss various lumped parameter models in brief, and describe various heat transfer mechanisms that would be incorporated in such models.

1. Compartmental Approach

In general, lumped parameter models describing the mammalian thermal system have focused on either specific organs or the whole body (for review, see Volpe and Jain, 1982, 1983). We will first discuss the whole-body model developed by Huckaba and co-workers, and then our model for a tumor-bearing host (Jain, 1985b).

The whole-body lumped parameter model of Huckaba and co-workers is based on the distributed parameter models developed by Stolwijk, Hardy, and Wissler. In this model, the body is divided into one spherical and 10 cylindrical segments: head, neck, upper trunk, lower trunk, upper arms, forearms, hands, fingers, thighs, legs and feet. In the case of extremities (e.g., forearms and legs), single cylinders are used to represent corresponding pairs or segments together. Note that this symmetry assumption does not work for the tumor-bearing organs.

Each segment is further divided into four subsection: skin, fat, muscle and core. Unlike the distributed parameter model, each subsection is assumed to have spatially uniform temperature, which is given by an unsteady-state energy-balance equation:

$$\begin{array}{c}\text{Net accumulation of thermal}\\ \text{energy in each section}\end{array} = \begin{array}{l}[\text{Metabolic heat production}]\\ +[\text{Net heat gained by conduction}\\ \quad \text{from interacting subsection(s)}]\\ -[\text{Net heat lost to the environment}].\end{array}$$

In addition to the transient energy balance equation for each of the 44 subsections, the following balance is written for the central blood pool:

$$\begin{array}{c}\text{Net accumulation of thermal}\\ \text{energy in blood pool}\end{array} = \begin{array}{l}[\text{Energy brought in with the venous blood}]\\ -[\text{Energy carried away with the arterial blood}].\end{array}$$

These 45 equations, after substituting appropriate parameter values, are solved numerically to obtain transient temperature distributions in humans during hypo- and hyperthermia (Huckaba and Tam, 1980; Volpe and Jain, 1982, 1983).

In our analysis, a mammalian species is considered to be composed of a tumor and of normal tissues, represented by compartments interconnected in an anatomical fashion. Because of our focus on interaction between the tumor and the surrounding tissues, we lump all the normal tissues, except those next to the tumor, into a single compartment. For example, for a rat carrying a subcutaneous tumor, the model consists of the following seven compartments: the tumor, the surrounding normal tissue, the body (which represents the remaining normal tissues), the skin directly above the tumor, the skin above the surrounding normal tissue, the rest of the skin, and the central blood pool. For predictions of intra-tumor temperature distributions, it is necessary to subdivide the neoplastic tissue and the skin above it into N equal compartments, where N is determined by the spatial resolution and precision desired in the computed temperature field. While dividing compartments further in this model increases the spatial resolution, its advantages are offset by the greater number of parameters to be specified. In the limit of an infinite number of subcompartments, this model is equivalent to a distributed parameter model. The detailed schematic diagrams of various versions of our models are given elsewhere for the rat, rabbit, swine, dog, baboon, and humans (Jain, 1980; Sien and Jain, 1979; Chrysanthopoulos and Jain, 1980; Volpe and Jain, 1982, 1983).

Once the number of compartments has been specified, the analysis consists of applying unsteady-state energy balance equations to each compartment. Upon substitution of suitable numerical values for the various parameters and heat flux terms, the set of coupled, nonlinear ordinary differential equations is solved numerically.

2. *Heat Transfer Mechanisms*

Under normal physiological conditions, the following heat transfer terms should be incorporated in a lumped or distributed parameter model: metabolic heat generation; conduction and convection within the body; heat exchange with the environment by radiation, conduction and convection; heat loss from the skin by evaporation of sweat and water diffused across the skin; and respiratory heat loss. Expressions for each of these terms, along with the parameter values, are given elsewhere (Cooney, 1976).

During hyperthermia, terms representing the heat input to a specific tissue or whole body must be added to the proper system equation(s). For example, during whole-body or local hyperthermia induced by radiofrequency currents, microwaves, or ultrasound, a heat-generation term is added to the section of the body being heated. During hyperthermia with blood perfusion, the afferent blood temperature is set at a desired value, and the efferent blood is circulated to the central blood pool, or to the extracorporeal device used for heating the blood. Suitable numerical values for the various parameters involved in these heat flux terms are given elsewhere (Sien and Jain, 1979, 1980; Chrysanthopoulos and Jain, 1980; Volpe and Jain, 1982, 1983).

It remains to comment upon the incorporation of thermoregulation in normal and neoplastic tissues in such a model. The first reaction of an animal exposed to high ambient temperature is to increase the blood flow to the skin, which in turn increases the heat flux from the skin to the surroundings. This type of physical thermoregulation is effective only when the skin temperature is higher than the ambient temperature; when the ambient temperature is higher than the body temperature, more drastic means of cooling are needed. Animals such as the rat, rabbit, dog, and swine increase their evaporative cooling by panting. Shallow breathing occurs, which increases the ventilation rate in the upper parts of the respiratory system only and which provides the desirable increase in evaporation. Perspiration, which is a major heat loss modality in human systems, does not constitute a significant cooling mechanism in these animals (Altman and Ditmer, 1954; Shitzer and Eberhart, 1985; Schmidt-Nielsen, 1990).

There are two ways in which thermoregulation can be included in such a model: feedforward and feedback controls (Huckaba and Tam, 1980). While the latter model is more sophisticated and realistic, several investigators have used the former approach in their analyses because of its simplicity and because of our lack of understanding of the physiological feedback control system. In panting animals, thermoregulation is introduced by an increase in the respiration rate as a function of temperature and time. Similar increases are incorporated in the blood flow rates and the metabolic heat generation rates of various organs, as reported in the literature.

Unlike normal tissues, the physiological response of tumors is poorly understood. With our current understanding of tumor thermoregulation, the following points must be borne in mind while modeling tumor thermal behavior at elevated temperatures.

1. In the absence of any tumor data, the following assumption may be used in developing a mathematical model; most transplanted tumors show a moderate increase in their blood supply up to 40–41°C, and then their supply may be impaired. In normal tissues, the blood flow may increase up to 46°C, and then may decrease at higher temperatures and/or longer duration of heating. The thermal response of human tumors appears to be closer to normal tissues.

2. Each tumor is different, and therefore mathematical generalizations about tumors are hard to make. In addition to the differences among

tumors, heterogeneities within a tumor make the situation more complex for modeling purposes.

B. Distributed Parameter Approach

The temperature field in a tissue is determined by heat conduction and convection, metabolic heat generation, thermal energy transferred to the tissue from an external source or the surrounding tissue, and the tissue geometry. Thermal conduction is characterized by a thermal conductivity, k, at steady state and by a thermal diffusivity, α, in transient state. Thermal convection is characterized by the topology of the vascular bed and the blood flow rate, which is subject to the thermal regulation.

1. The Bio-heat Transfer Equation

The most common representation of the spatial and temporal distribution of temperature in living systems is the so-called "bio-heat transfer" equation (BHTE). It was first suggested by Pennes (1948) in the following form:

$$\rho C \frac{\delta T}{\delta t} = \nabla \cdot (k \nabla T) + Q_{\mathrm{b}} + Q_{\mathrm{m}}.$$

Here, T is the tissue temperature, C is the tissue heat capacity, ρ is the tissue density, k is the tissue thermal conductivity, Q_{m} is the rate of metabolic heat generation, and Q_{b} is the rate of heat exchange with blood. Q_{m} is generally small and is calculated from the oxygen consumption of the tissue (Jain, 1984). The estimation of Q_{b} is discussed next.

Within the vasculature of a tissue, blood flows in all directions, and the local direction of convection depends on the vascular morphology of the tissue. The situation is even more complex in tumors where the direction and magnitude of blood flow are not fixed. In tumors, blood flow is temporally and spatially inhomogeneous. Therefore, the local description of convective heat transfer term, Q_{b}, in tissues would include a time-dependent velocity vector—a problem which is enormously complex and has thus far proven mathematically intractable. In order to circumvent a mathematical description of the details and complexities of the microcirculation in a capillary bed, primarily two approaches have been taken by investigators in this area of research (Charny, 1992).

In the first approach, the convection term is replaced by a "diffusion type" of term, and the heat transfer in tissues is described in terms of an effective thermal conductivity (k_{eff}):

$$\rho C \frac{\delta T}{\delta t} = \nabla \cdot (k_{\text{eff}} \nabla T) + Q_{\text{m}}.$$

Implicit in this equation is the assumption that because of a large vascular surface area, the blood temperature equilibrates with the tissue temperature. The concept of effective thermal conductivity has been used by several investigators in thermal physiology (Shitzer and Eberhart, 1985). Jain and Wei (1977) also used this concept to describe the drug distribution in tumors.

In the second approach, the convective heat transfer term, Q_{b}, is replaced by the thermal energy brought in by the arterial blood minus the thermal energy carried away with the venous blood:

$$Q_{\text{b}} = \eta P \rho_{\text{b}} C_{\text{b}} (T_{\text{a}} - T_{\text{V}}).$$

Here, ρ_{b} is the blood density, C_{b} is the blood heat capacity, T_{a} and T_{V} are the arterial and venous blood temperatures, and η is a measure of the effectiveness of heat transfer between the tissue and venous blood ($0 \leq \eta \leq 1$); η is equal to 1 when venous blood is in complete equilibrium with tissue ($T_{\text{V}} = T$). It is reasonable to expect that because of slow blood flow, η will be close to 1. Although it is possible to introduce a value of η different from 1, it introduces no new insight and changes the numerical value of the blood flow rate slightly.

The bio-heat transfer equation with both of these assumptions has been solved for various tissue geometries and initial and boundary conditions (Shitzer and Eberhart, 1985). Because of scalar treatment of the convective heat transport by blood, the use of the bio-heat transfer equation has been questioned repeatedly (Charny, 1992). Considering tissue as porous media, Wulff (1974, 1980) introduced the blood velocity vector $\overline{u}_{\text{b}}$, in the bio-heat transfer equation. Unfortunately, the complex nature of the system defies any attempt to specify the circulation vector at the microscopic level. As non-invasive technologies (e.g., MRI) provide improved spatial resolution, it may be possible to incorporate such data numerically (Dutton *et al.*, 1992).

A second criticism of the bio-heat transfer equation originates from the fact that it does not account for the countercurrent heat exchange in the capillary bed. Assuming that the velocity vector is one-dimensional, Mitchell and Myers (1968), and later, Keller and Seiler (1971), analyzed the countercurrent heat transfer in tissues. While the model of Keller and Seiler attempts to account for the continuous change in temperature of the arterial and venous networks as one moves from the body core to the skin, the model does not account for the heterogeneous structure of the vascular network or the continuous variations between the arterial and venous temperature in the tissue. To this end, Weinbaum and co-workers (Weinbaum *et al.*, 1984; Jiji *et al.*, 1984; Weinbaum and Jiji, 1985; Charny, 1992) proposed a two-phase model which provides the temperature distribution along the arterial and venous networks, as well as the temperature variation in the extravascular space as a function of the distribution of the collateral circulation and a simple vessel branching law. While their model is elegant conceptually, it is impractical for most tissues where the vascular morphology is much more complex, and the velocity vector changes its magnitude and direction randomly.

Klinger (1974, 1980) used the Green's function to obtain an exact analytical solution of the diffusion equation with convection terms without making any special assumptions concerning the velocity field. The absence of a detailed knowledge of the convection field makes this approach of limited use as well.

Chen and Holmes (1980) showed that in addition to the blood perfusion term, the blood flow in the microvasculature may have at least two contributions to heat transfer: a contribution proportional to the local blood flow velocity vector $\overline{u_b}$, and a contribution proportional to the temperature gradient similar to the effective thermal conduction term. They also suggest that in some circumstances, these two additional contributions may be negligible compared to the perfusion term.

Recently, Baish (1994) has developed a model for heat transfer which predicts a probability density function for the tissue temperature, as opposed to a local average. The model includes information on the most probable temperature at a given point, as well as its uncertainty due to the proximity of thermally significant vessels (Chen and Holmes, 1980; Chato, 1980; Weinbaum *et al.*, 1984; Baish *et al.*, 1986). The model is based on the use of an algorithm for tumor and vascular growth to generate a sample network of thermally significant vessels (Baish, 1994). The heat conduction equation is then solved in the resulting interstitial space, with statistical sampling of the solution to generate the probability density function for temperature.

While these various improvements in the bio-heat transfer equation provide new insight into the heat transfer process in the microvascular bed, mathematical complexity in describing the microcirculation and vascular topology makes their application to normal and neoplastic tissues nearly impossible. Therefore, most investigators use the bio-heat transfer equation of Pennes to describe heat transfer and temperature distribution in tissues.

2. *Tissue Geometry*

Once all the model parameter values are specified, the geometry of the model system must be defined. Depending upon the information desired, either a particular organ (or tissue region) or the whole mammalian body may be considered as the region in which the bio-heat transfer equation must be solved. Both of these approaches have been discussed in depth elsewhere (Shitzer and Eberhart, 1985) for application in the normal tissues; therefore, we will focus our attention on tumors.

The situation for tumors is more complex. It is known that a tumor may infiltrate the surrounding tissue in a complex geometrical fashion. However, for simple geometries (i.e., cylinder, sphere), it is possible to obtain analytical solutions. For more complex geometries, finite difference or finite element methods are necessary to calculate the temperature field in the tumor and the surrounding normal tissues.

3. *Boundary Conditions*

In order to solve the BHTE for a given geometry, the following boundary conditions must be specified. Within the tissue region or an organ, heat flux and temperature at various interfaces must be continuous. If the tissue or organ containing the tumor is exposed to the ambient, heat exchange with the external environment by conduction, convection, radiation, and evaporation must be accounted for.

Heat source terms must be added either in the bio-heat equation or the boundary conditions, depending upon the method used for inducing hyperthermia. During surface heating by hot air or water or molten wax bath, heat transfer by conduction and convection to the overlaying skin must be added to the boundary condition. During infrared or visible radiation–induced heating, a radiation term must be added to the skin boundary condition. During hyperthermic perfusion, the arterial temperature T_a must be set equal to the experimentally set afferent blood temperature in the BHTE. During volume heating by ultrasound, microwaves, or radiofrequency currents, an additional term describing temporal and spatial distribution of absorbed energy must be added to the right-hand side of the BHTE (Jain, 1985a).

C. Temperature Distribution during Normothermia

The proper knowledge of temperature distribution during normothermia may be useful for improving thermography for cancer detection (Jain and Gullino, 1980; Jain, 1985a).

If the tumor were considered infinite and system parameters were constant, the temperature of the tumor, T, would equal the arterial blood temperature, T_a, plus the temperature rise due to metabolic heat generation, T_m:$T = T_a + T_m$, where $T_m = Q_m/(\rho_b C_p P)$. It is of interest to note that T_m is less than 0.25°C and does not change significantly with tumor weight (Sien and Jain, 1979).

For tumors of finite radii, which interact thermally with the surroundings at temperature T_s, the calculated profiles depend on tumor size. The results indicate that the temperature throughout a small tumor is lower than that in large tumors for a fixed, uniform blood flow rate. This result is not surprising if one realizes that the temperature profile is determined by both the total metabolic heat generation rate (which is proportional to tumor volume) and heat loss (which is proportional to the outer surface area). Consequently, for a fixed P, Q_m, and T_s, a higher total heat generation rate per unit surface area in large tumors leads to a higher temperature in large tumors when compared to small ones (Jain, 1978).

Figure 11 shows the temperature distribution in a human breast tumor measured by Gautherie and co-workers (1972). These data suggest that the temperature is maximum in the center of these tumors and is in qualitative

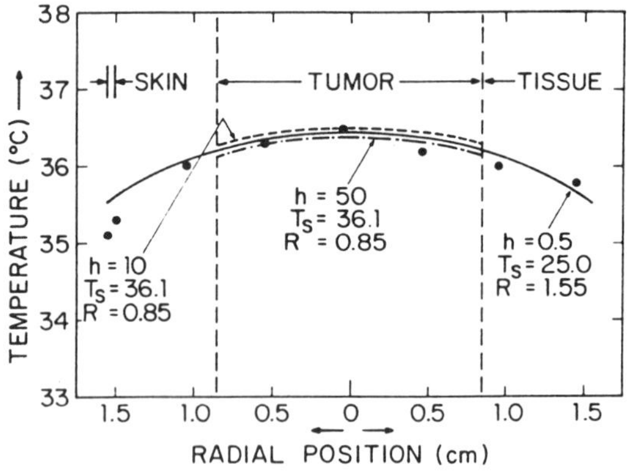

Fig. 11. Comparison of model predictions with the data on temperature distribution in the breast cancer and the surrounding tissue in a woman. Solid line refers to the first approach, and dotted lines refer to the second approach discussed in the text. Note that two different dotted lines represent different values of the heat transfer coefficients (h). T_S refers to the surface temperature, and R refers to the tissue radius. (Adapted from Jain, 1979.)

agreement with our analysis (Jain, 1978). For a quantitative comparison, some additional assumptions must be made about the thermal symmetry of the system. In reality, the tumor is located between the skin exposed to the ambient air at 25°C, and the chest at 36–37°C. Hence, the temperature of surroundings, T_s, is not uniform. However, it is possible to set bounds on the temperature distributions in the tumor by considering two limiting cases: (i) the tumor and the surrounding tissue can be considered a sphere of radius $R = 1.55$ cm, exposed to ambient air temperature (25°C), or (ii) the tumor alone ($R = 0.85$ cm) is surrounded by a tissue at 36.1°C. The results of computation using these two approaches are compared with data in Fig. 11.

Nonuniformities in the perfusion rate have interesting effects on the temperature profile. Because of its large blood flow rate and higher rate of metabolism, the temperature in the periphery of a necrotic tumor is higher than that in a tumor which has a uniform blood flow rate, although both tumors have the same average perfusion rate. Inhomogeneities in blood flow rate, therefore, tend to make the temperature profile flat (Jain, 1978). Future efforts should be directed towards improving this analysis by considering thermal asymmetry of tumors.

D. Temperature Distribution during Hyperthermia

Currently available "physical" methods of producing hyperthermia can be divided into two categories: surface heating and volume heating. In surface heating, the temperature is increased using one or more of the following methods: immersion in hot water bath or hot air incubator, exposure to visible or infrared radiation, or direct contact with an interface at a higher temperature. Heat transfer, then, takes place from the skin to the underlying tissue by conduction and convection. In volume heating, the temperature of underlying tissue is brought to an elevated temperature either by perfusing the tissue with preheated blood or by exposing it to ultrasound, microwaves, or radiofrequency currents. The only "non-physical" method of inducing hyperthermia is the injection of "mixed bacterial toxins" (MBT) or some other pyrogenic agents to the host.

Depending upon the surface area or volume heated, hyperthermia can be divided into three categories: (i) local, (ii) regional, and (iii) whole-body. In local hyperthermia, tumor mass and minimum surrounding tissue are heated; in regional hyperthermia, usually the limb containing the tumor mass is heated; and in whole-body hyperthermia (WBH), the temperature of the host is elevated.

No matter which of the preceding methods is used to induce hyperthermia, it is essential to monitor the resulting temperature distributions in the normal and neoplastic tissues continually, and to control the power input and position of the heating source so that the temperatures are maintained in the desired range for optimal time. This type of control can be achieved either manually or automatically and is incorporated in most commercial or in-house-built hyperthermia systems used currently.

Since it is nearly impossible to measure detailed temperature distribution in human tumors, current efforts in this field are directed towards calculating the complete temperature profile based on a limited number of spot measurements.

E. Summary and Recommendations

The objective of this section was to present various theoretical frameworks that may be used to describe temperature distributions in normal and neoplastic tissues during hyperthermia. The emphasis in this review has been on the physical factors involved in hyperthermia. To this end, two approaches—distributed and lumped—were presented for modeling the thermal distribution between the normal and neoplastic tissues of various mammals. The theoretical considerations were summarized according to the method used for heating. Several important and not well-understood problems were pointed out in the text in the hope of stimulating interest in this multidisciplinary research.

Some heat transfer–related areas that deserve further attention, in my view, are listed here:

1. While the bio-heat transfer equation, as it stands, appears to give adequate results in several applications, a precise description of heat transfer in tissues remains a tedious but challenging problem.

2. As pointed out throughout this article, data on the thermal, electrical, and acoustic properties, intratumor blood flow rates, and metabolism of human tumors are absent or limited. These parameters should be measured over a wide range of temperatures and stages of growth and regression. Physiological studies in animals and humans are needed to understand thermoregulation during hyperthermia. This information should then be incorporated into the mathematical models of the type described in this review.

3. It is essential to provide accurate measurements of intratissue temperature distributions during normothermia and hyperthermia. New developments in the noninvasive thermometric techniques using MRI and microwave should alleviate some of these problems.

4. Analysis of heat transfer and temperature distributions during US, MW, and RF diathermy is imperative for the proper use of these techniques. Such efforts must go hand-in-hand with the development of new heating methods. The field of hyperthermia has reached a plateau in recent years because of the inability to heat human tumors adequately. Quantitative comparison of various methods of inducing hyperthermia should be made on the basis of temperatures reached in various parts of normal and neoplastic tissues. This type of analysis will help in deciding the "best" modality of heating a given tumor and will help in designing feedback control mechanisms and heating protocols for maintaining desired temperatures in normal and neoplastic tissues.

VII. Future Perspective

Spectacular progress in the molecular and cellular biology of cancer has led to the identification of genes whose activation and/or inactivation is associated with tumor growth and metastasis. These advances have also contributed to the development of various genetically engineered agents, potentially useful for cancer treatment. These agents include molecules such as monoclonal antibodies, immunotoxins, tumor necrosis factor, interferons, interleukins, antisense agents, and cells such as activated macrophages, lymphokine-activated killer cells, and tumor-infiltrating lymphocytes. Because of their potent toxicity to cancer cells in Petri dishes and in a limited number of patients, some of these agents were heralded as "magic bullets" or "breakthrough drugs." Although the potential use of these agents remains attractive, they have had, in fact, minimal impact on the most common solid tumors (for example, lung, breast, colon, rectum, prostate, brain) accounting for the majority of adult cancer-related deaths. Similarly, the conventional anticancer drugs, which have shown impressive results in the treatment of hematologic cancer (for example, leukemias and lymphomas) and pediatric cancers, have not had as much success in the treatment of common solid tumors. While advances in treatment have improved quality of life for some cancer patients, the actual incidence and mortality from cancer have continued to rise, and the cure rates have increased slowly in the past 20 years (Fig. 12). What is the reason that these conventional and novel agents, which are so effective in killing cancer cells in a Petri dish or in our bloodstream, are not able to eradicate cancer cells when these cells form a large solid tumor mass in our body? The answer to this question is not known completely. Our hypothesis is that the effectiveness of these agents is currently limited by physiological resistance and by intrinsic or acquired cellular resistance. The former

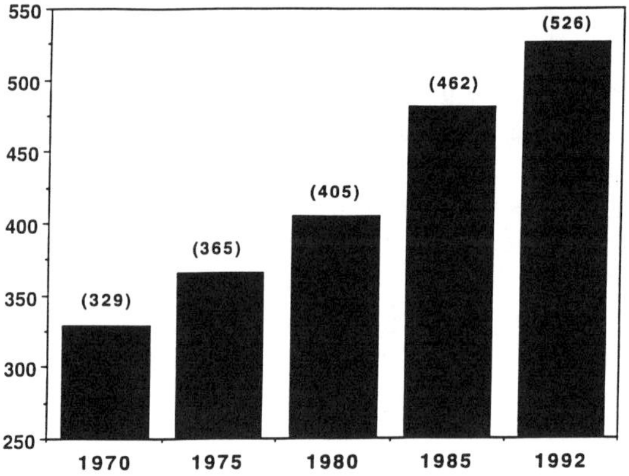

FIG. 12. Although advances in cancer treatment have improved quality of life for patients, the actual incidence and death rates in the United States from cancer have continued to increase in the past 20 years. (Source: American Cancer Society.) Our hypothesis is that the effectiveness of current treatment methods is limited by physiological resistance and by intrinsic or acquired cellular resistance. The former impedes the delivery of blood-borne agents to solid tumors, and the latter reduces their effectiveness once these agents have reached the target cells. A better understanding of transport in tumors may help develop strategies to overcome or to exploit the physiological resistance for improved cancer treatment (Jain, 1994).

impedes the delivery of blood-borne agents to solid tumors, and the latter reduces their effectiveness once these agents have reached the target cells. In this article I have discussed the problem of the physiological resistance in solid tumors from a chemical engineer's point of view.

In light of these problems in delivering anticancer therapy, what do we do to improve the situation? Early detection of cancer would continue to be helpful. In addition to improved operability at this stage, the physiological barriers may not yet exist or may be easier to overcome. With improved local control of cancer through surgery and radiation therapy, improved survival and quality of life may be achieved. Conventional and novel systemic therapies may also be more effective at this stage. Treatment of established tumors would benefit from the continued development of more selective agents. Because of their selectivity, they would either not penetrate into the normal tissue, or if they did, they would be nontoxic to normal host tissues. While agents with such exquisite sensitivity are being sought after and developed, an important approach would be to overcome or alter these transport barriers for improved delivery of available agents, or use the barriers themselves as the target of cancer therapy.

A prerequisite for reproducible and predictable modification of tumor physiology is a fundamental understanding of the parameters which govern blood flow and transport in tumors. Since there are a limited number of investigators in this area, there is a paucity of data on these basic parameters. The ability to grow transparent and tissue-isolated human tumors in immunodeficient mice and to perfuse human tumors with a single artery and a single vein, and the advances in noninvasive technologies such as nuclear magnetic resonance and positron emission tomography, should allow us and others to obtain these data for human tumors in the next decade. This should permit development of novel strategies for increasing blood flow, vascular permeability, and interstitial diffusion, and for lowering tumor pressure. For example, we have recently found that radiation therapy may lower interstitial pressure in cervical cancer in women who respond to therapy (Roh *et al.*, 1991). Furthermore, we have shown that agents such as pentoxifylline and nicotinamide, a vitamin B_3 derivative, may also lower pressure and increase tumor oxygenation (Lee *et al.*, 1992, 1994a, b). Our hope is that by lowering the pressure in tumors locally by radiation, or systemically by drugs such as nicotinamide or pentoxifylline, we may be able to deliver more therapeutic agents to solid tumors. While these data are limited, several studies in the literature which show an increased uptake of antibody in tumors after radiation support this hypothesis. Extensive studies are needed to optimize these physiological strategies prior to their use in the clinic.

Another approach would be to design drug delivery strategies that take the peculiar physiology of tumors into account. As discussed earlier, these include various two- or three-step approaches to delivering a low molecular-weight agent to the tumor so that pressure and slow interstitial diffusion are not a problem. Another approach is to use liposomes and nanoparticles that have a long half-life in blood so that they cross the leaky vessels of tumors and then release low molecular-weight agents outside the blood vessels (Langer and Vacanti, 1993; Saltzman, 1993; Yuan *et al.*, 1994). Finally, intratumor injection to increase convective movement of the agent has the potential to improve the treatment of local diseases. As our understanding of tumor physiology and transport improves, these approaches are likely to give better results.

Alternatively, if the tumor vasculature could be made the target, then the drugs would not have to cross the vessel wall or the interstitium. Anti-angiogenesis therapy, pioneered by Judah Folkman (1993), whose aim is to stop the growth of new vessels of a tumor, is a successful example of such an approach. Hyperthermia, photodynamic therapy, and cytokines such as TNF are other approaches which may also impair the tumor blood supply. One attractive hypothesis is that when several of the current cytotoxic therapies work, it is not only because they destroy cancer cells, but also because they may destroy a solid tumor by impairing its blood supply. Thus judiciously combining anti-vascular therapies with anti-cellular therapies may lead to synergistic results. Our recent study with lymphokine-activated killer cells, which shows that these cells adhere to the tumor vasculature and cause blood flow impairment, is in concert with this hypotheses (Sasaki *et al.*, 1991; Melder *et al.*, 1993). Development of monoclonal antibodies and other biologicals directed against the vascular endothelium or the subendothelial matrix of tumors should help the antivascular therapy. Since a tumor depends on both existing *and* newly formed blood vessels for survival, growth, and metastasis, these approaches seem rational. As our basic knowledge of the tumor vasculature and interstitium increases, these approaches are likely to yield promising results in clinical applications.

In summary, I have attempted to explain why various potentially useful therapeutic agents are not effective in the treatment of some common solid tumors. We have shown that there are several transport barriers that lead to compromised metabolic microenvironment in tumors (e.g., low pO_2, pH) and make it difficult to deliver a drug to all regions of a solid tumor. Since the delivery of a therapeutic agent is governed by tumor physiology, it makes sense to understand the fundamental nature of the transport barriers and to develop strategies to overcome them or to exploit them for cancer treatment. It is our hope that such research will help in realizing the clinical potential of existing and novel compounds developed in the future.

Acknowledgments

The work discussed in this review article was supported by grants from the National Science Foundation, National Cancer Institute, American Cancer Society, Guggenheim Foundation, Alexander von Humbolt Foundation, Hybritech Corporation, and the Edwin L. Steele Endowment.

I am grateful to Drs. Pietro M. Gullino and James Wei for introducing me to the field of tumor pathophysiology, and to my former and current co-workers for participating in this research. I would like to thank Drs. James Baish, Larry Baxter, David Berk, Yves Boucher, William Deen, Robert Dedrick, Marc Dellian, Paul Kristjansen, Robert Melder, Lance Munn, Paolo Netti, and Fan Yuan for many helpful comments on this manuscript; Dr. Larry Baxter for his help with the references; and Dawn Baxter, Gerry Mullowney, and Carol Lyons for help in preparing this manuscript.

This article is an update of my previous reviews published in *Advances in Transport Processes* (1984) and in the *Journal of the National Cancer Institute* (1989).

References

Aisenberg, A. C., "The Glycolysis and Respiration of Tumors." Academic Press, New York, 1961.

Algire, G. H., and Chalkley, H. W., *J. Natl. Cancer Inst.* (*U.S.*) **6**, 73 (1945).

Altman, P., and Ditmer, D., "Biology Data Book." Fed. Am. Soc. Exp. Biol., Bethesda, MD, 1954.
Astarita, G., "Mass Transfer with Chemical Reactions." Elsevier, Amsterdam, 1967.
Baish, J. W., *J. Biomech. Eng.* in press (1994).
Baish, J. W., Ayyaswamy, P. S., and Foster, K. R., *J. Biomech. Eng.* **106**, 321 (1986).
Baker, C. H., and Nastuk, W. L., "Microcirculatory Technology." Academic Press, Orlando, FL, 1986.
Baxter, L. T., and Jain, R. K., *Microvasc. Res.* **37**, 77 (1989).
Baxter, L. T., and Jain, R. K., *Microvasc. Res.* **40**, 246 (1990).
Baxter, L. T., and Jain, R. K., *Microvasc. Res.* **41**, 5 (1991a).
Baxter, L. T., and Jain, R. K., *Microvasc. Res.* **41**, 252 (1991b).
Baxter, L. T., Yuan, F., and Jain, R. K., *Cancer Res.* **52**, 5838 (1992).
Baxter, L. T., Zhu, H., Mackensen, D. G., and Jain, R. K., *Cancer Res.* **54**, 1517 (1994a).
Baxter, L. T., Zhu, H., Mackensen, D. G., Butler, W. F., and Jain, R. K., submitted for publication (1994b).
Beardsley, T., *Sci. Am.* **270**, 130 (1994).
Begg, R. W., *Adv. Cancer Res.* **5**, 1 (1961).
Berk, D., Yuan, F., Leunig, M., and Jain, R. K., *Biophys. J.* **65**, 2428 (1993).
Bischoff, K. B., and Dedrick, R. L., *J. Pharm. Sci.* **57**(8), 1346 (1968).
Bischoff, K. B., and Dedrick, R. L., *J. Theor. Biol.* **29**, 63 (1970).
Bischoff, K. B., Dedrick, R. L., and Zaharko, D. S., *J. Pharm. Sci.* **59**, 149 (1970).
Bischoff, K. B., Dedrick, R. L., Zaharko, D. S., and Longstreth, J. A., *J. Pharm. Sci.* **60**, 1128 (1971).
Bladel, van J., "Electromagnetic Fields." McGraw Hill, New York, 1964.
Boucher, Y., and Jain, R. K., *Cancer Res.* **52**, 5110 (1992).
Boucher, Y., Baxter, L. T., and Jain, R. K., *Cancer Res.* **50**, 4478 (1990).
Boucher, Y., Kirkwood, J. M., Opacic, D., DeSantis, M., and Jain, R. K., *Cancer Res.* **51**, 6691 (1991).
Burton, A. C., *Growth* **30**, 157 (1966).
Busch, W., *Verhdlgs. Naturhist. Preuss., Rhein., Westphal.* **23**, 28 (1866).
Butler, T. P., Grantham, F. H., and Gullino, P. M., *Cancer Res.* **35**, 3084 (1975).
Capecci, M. R., *Sci. Am.* **270**, 52 (1994).
Cavaliere, R., Ciocatto, E. C., Giovannela, B. C., Heidelberger, C., Johnson, R. O., Martotini, M., Mondovi, B., Moricca, G., and Rossi-Fanelli, A., *Cancer (Philadelphia)* **20**, 1351 (1967).
Chaplain, M. A. J., and Sleeman, B. D., *J. Math. Biol.* **31**, 431 (1993).
Charny, C. K., *Adv. Heat Transfer* **22**, 19 (1992).
Chary, S. R., and Jain, R. K., *Chem. Eng. Commun.* **55**, 235 (1987).
Chary, S. R., and Jain, R. K., *Proc. Natl. Acad. Sci. U.S.A.* **86**, 5385 (1989).
Chato, J., *J. Biomech. Eng.* **102**, 110 (1980).
Chen, M. M., and Holmes, K. R., *Ann. N.Y. Acad. Sci.* **335**, 137 (1980).
Chrysanthopoulos, G., and Jain, R. K., *Med. Phys.* **7**, 529 (1980).
Clauss, M. A., and Jain, R. K., *Cancer Res.* **50**, 3487 (1990).
Coley, W. B., *Am. J. Med. Sci.* **105**, 487 (1893).
Cooney, D. O., "Biomedical Engineering Principles." Dekker, New York, 1976.
Cooper, T. E., and Trezek, G. J., *Aerosp. Med.* **42**, 24 (1971).
Covell, D. G., Barbet, J., Holton, O. D., Black, C. D. V., Parker, R. J., and Weinstein, J. N., *Cancer Res.* **46**, 3969 (1986).
Deakin, A. S., *Growth* **39**, 159 (1975).
Dedrick, R. L., *J. Pharmacokinet. Biopharm.* **1**, 435 (1973).
Dedrick, R. L., *J. Natl. Cancer Inst.* **80**, 84 (1988).

Dedrick, R. L., Bischoff, K. B., and Zaharko, D. S., *Cancer Chemother. Rep.* **54**(2), 95 (1970).

Dedrick, R. L., Forrester, D. D., Cannon, J. N., El Dareer, S. M., and Mellett, L. B., *Biochem. Pharmacol.* **22**, 2405 (1973a).

Dedrick, R. L., Lutz, R. J., and Zaharko, D. S., *J. Pharm. Sci.* **62**, 882 (1973b).

Dedrick, R. L., Zaharko, D. S., Bender, R. A., Bleyer, W. A., and Lutz, R. J., *Cancer Chemother. Rep.* **59**, 795 (1975).

Dedrick, R. L., Myers, C. E., Bungay, P. M., and DeVita, V. T., Jr., *Cancer Treat. Rep.* **62**, 1 (1978).

Deen, W., *AIChE J.* **33**, 409 (1987).

DeVita, V. T., Jr., Hellman, S., and Rosenberg, S. A., eds., "CANCER: Principles and Practice of Oncology," 4th ed. Lippincott, Philadelphia, 1993.

Dickinson, R. B., McCarthy, J. B., and Tranquillo, R. T., *Ann. Biomed. Eng.* **21**, 679 (1993).

Diller, K. R., *Adv. Heat Transfer* **22**, 157 (1992).

Dudar, T. E., and Jain, R. K., *Microvasc. Res.* **25**, 1 (1983).

Dudar, T. E., and Jain, R. K., *Cancer Res.* **44**, 605 (1984).

Dutton, A. W., Darkazanli, A., Heinrich, J. C., and Roemer, R. B., *Bioelectromagnetics* **13**, 567 (1992).

Dvorak, H. F., Nagy, J. A., Dvorak, J. T., and Dvorak, A. M., *Am. J. Pathol.* **133**, 95 (1988).

Endrich, B., Intaglietta, M., Reinhold, H. S., and Gross, J. F., *Cancer Res.* **39**, 17 (1979a).

Endrich, B., Reinhold, H. S., Gross, J. F., and Intaglietta, M., *JNCI, J. Natl. Cancer Inst.* **62**, 387 (1979b).

Eskey, C. J., Koretsky, A. P., Domach, M. M., and Jain, R. K., *Cancer Res.* **52**, 6010 (1992).

Eskey, C. J., Koretsky, A. P., Domach, M. M., and Jain, R. K., *Proc. Natl. Acad. Sci. U.S.A.* **90**, 2646 (1993).

Eskey, C. J., Wolmark, N., McDowell, C. L., Domach, M. M., and Jain, R. K., *J. Natl. Cancer Inst. (U.S.)* **16**, 293 (1994).

Finkelstein, A., "Water Movement Through Lipid Bilayers, Pores, and Plasma Membranes." Wiley, New York, 1987.

Flessner, M. F., Dedrick, R. L., and Reynolds, J. C., *Am. J. Physiol.* **263**, F15 (1992).

Folkman, J., *N. Engl. J. Med.* **285**, 1182 (1971).

Folkman, J., *in* "Cancer Medicine" (J. F. Holland, ed.), pp. 153–170. Lea Febiger, Philadelphia, 1993.

Folkman, J., Long, D. M., and Becker, F. F., *Surg. Forum* **13**, 81 (1962).

Folkman, J., Long, D. M., and Becker, F. F., *Cancer (Philadelphia)* **16**, 453 (1963).

Folkman, J., Cole, P., and Zimmerman, S., *Ann. Surg.* **164**, 491 (1966).

Forbes, H. S., *Arch. Neurol. Psychiatry* **19**, 751 (1928).

Foster, K. R., and Cheever, E. A., *Bioelectromagnetics* **13**, 567 (1992).

Fujimori, K., Covell, D. G., Fletcher, J. E., and Weinstein, J. N., *Cancer Res.* **49**, 5656 (1989).

Fung, Y. C., "Biomechanics: Motion, Flow, Stress, Growth." Springer-Verlag, New York, 1990.

Gautherie, M., Bourjal, P., Quenneville, Y., and Gros, C., *Rev. Eur. Etud. Clin. Biol.* **17**, 776 (1972).

Gerlowski, L. E., and Jain, R. K., *J. Pharm. Sci.* **72**, 1103 (1983).

Gerlowski, L. E., and Jain, R. K., *Intern. J. Microchir.* **4**, 336 (1985).

Gerlowski, L. E., and Jain, R. K., *Microvasc. Res.* **31**, 288 (1986).

Gompertz, B., *Philos. Trans. R. Soc. London* 513 (1825).

Grantham, F., Hill, D., and Gullino, P. M., *J. Natl. Cancer Inst. (U.S.)* **50**, 1381 (1973).

Greenspan, H. P., *Stud. Appl. Math.* **51**, 317 (1972).

Greenspan, H. P., *Growth* **38**, 81 (1974).

Gullino, P. M., *in* "Organ Perfusion and Preservation" (J. C. Norman, J. Folkman, W. G. Hardison *et al.*, eds.), pp. 877–898. Appleton-Century-Crofts, New York, 1968.
Gullino, P. M., *in* "Methods in Cancer Research" (H. Busch, ed.), pp. 45–91. Academic Press, New York, 1970.
Gullino, P. M., *in* "Cancer" (F. F. Becker, ed.), pp. 327–354. Plenum, New York, 1975.
Gullino, P. M., *in* "Oxygen Transport to Tissue, 2" (J. Grote, D. Reneau, and G. Thews, eds.), pp. 521–536. Plenum, New York, 1976.
Gullino, P. M., and Grantham, F. H., *J. Natl. Cancer Inst. (U.S.)* **27**, 679 (1961).
Gullino, P. M., and Grantham, F. H., *Cancer Res.* **24**, 1727 (1964).
Gullino, P. M., Jain, R. K., and Grantham, F. H., *JNCI, J. Natl. Cancer Inst.* **68**, 519 (1982).
Gutmann, R., Feyh, J., Goetz, A. E., Leunig, M., Messmer, K., Kastenbauer, E., and Jain, R. K., *Cancer Res.* **52**, 1993 (1992).
Hall, E. J., "Radiobiology for the Radiologist." Lippincott, Philadelphia, 1988.
Hammer, D. A., and Apte, S. M., *Biophys. J.* **63**, 35 (1992).
Holland, J. F., Frei, E., Bast, R. C., Kufe, D. W., Morton, D. L., and Weichselbaum, R. R., eds., "Cancer Medicine," 3rd ed. Lea a Febiger, Philadelphia, 1993.
Huckaba, C. E., and Tam, H. S., *in* "Advances in Biomedical Engineering. Part 1" (D. O. Cooney, ed.). Dekker, New York, 1980.
Jain, R. K., *J. Biomech. Eng.* **100**, 235 (1978).
Jain, R. K., *J. Biomech. Eng.* **101**, 82 (1979).
Jain, R. K., *Ann. N.Y. Acad. Sci.* **335**, 48 (1980).
Jain, R. K., *Adv. Transp. Processes* **3**, 205 (1984).
Jain, R. K., *in* "Heat Transfer in Medicine and Biology" (A. Shitzer and R. Eberhart, eds.). Plenum, New York, 1985a.
Jain, R. K., *Biotechnol. Prog.* **1**, 81 (1985b).
Jain, R. K., *Cancer Metastasis Rev.* **6**, 559 (1987a).
Jain, R. K., *Cancer Res.* **47**, 3039 (1987b).
Jain, R. K., *Cancer Res.* **48**, 2641 (1988).
Jain, R. K., *J. Natl. Cancer Inst.* **81**, 570 (1989).
Jain, R. K., *in* "Drug Resistance in Oncology" (B. Teicher, ed.). Dekker, New York, 1993.
Jain, R. K., *Sci. Am.* **271**, 58 (1994).
Jain, R. K., and Baxter, L. T., *Cancer Res.* **48**, 7022 (1988).
Jain, R. K., and Gullino, P. M., *Chem. Eng. Commun.* **4**, 95 (1980).
Jain, R. K., and Ward-Hartley, K. A., *IEEE Trans. Sonics Ultrason.* **SU-31**, 504 (1984).
Jain, R. K., and Ward-Hartley, K., *Biorheology* **24**, 117 (1987).
Jain, R. K., and Wei, J., *J. Bioeng.* **1**, 313 (1977).
Jain, R. K., Grantham, F. H., and Gullino, P. M., *JNCI, J. Natl. Cancer Inst.* **62**, 927 (1979a).
Jain, R. K., Wei, J., and Gullino, P. M., *J. Pharmacokin. Biopharmac.* **7**, 181 (1979b).
Jain, R. K., Gerlowski, L., Weissbrod, J., Wang, J., and Pierson, R. N., *Ann. Biomed. Eng.* **9**, 345 (1981).
Jain, R. K., Shah, S. A., and Finney, P. L., *JNCI, J. Natl. Cancer Inst.* **73**, 429 (1984).
Jain, R. K., Stock, R. J., Chary, S. R., and Rueter, M., *Microvasc. Res.* **39**, 77 (1990).
Jiji, L. M., Weinbaum, S., and Lemons, D. E., *J. Biomed. Eng.* **106**, 331 (1984).
Kallman, R. F., ed., "Rodent Tumor Models in Experimental Cancer Therapy." Pergamon, New York, 1987.
Kaufman, E. N., and Jain, R. K., *Biophys. J.* **58**, 873 (1990).
Kaufman, E. N., and Jain, R. K., *Biophys. J.* **60**, 596 (1991).
Kaufman, E. N., and Jain, R. K., *Cancer Res.* **52**, 4157 (1992a).
Kaufman, E. N., and Jain, R. K., *J. Immunol. Methods* **155**, 1 (1992b).

Keller, K. H., and Seiler, L., *J. Appl. Physiol.* **30**, 187 (1971).
Klinger, H. G., *Bull. Math. Biol.* **36**, 403 (1974).
Klinger, H. G., *Ann. N.Y. Acad. Sci.* **335**, 133 (1980).
Kristjansen, P. E. G., Boucher, Y., and Jain, R. K., *Cancer Res.* **53**, (1993).
Kristjansen, P. E. G., Roberge, S., Lee, I., and Jain, R. K., *Microvas. Res.* (1994) (in press).
Krogh, A., *J. Physiol. (London)* **52**, 409 (1919).
Kushmerick, M. J., and Podolsky, R. J., *Science* **166**, 1297 (1969).
Langer, R., and Vacanti, J. P., *Science* **260**, 920 (1993).
Lauffenburger, D. A., and Linderman, J. J., "Receptors: Models for Binding, Trafficking, and Signaling." Oxford Univ. Press, New York, 1993.
Lee, I., Boucher, Y., and Jain, R. K., *Cancer Res.* **52**, 3237 (1992).
Lee, I., Boucher, Y., Demhartner, T. J., and Jain, R. K., *Br. J. Cancer* **69**, 492 (1994a).
Lee, I., Demhartner, T. J., Boucher, V., Jain, R. K., and Intaglietta, M., *Microvasc. Res.* (in press) (1994b).
Less, J., Skalak, T., Sevick, E. M., and Jain, R. K., *Cancer Res.* **51**, 265 (1991).
Less, J. R., Posner, M. C., Boucher, Y., Borochovitz, D., Wolmark, N., and Jain, R. K., *Cancer Res.* **52**, 6371 (1992).
Less, J. R., Posner, M. C., Wolmark, N., and Jain, R. K., *Cancer Res.* (submitted) (1994).
Leunig, M., Goetz, A. E., Dellian, M., Zetterer, G., Gamarra, R., Jain, R. K., and Messmer, K., *Cancer Res.* **52**, 487 (1992a).
Leunig, M., Yuan, F., Menger, M., Boucher, Y., Goetz, A., Messmer, K., and Jain, R. K., *Cancer Res.* **52**, 6553 (1992b).
Leunig, M., Goetz, A. E., Gamarra, F., Zetterer, G., Messmer, K., and Jain, R. K., *Br. J. Cancer* **69**, 101 (1994a).
Leunig, M., Yuan, F., Gerweck, L., and Jain, R. K., *Lab. Invest.* **71**, 300 (1994b).
Licht, S., *in* "Therapeutic Heat and Cold." Waverly Press, Baltimore, MD, 1965.
Lieblet, A. G., and Lieblet, R. A., *in* "Transplatation of Tumors." 1967.
Liotta, L. A., Kleinerman, J., and Saidel, G. M., *Cancer Res.* **34**, 999 (1974).
Liotta, L. A., Saidel, G. M., and Kleinerman, J., *Bull. Math. Biol.* **39**, 117 (1977).
Lutz, R. J., Dedrick, R. L., Straw, J. A., Hart, M. M., Klubes, P., and Zaharko, D. S., *J. Pharmacokinet. Biopharm.* **3**, 77 (1975).
Lutz, R. J., Dedrick, R. L., and Zaharko, D. S., *Pharmacol. Ther.* **11**, 559 (1980).
Martin, G. R., and Jain, R. K., *Microvasc. Res.* **46**, 216 (1993).
Martin, G. R., and Jain, R. K., *Cancer Res.* (in press) (1994).
Matsuda, T., "Cancer Treatment by Hyperthermia, Radiation and Drugs." Taylor & Francis, Bristol, PA, 1992.
Mayneord, W. V., *Am. J. Cancer* **16**, 841 (1932).
McElwain, D. L. S., and Ponzo, P. J., *Math. Biosci.* **35**, 267 (1977).
McFadden, R., and Kwok, C. S., *Cancer Res.* **48**, 4032 (1988).
McIntire, L. V., *in* "Cellular Mechanics and Cellular Engineering" (V. C. Mow, ed.), pp. 202–207. Springer-Verlag, New York, 1994.
Melder, R. J., and Jain, R. K., *Cell Biophys.* **20**, 16 (1992).
Melder, R. J., and Jain, R. K., *in* "Recent Advances in Cancer Research" (J. G. Park, ed.), pp. 202–207. Seoul National University, Seoul, 1993.
Melder, R. J., Brownell, A. L., Shoup, T. M., Brownell, G. L., and Jain, R. K., *Cancer Res.* **53**, 5867 (1993).
Mitchell, J. W., and Myers, G. E., *Biophys. J.* **8**, 897 (1968).
Munn, L., Melder, R. J., and Jain, R. K., *Biophys. J.* **67**, 889 (1994).
Nakagawa, H., Groothuis, D. R., Owens, E. S., Fenstermacher, J. D., Patlak, C. S., and Blasberg, R. G., *J. Cereb. Blood Flow Metab.* **7**, 687 (1987).

Nugent, L. J., and Jain, R. K., *Cancer Res.* **44**, 238 (1984a).
Nugent, L. J., and Jain, R. K., *Am. J. Physiol.* **246**, H129 (1984b).
Ohkubo, C., Bigos, D., and Jain, R. K., *Cancer Res.* **51**, 1561 (1991).
Pass, H. I., *J. Natl. Cancer Inst.* **85**, 443 (1993).
Patlak, C. S., Goldstein, D. A., and Hoffman, J. F., *J. Theor. Biol.* **5**, 426 (1963).
Peloso, R., Tuma, D. T., and Jain, R. K., *IEEE Trans. Biomed. Eng.* **BME-31**, 725 (1984).
Pennes, H. H., *J. Appl. Physiol.* **1**, 93 (1948).
Pierson, R. N., Price, D. C., Wang, J., and Jain, R. K., *Am. J. Physiol.* **235**, 254 (1978).
Rippe, B., and Haraldsson, B., *Acta Physiol. Scand.* **131**, 411 (1987).
Roh, H. D., Boucher, Y., Kalnicki, S., Buckshaum, R., Bloomer, W. D., and Jain, R. K., *Cancer Res.* **51**, 6695 (1991).
Rosenberg, S., *Sci. Am.* **262**, 62 (1990).
Saidel, G. M., Liotta, L. A., and Kleinerman, J., *J. Theor. Biol.* **56**, 417 (1975).
Saidel, G. M., Liotta, L. A., and Kleinerman, J., *Bull. Math. Biol.* **39**, 117 (1977).
Saltzman, W. N., *Crit. Rev. Ther. Drug Carrier Syst.* **10**, 111 (1993).
Sandison, J. C., *Anat. Rec.* **28**, 281 (1924).
Sands, H. J., *J. Nuc. Med.* **33**, 29 (1992).
Sasaki, A., Jain, R. K., Maghazachi, A. A., Goldfarb, R. H., and Herberman, R. B., *Cancer Res.* **49**, 3742 (1989).
Sasaki, A., Melder, R. J., Whiteside, T. L., Herberman, R. B., and Jain, R. K., *J. Natl. Cancer Inst.* **83**, 433 (1991).
Schmidt-Nielsen, K., "Animal Physiology: Adaptation and Environment." Cambridge Univ. Press, New York, 1990.
Schwan, H. P., *in* "Therapeutic Heat and Cold" (S. Licht, ed.), pp. 63–125. E. Licht Publications, New Haven, CT, 1965.
Secomb, T. W., Hsu, R., Dewhirst, M. W., Klitzman, B., and Gross, J. F., *Int. J. Radiat. Oncol. Biol. Phys.* **25**, 481 (1993).
Sevick, E. M., and Jain, R. K., *Cancer Res.* **48**, 1201 (1988).
Sevick, E. M., and Jain, R. K., *Cancer Res.* **49**, 3506 (1989a).
Sevick, E. M., and Jain, R. K., *Cancer Res.* **49**, 3513 (1989b).
Sevick, E. M., and Jain, R. K., *Cancer Res.* **51**, 1352 (1991a).
Sevick, E. M., and Jain, R. K., *Cancer Res.* **51**, 2727 (1991b).
Shitzer, A., and Eberhart, R., "Heat Transfer in Medicine and Biology," Vols. 1 and 2. Plenum, New York, 1985.
Shymko, R. M., and Glass, L., *J. Theor. Biol.* **63**, 355 (1976).
Sien, H. P., and Jain, R. K., *J. Therm. Biol.* **4**, 157 (1979).
Sien, H. P., and Jain, R. K., *J. Therm. Biol.* **5**, 127 (1980).
Skalak, R., Dasgupta, G., Moss, M., Otten, E., Dullemeijer, P., and Vilmann, H., *J. Theor. Biol.* **94**, 555 (1982).
Smith, S. R., Foster, K. R., and Wolf, G. L., *IEEE Trans. Biomed. Eng.* **BME-33**, 522 (1986).
Steel, G. G., "Growth Kinetics of Tumours." Oxford Univ. Press, Oxford, 1977.
Stehlin, J. S., *Surg. Gynecol. Obstet.* **129**, 305 (1969).
Stein, W. D., "Transport and Diffusion Across Cell Membranes." Academic Press, Orlando, FL, 1986.
Straw, J. A., Hart, M. M., Klubes, P., Zaharko, D. S., and Dedrick, R. L., *JNCI, J. Natl. Cancer Inst.* **52**, 1327 (1974).
Summers, W. C., *Nature (London)* **205**, 414 (1965).
Sung, C., Youle, R. J., and Dedrick, R. L., *Cancer Res.* **50**, 7382 (1990).
Sung, C., Dedrick, R. L., Hall, W. A., Johnson, P. A., and Youle, R. J., *Cancer Res.* **53**, 2092 (1993).

Surowiec, A. J., Stuchly, S. S., Barr, J. R., and Swarup, A., *IEEE Trans. Biomed. Eng.* **BME-35**, 257 (1988).

Sutherland, R. M., *Science* **240**, 177 (1988).

Swabb, E. A., Wei, J., and Gullino, P. M., *Cancer Res.* **34**, 2814 (1974).

Swan, G. W., "Some Current Mathematical Topics in Cancer Research." University Microfilms Int., Ann Arbor, MI, 1977.

Sylvén, B., and Bois, I., *Cancer Res.* **20**, 831 (1960).

Tannock, I. F., *Br. J. Cancer* **22**, 258 (1968).

Tannock, I. F., *Cancer Res.* **30**, 2470 (1970).

Torres-Filho, I. P., Leunig, M., Yuan, F., Intaglietta, M., and Jain, R. K., *Proc. Natl. Acad. Sci. U.S.A.* **91**, 2081 (1994).

van Osdol, W. W., Sung, C., Dedrick, R. L., and Weinstein, J., *J. Nucl. Med.* **34**, 1552 (1993).

Vaupel, P., and Jain, R. K., "Tumor Blood Supply and Metabolic Microenvironment: Characterization and Therapeutic Implications." Fischer, Stuttgart, 1991.

Vaupel, P., Kallinowski, F., and Okunieff, P., *Cancer Res.* **49**, 6449 (1989).

Volpe, B. T., and Jain, R. K., *Med. Phys.* **9**, 506 (1982).

Volpe, B. T., and Jain, R. K., *AIChE Symp. Ser.* **277**, 116 (1983).

Wagner, J. C., "Biopharmaceutics and Relevant Pharmacokinetics." Drug Intelligence Publications, Hamilton, IL, 1971.

Ward, K. A., and Jain, R. K., *Int. J. Hyperthermia* **4**, 223 (1988).

Ward-Hartley, K. A., and Jain, R. K., *Cancer Res.* **47**, 371 (1987).

Weinbaum, S., and Jiji, L. M., *J. Biomed. Eng.* **107**, 131 (1985).

Weinbaum, S., Jiji, L. M., and Lemons, D. E., *J. Biomed. Eng.* **106**, 321 (1984).

Weiss, P., and Kavanau, J. L., *J. Gen. Phys.* **41**, 1 (1957).

Weissbrod, J. M., Jain, R. K., and Sirotnak, F. M., *J. Pharmacokinet. Biopharm.* **6**, 487 (1978).

Wette, R., Katz, I. N., and Rodin, E. Y., *Math. Biosci.* **19**, 231 (1974a).

Wette, R., Katz, I. N., and Rodin, E. Y., *Math. Biosci.* **21**, 311 (1974b).

Wike-Hooley, J. L., Haveman, J., and Reinhold, H. S., *Radiother. Oncol.* **2**, 343 (1984).

Wulff, W., *IEEE Trans. Biomed. Eng.* **BME-21**, 494 (1974).

Wulff, W., *Ann. N.Y. Acad. Sci.* **335**, 151 (1980).

Yang, K. H., Fung, W. P., Lutz, R. J., Dedrick, R. L., and Zaharko, D. S. C., *J. Pharm. Sci.* **68**, 941 (1979).

Young, J. S., Lumsden, C. E., and Stalker, A. L., *J. Pathol. Bacteriol.* **62**, 313 (1950).

Yuan, F., Baxter, L. T., and Jain, R. K., *Cancer Res.* **51**, 3119 (1991).

Yuan, F., Leunig, M., Berk, D., and Jain, R. K., *Microvasc. Res.* **45**, 269 (1993).

Yuan, F., Leunig, M., Huang, S. K., Berk, D. A., Papahadjopoulos, D., and Jain, R. K., *Cancer Res.* **54**, 3352 (1994).

Zaharko, D. S., Dedrick, R. L., Peale, A. L., Drake, J. C., and Lutz, R. J., *J. Pharmacol. Exp. Ther.* **189**, 585 (1974).

Zawicki, D. F., Jain, R. K., Schmid-Schoenbein, G. W., and Chien, S., *Microvasc. Res.* **21**, 37 (1981).

Zhu, H., Baxter, L. T., and Jain, R. K., submitted (1994a).

Zhu, H., Jain, R. K., and Baxter, L. T., submitted (1994b).

Zlotecki, R. A., Boucher, Y., Lee, I., Baxter, L. T., and Jain, R. K., *Cancer Res.* **53**, 2466 (1993).

Zlotecki, R. A., Baxter, L. T., Boucher, Y., and Jain, R. K., submitted for publication (1994).

Zywietz, F., and Knöchel, R., *Phys. Med. Biol.* **31**, 1021 (1986).

A SYSTEMS APPROACH TO MULTIPHASE REACTOR SELECTION

R. Krishna

Department of Chemical Engineering
University of Amsterdam
1018 WV Amsterdam, The Netherlands

I. Introduction

For carrying out multiphase reactions (gas–solid, gas–liquid, gas–liquid–solid, liquid–liquid, gas–liquid–solid, liquid–liquid–solid, . . .), the number of reactor configurations that are possible is extremely large. There is therefore a need to give careful consideration to the choice of the "ideal" reactor configuration that meets fully with all the process "musts" and, to the maximum possible extent, the process "wants." The process "musts" could be:

- operability within technologically feasible reaction coordinates of temperature, pressure, and residence time;

- intrinsically safe operation, freedom from instabilities, runaways, etc.;
- environmental acceptability; and
- feasibility of scale-up to economically justified size.
- maximum possible conversion of the feedstocks;
- maximum selectivity of reaction to desired products; and
- lowest capital and operating costs, stemming from, e.g., the desire to maintain low pressure drop.

Figure 1 pictures the central question addressed in this article.

Typically, in the petroleum and petrochemical industry, even small percentage improvements, say of the order of 0.5%, with respect to selectivity can be extremely significant. For example, improvement of gasoline selectivity in fluid catalytic cracking (FCC) operations by 0.5% would mean an increased revenue of $2.5 million per day on a global basis. Improved yield and selectivity can be crucial for process licensors. A 1% selectivity advantage in the manufacture of ethene oxide (obtained by air oxidation of ethene) could be significant enough for a process licensor to gain a marketing edge over a competitor. While the major process improvements will no doubt stem from improved reaction "chemistry" and catalyst design, there is a further scope for effecting improved performance by clever choice of the reactor configuration. In the FCC riser reactor, improved feed atomization, better gas–solids contacting at inlet (e.g., by pre-fluidization with steam), and closer approach to plug flow of gas and catalyst phases are known to lead to great economic benefits. For ethene oxide manufacture, if we are able to develop a packed bed reactor

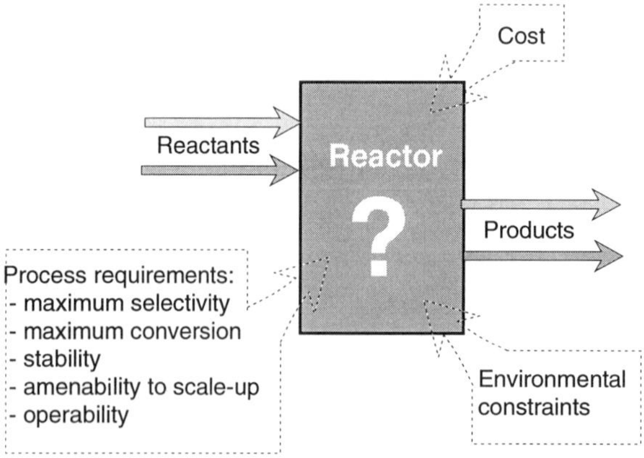

FIG. 1. The problem of reactor selection to meet the desired process requirements and constraints.

that operates under substantially isothermal conditions, this will result in significant selectivity advantages due to suppression of the combustion reaction.

During the development of new processes involving first-of-a-kind technology, the choice of the reactor assumes added importance because of the lack of prior art. This is exemplified by the relatively recent development of the hydrodemetalization (HDM) process; in this case, major companies have adopted widely different configurations, e.g., three-phase fluidized beds slurry reactors, (fixed) trickle beds, co-current down flow moving bed, and countercurrent upflow moving bed. The Shell HYCON process employing the co-current downflow moving bed concept is an example of a novel first-of-a-kind technology.

In the Shell Middle Distillates Synthesis (SMDS) process, which converts natural gas to synthetic liquid hydrocarbons via advanced Fischer–Tropsch synthesis, the synthesis reactor configuration chosen for the first commercial unit in Malaysia, started up in 1993, is the multi-tubular downflow trickle bed with catalyst inside the tubes (Sie *et al.*, 1991). Because of the enormous exothermicity of the synthesis reaction and the relatively poor heat transfer, a very large heat transfer area is required. The reactor volume and weight are largely governed by the installable heat transfer area in a vessel of given volume. Use of the multi-tubular bubble column slurry provides much better heat transfer characteristics (an improvement of a factor of about five over fixed bed units) and could lead to considerably lower reactor volumes. However, the anticipated scale-up problems with bubble column operation were of overriding concern for Shell, who decided to adopt the fixed-bed technology due mainly to a quicker development scenario which allowed the time plans of the business to be met. The lead time for development of processes in the petroleum and petrochemical industries is usually of the order of a decade, and for first-of-a-kind technology such as the SMDS process, there is an incentive to adopt a sure, safe, and quicker process development route. It is interesting to note that other companies, e.g., Sasol and Exxon, have more recently opted for the slurry reactor configuration. These companies apparently did not consider the long lead time for development of the bubble column slurry reactor to be an insurmountable problem.

The preceding discussions serve to underline not only the importance of choosing the reactor with the promise of best performance, but also the need to anticipate scale-up difficulties. The approach we advocate in this article is to attack the problem of reactor selection in a systematic, structured manner, using some concepts borrowed from management sciences. We develop the arguments leading to our general systems approach by first considering a case study involving recovery of oil from oil shale.

II. Case Study: Recovery of Oil from Oil Shale

Oil shale contains an aromatic component called kerogen, which on heating, in the temperature range 400–500°C, decomposes to yield oil, coke, and gas. At temperatures below 400°C, the reaction is extremely slow, and at temperatures exceeding about 550°C, excessive cracking of the oil vapor, liberated during reaction, takes place. Burning off the coke from the spent shale in a combustor provides a source of energy for the endothermic pyrolysis reaction; see Fig. 2. The choice of the ideal reactor configuration is the topic addressed here. There are numerous processes and reactor configurations that have been suggested for carrying out the thermal pyrolysis reaction (Synthetic Fuels Data Handbook, 1978); these are sketched in Fig. 3. The various technologies have apparently little in common. For example, on the basis of particle size used in the process, we have: (a) large-sized ($\cong$ 50 mm) particles, (b) medium-sized ($\cong$ 5–10 mm) particles, and (c) small-sized ($<$ 3 mm) particles. Further, both packed beds [groups (a) and (b)] and fluidized operations [group (c)] are encountered. The contacting pattern between the oil vapor (+stripping gas) and

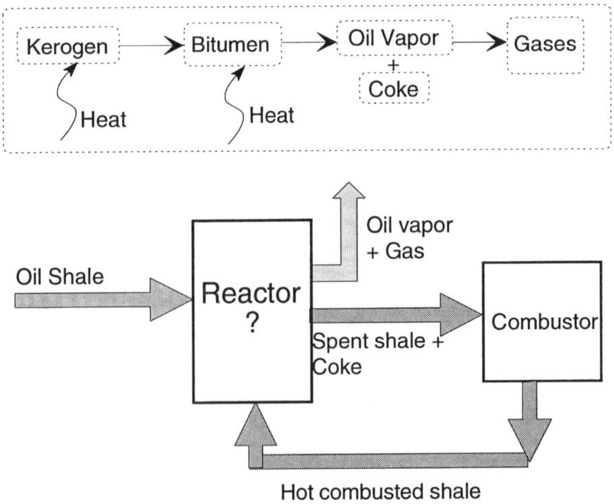

FIG. 2. Schematic process flow diagram for the recovery of oil from oil shale.

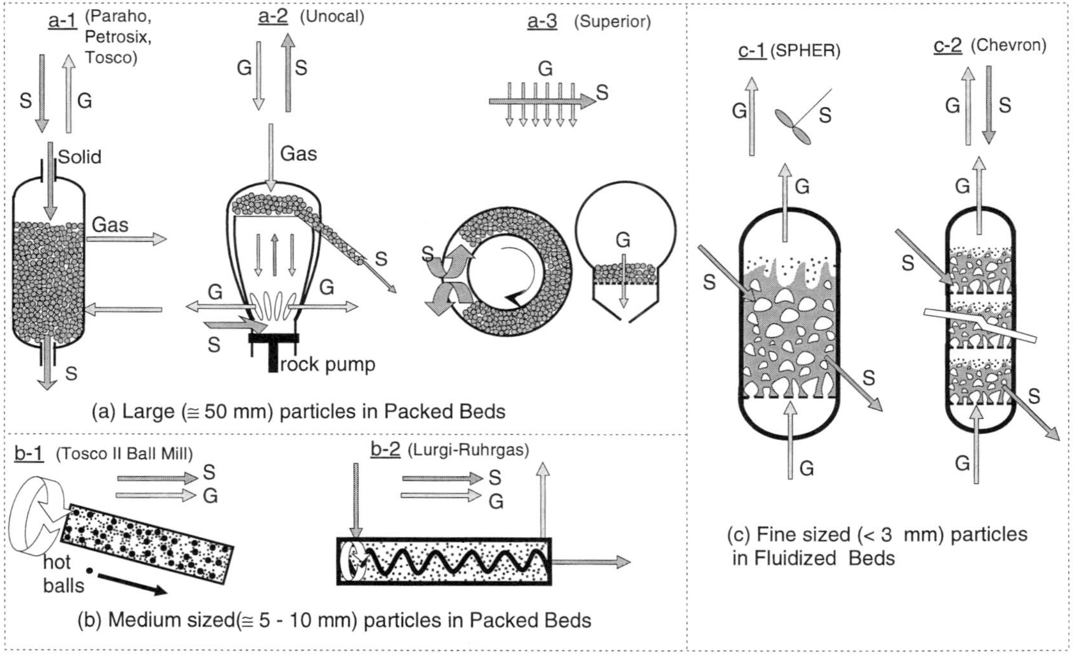

FIG. 3. Various reactor configurations used in oil shale processing technologies. Adapted from Levenspiel (1988).

the solid phase used in these technologies also varies widely: (i) countercurrent in a-1, a-2, and c-2; (ii) co-current in technologies b-1 and b-2; and (iii) cross-current in a-3. The solids phase is more or less well mixed in the SPHER process c-1, whereas in the other technologies there is staging of the solids phase. The Unocal process involves another unique technology in which the shale particles are moved upwards, countercurrent to the vapors, by means of a rock pump. For a reactor engineer involved in developing a shale oil recovery process, the diversity of the reactor configurations shown in Fig. 3 is more than a little disconcerting. How is one to make a choice among the various options? We shall demonstrate our suggested systems approach by attempting to derive the ideal oil-shale reactor configuration.

A. The Process Wish List

Any systematic approach to reactor selection must begin with a "wish" list of features:

Wish 1: The reactor must be capable of maximum recovery of oil. Oil recovery can be maximized by making sure that high (say, 99% +) conversion of kerogen is obtained and that the oil vapor once produced does not suffer further cracking and degradation to light gases.

Wish 2: The reactor design should allow scale-up to large scale units capable of handling, say, 50,000 tons per day of oil shale in one processing train; this is important for economy of scale.

Wish 3: In view of the large quantities of shale rock to be handled, of the order of 500 kg/s, there is need to restrict the reactor volumes in order to reduce the investment costs.

Wish 4: During grinding operation there is inevitable production of fines, and the chosen reactor should be capable of handling these fines, both from economic as well as environmental considerations.

B. Gas–Solid Reactor Selection Subsets

We split up the problem of reactor selection into three sub-problems. By making decisions regarding these three separate attributes of the reactor, we obtain the final reactor choice. These three subsets of the reactor are discussed next.

1. Subset I: Particle Size

The "ideal" particle size to use in the reactor should meet the requirements in the wish list; concretely put, should we use small particles, medium-sized particles, or coarse particles? (See Fig. 4.)

2. Subset II: Gas–Solid Contacting Flow Pattern

Here we have to decide among the following three contacting patterns between the gas (= oil vapor + liberated light gases + stripping gas) and the (hot) shale particles (see Fig. 4).

(a) *Countercurrent contacting*,
(b) *Co-current contacting*, and
(c) *Cross-current contacting*.

Each of the two contacting phases (gas and solid) can be either in plug flow (perfectly staged) or backmixed (perfectly mixed) condition. At this stage of reactor selection it is only necessary to specify what the ideal contacting pattern ought to be; the technical limits of feasibility are taken into account in a subsequent analysis.

3. Subset III: Gas–Solid Fluidization Regime

Even when the above two subsets I and II have been decided, the definition of the reactor configuration is not complete; there remains the choice of the appropriate gas–solid fluidization regime. Basically we have to choose between the following six modes of operation; see Fig. 4.

1. *Packed bed regime* (fixed or moving bed operation). Here the particle hold-up is typically in the region 0.5–0.7. The particle size suitable in the packed bed regime is usually larger than 1 mm because smaller particle sizes result in unacceptably high pressure drops.
2. *Fluidized bed* operating under *homogeneous fluidization* conditions (i.e., just above the minimum fluidization velocity). This regime of operation is only prevalent for fine particles, and the operating window is extremely limited. It is not possible to design a gas–solid fluidized bed commercial-scale reactor to operate under this regime in a stable manner because it is difficult to prevent the onset of bubbles due *inter alia* to flow instabilities resulting from, say, improper gas distribution at the inlet.
3. *Bubbling bed* operation. The particle hold-up in this regime is typically 0.4–0.5, and this regime is characterized by the presence of fast-moving bubbles that tend to churn the system, resulting in an almost completely backmixed solids phase.

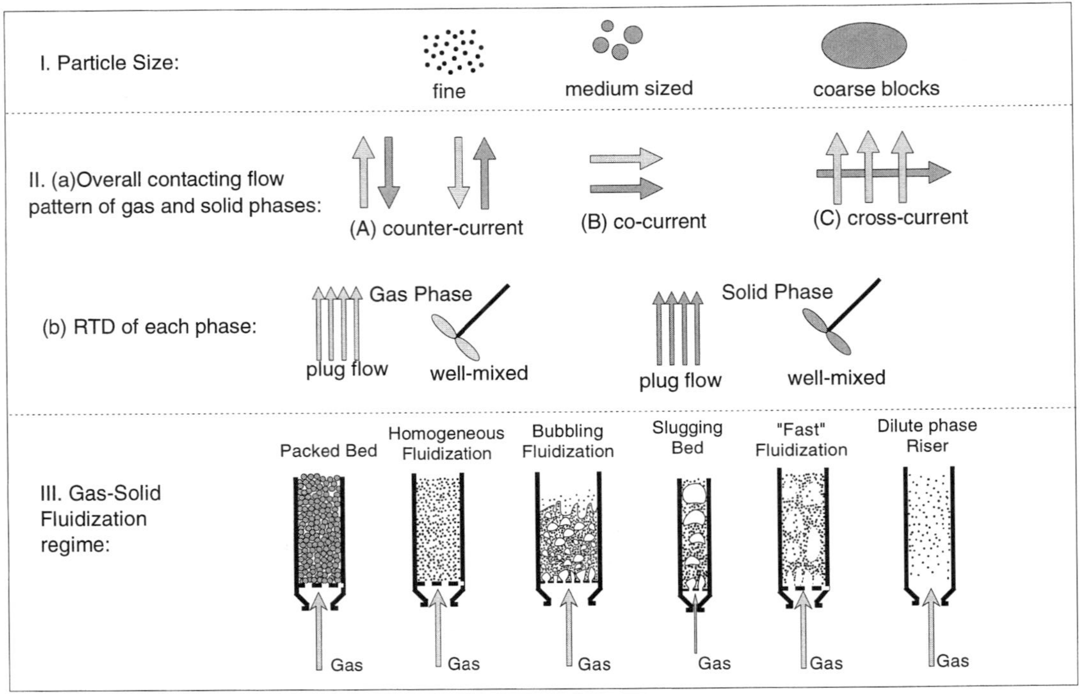

FIG. 4. The three subsets, or attributes, of a gas–solids reactor.

4. *Slugging bed*. For relatively small-diameter columns, e.g., typically of the order of 0.1 m, the size of the bubbles attains the dimensions of the vessel and slugging conditions prevail. This regime of gas–solids flow is quite common in pilot plants operating at high velocity. For commercial-scale units with diameters larger than 0.5 m, it is usually not possible to attain slug flow conditions.

5. *Turbulent regime* and "*fast*" *fluidization*. If the gas velocity is increased further beyond the bubbling fluidization regime, the *turbulent* regime of fluidization is reached. In this regime the bubbles are of indistinguishable and ever-changing shape. The particle hold-up is typically in the range 0.3–0.45. There is heavy entrainment of the solids, and bed inventory is lost without solids recycle by means of a cyclone. If the gas velocity is increased still further, the bed can be transported, and this mode of operation is commonly termed "*fast*" *fluidization* or *dense-phase riser transport*. The particle hold-ups in this regime are typically 0.1–0.2.

6. *Dilute phase riser transport*. As the gas velocity is increased still further, the dilute phase riser transport regime is reached. The particle hold-up in this regime is of the order of 0.05 or smaller.

Besides significant differences in the particle hold-ups in the foregoing modes of fluidization, there are other differences, e.g., in gas–solids contacting efficiency, solids mixing, gas-phase mixing, and heat and mass transfer characteristics.

We now analyze each of the three subsets above in turn.

C. Particle Size Selection

As already seen in Fig. 3, existing oil shale processes display a wide range of particle size specifications. In order to arrive at the decision regarding the ideal particle size, we need to analyze the transport and chemical reaction processes inside the particle. The kinetic scheme for the thermal pyrolysis reaction is depicted in Fig. 5, following Wallman *et al.* (1980). For a temperature of 482°C, the residence time requirements for 99% conversion of kerogen can be calculated using the kinetic data of Wallman *et al.* (1980). The residence time requirements for the limiting cases of plug flow of solids (perfectly staged) and backmixed solids (perfect mixing) are shown in Fig. 6; for plug flow of solids $\tau = 8$ min, whereas for a backmixed reactor $\tau = 174$ min. Also shown in Fig. 6 is the time required to heat up the particle of shale to within 95% of the surrounding temperature. We can distinguish three distinct ranges of particle sizes in Fig. 6. For particles smaller than 20 mm (Range I), the heating-up times

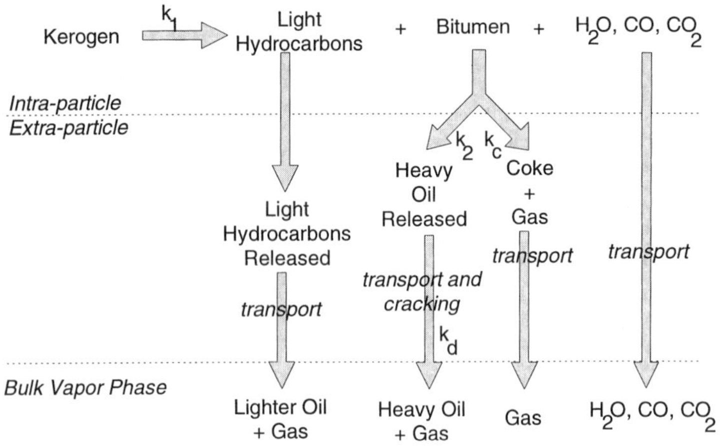

FIG. 5. Oil shale pyrolysis kinetic scheme according to Wallman *et al.* (1980). The first-order reaction rate constant for kerogen decomposition is $k_1 = 9.633 \times 10^{10} \exp(-21943/T)$ [s^{-1}]. The first-order reaction rate constant for heavy oil production is $k_2 = 3 \times 10^3 \exp(-11370/T)$ [s^{-1}]. The first-order reaction rate constant for coking is $k_2 = A_c \times 10^3 \exp(-11370/T)$ [s^{-1}], where $A_c = 30$ for $d_p = 3$ mm; $A_c = 15$ for d_p 2 mm; $A_c = 6.667$ for $d_p = 1$ mm; $A_c = 5$ for $d_p = 0.4$ mm.

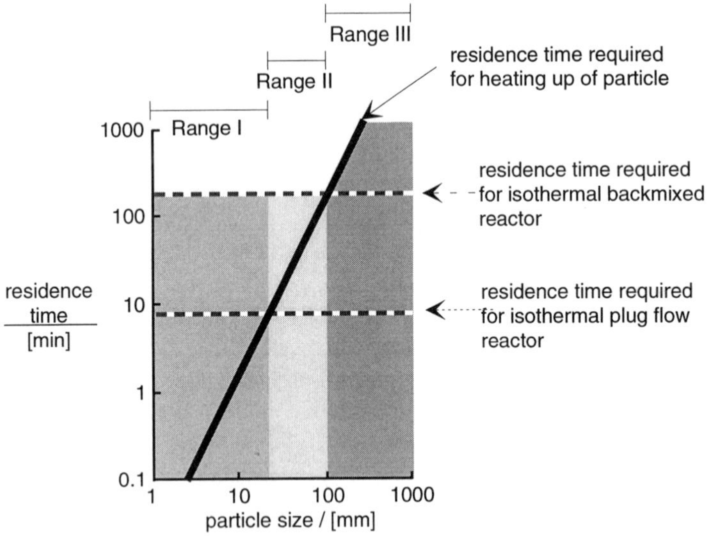

FIG. 6. Particle residence time requirements for isothermal oil shale reactor operating at 482°C. The residence time requirements for achieving the desired degree of conversion were obtained from the kerogen decomposition kinetics of Wallman *et al.* (1980); see Fig. 5. The heating-up requirements of the shale particles were calculated assuming an effective thermal diffusivity inside the particle of 2.7×10^{-7} [$m^2\ s^{-1}$].

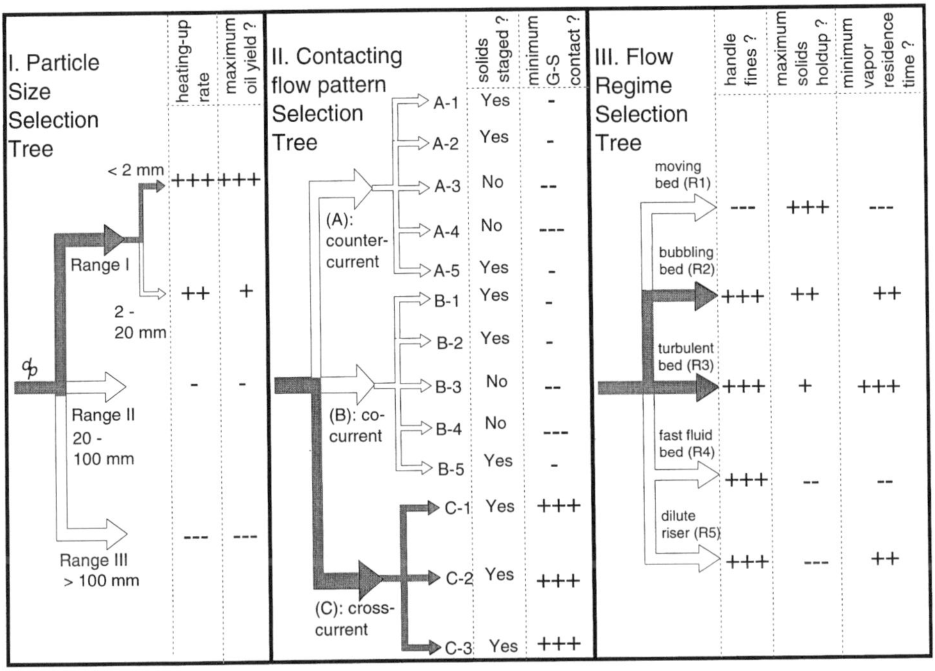

FIG. 7. Decision tree analysis for oil shale reactor selection.

are insignificant compared to the time required for converting the kerogen. The residence time requirement of particles is therefore governed purely by backmixing characteristics of the solids. For particles larger than 100 mm in size (Range III), the heating up time becomes dominant and it does not matter whether the solids are backmixed or not. For particles of size between 20 and 100 mm (Range II), both heating-up and backmixing characteristics play important roles.

A typical large oil shale complex will have a solids flow rate of 500 kg/s, and there is a great incentive to keep the required residence time of shale particles to the minimum possible level (Wishes 1, 2, and 3). This desire will be met if we choose a particle size below 20 mm (Range I) with no heating-up limitations and, further, ensure plug flow of the solids phase. This conclusion is summarized in the form of a decision tree in Fig. 7.

The oil vapor produced within the particle will have to be transported to the bulk vapor phase, and during this transport process it will suffer further degradation and cracking; this can be seen in the kinetic scheme in Fig. 5. The yield of heavy oil, which is the desired product, has been found to be dependent on the particle size, as evident from calculations on the

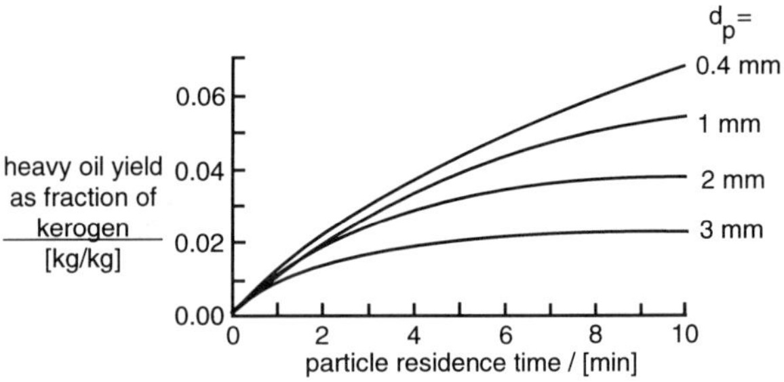

FIG. 8. Heavy oil yield as a function of particle residence time for a range of particle sizes. Data for oil shale reactor operating isothermally at 482°C. The yields are calculated using the Wallman *et al.* (1980) kinetic data in Fig. 5.

basis of Wallman kinetics; see Fig. 8. There is a significant yield improvement in using particles below 2 mm. Now in any grinding operation, if we specify 2 mm as the top size, there will be a significant proportion of particles smaller than this top size. To fulfill Wish 1, we further branch up the particle size decision tree by choosing a size smaller than 2 mm; see Fig. 7.

D. Contacting Flow Pattern

Several contacting flow patterns are possible; the important ones are pictured in Fig. 9. Scheme A-1 is used by Paraho, Petrosix, Tosco and Chevron. Scheme A-2 is used in the Unocal rock pump contactor with upwards flow of solids. Scheme A-3 corresponds to the SPHER process with a backmixed solids phase. The horizontal co-current contacting scheme B-5 is used in Lurgi-Ruhrgas and Tosco-II. The cross-current contacting schemes C-1 and C-2 are used in the Superior Oil traveling grate process, where the gaseous heating medium traverses up or down a packed bed of solids placed on a grate. The cross-current contacting scheme C-3 is used in the moving bed concept of Kiviter with radial outflow of gas.

In the contacting flow pattern selection tree (Fig. 7), we choose only those branches where the solids phase is in plug flow because of our desire to reduce the reactor volume requirements (Wish 3). There is a further factor that needs to be taken into account. The oil vapor that is formed during the process is in contact with other hot shale particles within the reactor, and the chance of further degradation of this oil increases with the gas phase residence time (*cf.* Fig. 5). Wilkins *et al.* (1981) have studied the oil vapor degradation kinetics, and calculations based on their kinetics

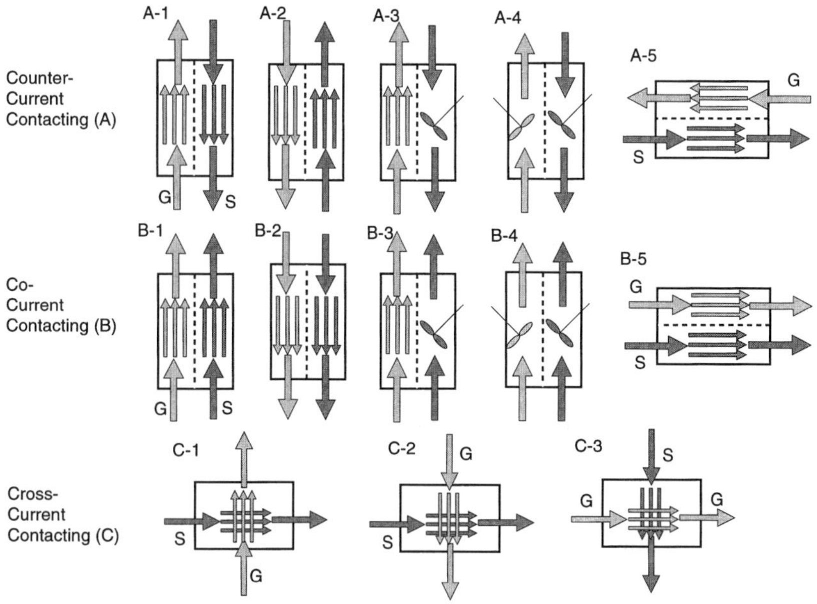

FIG. 9. The various possible gas–solid contacting flow patterns.

are shown in Fig. 10. It is noteworthy that 5% of the oil suffers further degradation for a vapor residence time of 2 s. Clearly, to reduce the chance of oil degradation (*cf.* Wish 1), it is necessary to remove the oil vapor from the reaction zone as soon as it is formed. The important conclusion to emerge from this analysis is that neither counter- nor co-current contacting is desired. What we require is cross-current contact-

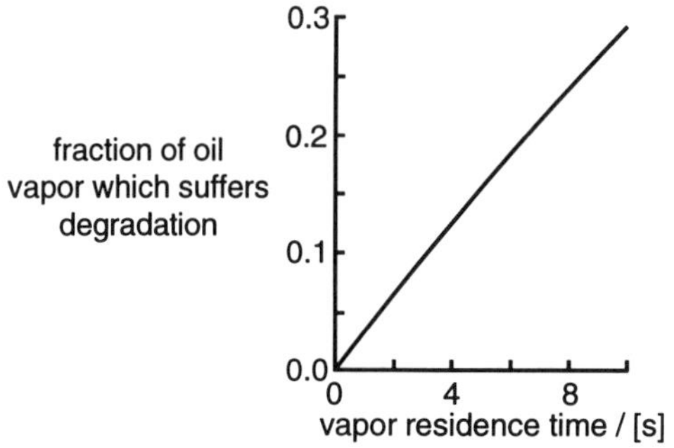

FIG. 10. The fraction of oil vapor formed which is degraded due to overcracking as function of oil vapor residence time. Data for isothermal operation at 482°C (Wilkins *et al.*, 1981). The calculations were carried out with a first-order reaction rate constant for oil degradation, $k_1 = 3 \times 10^3 \exp(-8700/T)$ [s^{-1}].

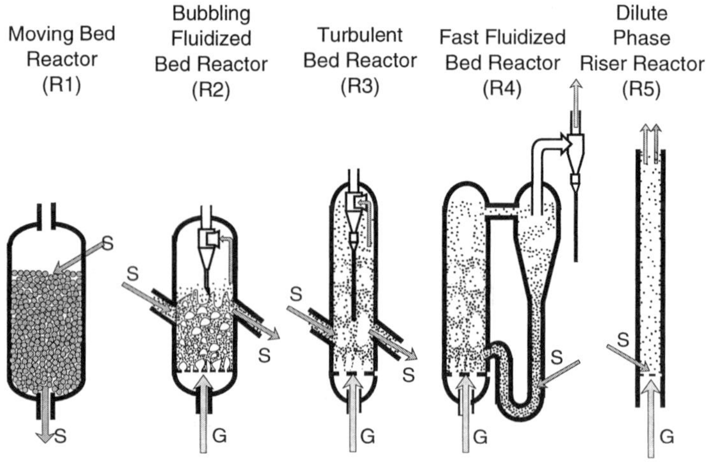

FIG. 11. Gas–solid reactor configurations involving operation with various regimes.

ing of oil vapor and hot solids, wherein the chance of contact between the phases is minimized. The favored contacting flow patterns are, therefore C-1, C-2, and C-3; this is incorporated into the contacting pattern selection tree in Fig. 7.

E. Gas–Solids Fluidization Regime

For commercial operations, the regimes of homogeneous fluidization and slug flow (see Fig. 4) are not feasible, and the practical implementation of the various fluidization regimes is shown in Fig. 11. A moving bed of packed shale particles (R-1), moving downwards, upwards, or horizontally, is the most commonly used flow regime in the existing processes. This packed bed flow regime has one serious disadvantage that fine particles (smaller, than, say, 0.5 mm), inevitably formed in the crushing operation, will block moving-bed operation or will be blown away by the gases. Existing moving-bed processes such as Paraho, Unocal, Petrosix, Superior, and Kiviter operate with lumps of particles of average size 50 mm and are not capable of handling fine powders (see Wish 4). Note that we have already discarded operation with large lumps of particles from oil yield and reactor volume considerations (Wish 1, 2, and 3).

Respecting the requirements of Wish 3, we aim to maximize the solids hold-up in the system. Using this criterion we have the hierarchy of choices, indicated by pulses and minuses, in Fig. 7. Dense- and dilute-phase riser transport operation, operating at solids hold-ups below 0.2, cannot therefore be serious contenders as oil-shale reactors.

There is another factor that needs to be taken into consideration: the need to reduce oil vapor degradation (Wish 1), requiring us to reduce the oil vapor residence time in the reactor. In bubbling fluidized beds (R-2) and turbulent fluid beds (R-3), the bubble rise velocities are of the order of 1.5 m/s, and in a shallow bed of, say, 2 m the oil vapor residence time may be restricted to below 2 s.

The flow regime selection tree has been summarized in Fig. 7. On the basis of the qualitative reasoning, we may conclude that the best operating regime for the oil shale retort is a bubbling or turbulent bed operation.

F. Summary of Oil Shale Reactor Configuration Decisions

The various decisions on the reactor subsets, outlined in Fig. 7, can be summarized in words as follows. The ideal oil shale reactor, respecting all items in the wish list, is one in which fine particles, say smaller than 2 mm, are used in a reactor configuration wherein the overall gas solids contacting pattern corresponds to cross-flow of gas and solid. The solids phase in the reactor should be staged, and the oil vapor residence time is limited to a few seconds by use of the bubbling/turbulent fluidization regime. The resulting cross-flow fluid bed reactor configuration is shown in Fig. 12. This is the configuration of the Shell Shale Retorting Process that is under development by Shell Research. This process was developed using the decision analysis sketched earlier (see also Poll *et al.*, 1987). Raw shale

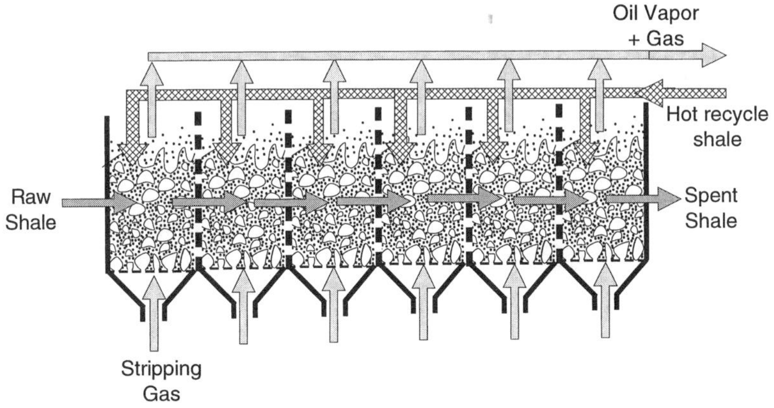

Fig. 12. The cross-flow multi-staged fluidized bed reactor concept used in the Shell Shale Retorting Process (Poll *et al.*, 1987).

enters the multi-compartment bed at the left. Baffles with large free area separate adjacent compartments, each of which may be considered to be well mixed. The flow of fluidized solids from one compartment to the next is by means of "hydrostatic" head, similar to the flow of water in a bathtub. If the number of horizontally disposed compartments exceeds about 10, we approach plug flow conditions of the solids. The overall contacting flow pattern for the reactor train as a whole is cross-flow. Within individual compartments, however, the gas (containing oil vapor) traverses up the bed in the form of bubbles virtually in plug flow, while the solids phase is almost completely backmixed.

A careful comparison of the Shell process with the existing technologies (Fig. 3) shows that none of the "ideal" subsets chosen is unique. Fine particles smaller than 3 mm are used in the SPHER and Chevron processes. Cross-current contacting is employed by Superior Oil and Kiviter technologies. The Chevron process uses a fluidized bed. However, the *combination* of these ideal subsets is apparently unique, and the promise of improved yield was sufficient to justify a substantial development effort (Poll *et al.*, 1987). There are also no scale-up problems envisaged in the multi-compartment fluidized bed approach; for scaling-up purposes it is sufficient to study in detail the hydrodynamics of one of the fluid bed compartments. In theory, to obtain sufficient solids-phase residence time, the number of compartments can be increased at will without running into any scale-up difficulties. A vertically disposed multi-compartment configuration (Chevron; see Fig. 3) poses scale-up problems in addition to the undesirable long gas–solid contact time implicit in countercurrent operation.

The benefits of employing a systems approach to the oil shale reactor selection example can be gleaned from the fact that the number of possible combinations of

- three particle size ranges (*cf*. Fig. 6),
- thirteen gas–solids contacting flow patterns (Fig. 9), and
- five gas–solids fluidization regimes (Fig. 11)

is $3 \times 13 \times 5 = 195$ reactor types! By adopting a *sequential* decision-making strategy, we have been able to arrive at the ideal reactor choice without brute-force evaluation of all the options.

III. General Selection Methodology for Multiphase Reactors

The oil shale reactor selection can now be generalized to the general case of multiphase reactors (gas–liquid, gas–solid, gas–liquid–solid, liquid–liquid, liquid–liquid–solid), retaining the essential structure of the methodology. The discussions of the various ingredients of the general methodology are illustrated next, using several practical examples of commercial reactor selection.

A. The Wish List

One of the most important aspects of the reactor selection example is the setting up of the wish list. This list may be crucial in arriving at the final decision. Omission of one item may in some cases lead to a completely different reactor choice. To take the example of the oil shale reactor, it was the "wish" to maximize yield of oil and prevent degradation of the oil vapor which culminated in the cross-flow configuration choice. On the other hand, in the interest of reducing process development costs, if we had wished for a simple, proven reactor configuration, the choice would perhaps have fallen on moving (packed) bed operation. For many organizations involved in process development, one common item in the wish list is that the reactor hardware choice should not constitute a major "step-out" in technology; such step-outs require huge development efforts. The cross-current multi-compartment fluid bed shale process does not constitute a major step out for Shell, which has considerable in-house expertise in fluid bed reactor design and scale-up (see, e.g., Van Swaaij and Zuiderweg, 1972, and Krishna, 1981).

Often the desire to maximize yield and selectivity of the reaction may lead to a reactor configuration that may pose operability problems; it is then the task of the experienced process developer to carefully weigh the alternatives and assign a hierarchy to the wish list. Operability, stability, and environmental constraints usually gain precedence. To give one example, the wish to maximize yield and selectivity may lead to the choice of 1–5 μm sized catalyst particles in a slurry reactor. This choice, though "ideal" from a transport phenomena–chemical kinetics analysis, will pose problems of separation from the product stream (operability problems). If the benefits of the use of 1–5 μm particles can provide a substantial competitive edge it may be worthwhile to examine the possibility of magnetizing the fine catalyst particles and employing an electromagnetic separation device. The net result of the systems approach could be a novel technology.

B. Reactor Subset I—(Volume/Surface Area) Selection

For multiphase reactors, the first important decision to be made concerns the choice of the (volume/surface area) ratio for each of the phases in the reactor. We discuss some general guidelines for arriving at this choice for specific reactor types.

1. Gas–Solid Systems

The solid phase could be a reactant, product, or catalyst. In general the decision on the choice of the particle size rests on an analysis of the extra- and intra-particle transport processes and chemical reaction. For solid-catalyzed reactions, an important consideration in the choice of the particle size is the desire to utilize the catalyst particle most effectively. This would require choosing a particle size such that the generalized Thiele modulus ϕ_{gen}, representing the ratio of characteristic intraparticle diffusion and reaction times, has a value smaller than 0.4; see Fig. 13. Such an effectiveness factor–Thiele modulus analysis may suggest particle sizes too small for use in packed bed operation. The choice is then either to consider fluidized bed operation, or to used shaped catalysts (e.g., spoked wheels, grooved cylinders, star-shaped extrudates, four-leafed clover, etc.). Another commonly used procedure for overcoming the problem of diffusional limitations is to have nonuniform distribution of active components (e.g., precious metals) within the catalyst particle.

Often an important reason to avoid intraparticle diffusion resistances is from selectivity considerations. To maximize the intermediate product in a consecutive reaction scheme, we should avoid intraparticle diffusional resistances. For butene dehydrogenation it can be seen in Fig. 14 that

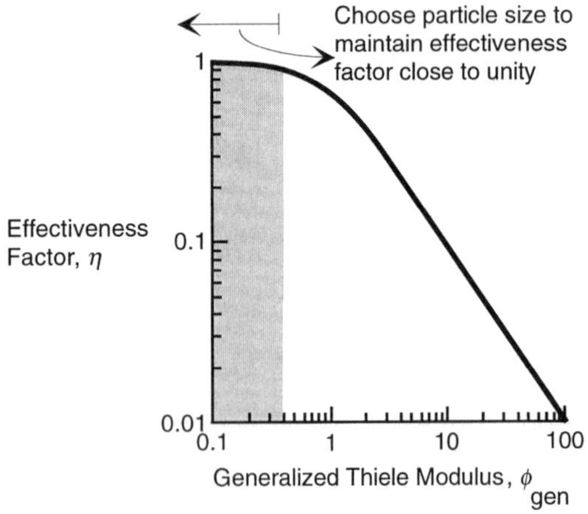

FIG. 13. Isothermal effectiveness factor, η, inside catalyst particles as function of the generalized Thiele modulus ϕ_{gen}.

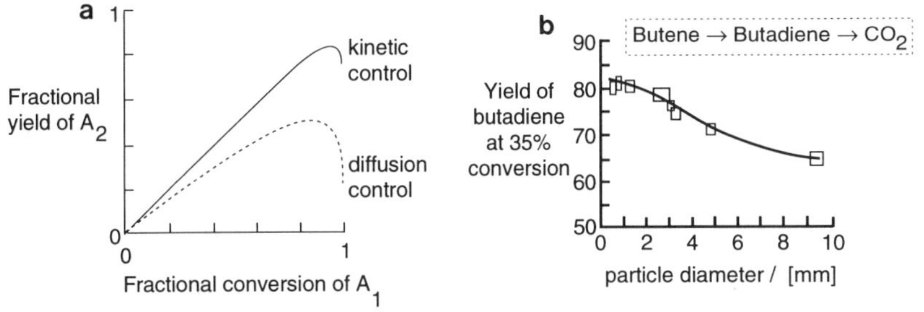

FIG. 14. Yield of intermediate product A_2 for the consecutive reaction scheme $A_1 \rightarrow A_2 \rightarrow A_3$. (a) Calculated fractional yield of A_2 as a function of conversion of A_1. (b) Dependence of the yield of butadiene on iron oxide catalyst particle size at 620°C (Adapted from Voge and Morgan, 1972).

increased particle size has a significant deleterious effect on the yield of the intermediate product butadiene (Voge and Morgan, 1972).

For highly exothermic reactions, under certain operation conditions the effectiveness factor may exhibit multiple steady-state values; see Fig. 15. The "hot" branch has a high effectiveness, while the "cold" branch exhibits relatively low effectiveness-factor values. From an operation viewpoint, it may be prudent to avoid the region exhibiting multiplicity altogether (see shaded region in Fig. 15). Steady-state multiplicity within a single catalyst pellet has been experimentally confirmed for the oxidation of ethene. Such multiplicity of steady states within a single catalyst pellet can lead to multiplicity of steady states for the reactor considered as a whole (Adaje and Sheintuch, 1990), leading to problems in operation and control.

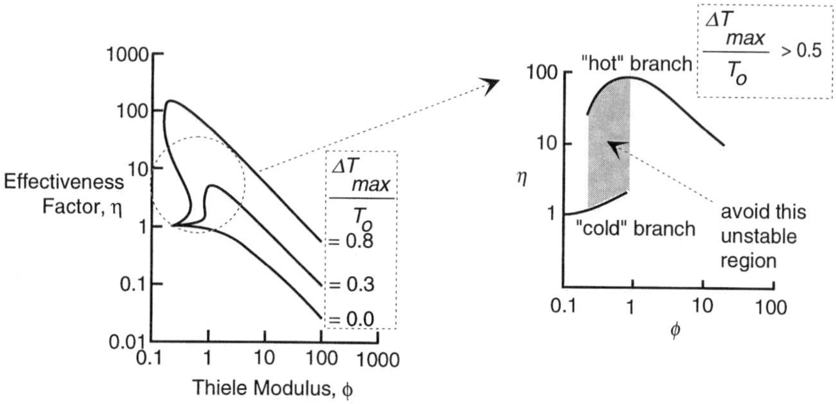

FIG. 15. Non-isothermal effectiveness factor for spherical particle as function of the Thiele modulus, ϕ. Adapted from Weisz and Hicks (1962) and Trambouze *et al.* (1988).

2. *Gas–Liquid Systems*

For a gas liquid system with reaction within the liquid phase, there are fundamentally three different modes of gas–liquid contact: (i) gas bubbles dispersed in liquid (as encountered in bubble columns), (ii) liquid droplets dispersed in gas (e.g., tray operating in the spray regime), and (iii) a thin flowing liquid film in contact with a gas (e.g., gas–liquid contacting in a packed column); see Fig. 16. The hydrodynamic and mass transfer characteristics for any system are reflected by the parameter β, which is the ratio of the liquid phase volume to the volume of the diffusion layer. The first major decision, reactor subset I, for a gas–liquid system is the choice for this parameter β; this choice is analogous to the particle size decision for a gas–solid reactor. The value of β takes on values in the range of 10–40 for liquid sprays and thin liquid films, whereas $\beta = 10^3$–10^4 for gas bubbles in liquid. The choice with regard to β depends on the relative rates of chemical reaction and mass transfer within the liquid phase, portrayed by the Hatta number. The choices for β are summarized in the enhancement factor–Hatta number diagram of Fig. 17, which diagram is entirely equivalent to the effectiveness factor–Thiele modulus diagram of Fig. 13. The overall aim is to choose the value of β such that the reactor volume is effectively utilized. Thus, for slow liquid–phase reactions we should aim to increase the bulk liquid volume at the expense of interfacial area. We achieve a high value of β by dispersing the gas in the form of bubbles (e.g., bubble columns and tray columns operating in the froth regime). To give an example, air oxidation of cyclohexane (in the liquid phase) is a slow reaction usually carried out in bubble contactors. In the fast pseudo first-order reaction regime, the reaction occurs predominantly in the diffusion film close to the gas–liquid interface, and we should choose a contactor with low value of β (e.g., spray towers and packed columns). Further, in the fast pseudo first-order reaction regime, the rate of transfer is independent of the liquid-phase hydrodynamics; there is no need to spend energy for increasing turbulence in the liquid phase. An example of

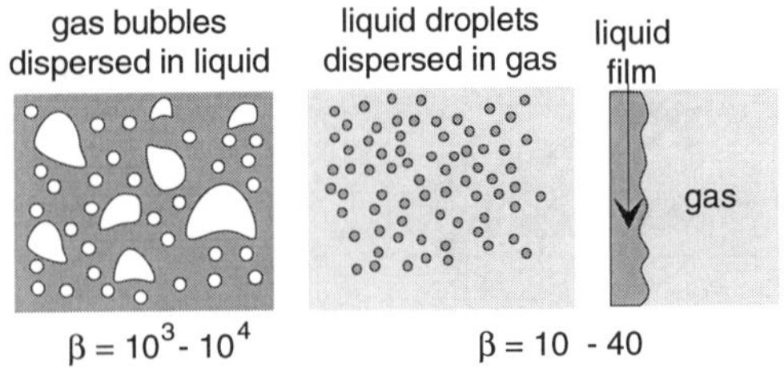

FIG. 16. Three fundamental procedures for contacting gases and liquids. β is the ratio of the liquid phase volume to the volume of the diffusion layer within the liquid phase.

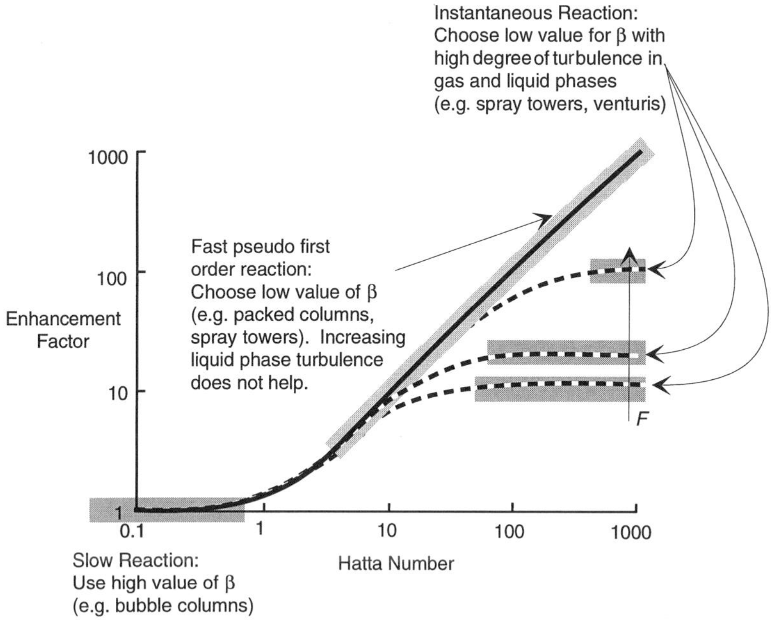

FIG. 17. Enhancement factor for gas–liquid reactions as function of the Hatta number; adapted from Trambouze *et al.* (1988).

process operating in the fast pseudo first-order reaction regime is absorption of carbon dioxide in aqueous caustic solutions; this is usually carried out in packed columns. The liquid phase flows down the column in thin liquid rivulets. If the gas–liquid reaction corresponds to the instantaneous reaction rate regime, our efforts, once again, should be to maximize the interfacial area at the expense of bulk liquid volume. In contrast to the fast pseudo first-order reaction regime, it generally pays to attempt to enhance the degree of turbulence in both the liquid and gas phases. Contactors that satisfy these requirements include tray columns operating in the spray regime and venturi scrubbers. The sulfonation of aromatics using gaseous sulfur trioxide is an instantaneous reaction and is controlled by gas-phase mass transfer. In the commercially used thin-film sulfonator, the liquid reactant flows down a tube as a thin film (low β) in contact with a highly turbulent gas stream (high k_g). A thin-film contactor is chosen in place of a liquid droplet system because of the desire to remove heat from the liquid phase; this heat is generated by the highly exothermic sulfonation reaction.

Often a more important aspect is the choice of β so as to maximize selectivity to a desired product. We shall illustrate this by considering the example of selective absorption of hydrogen sulfide from a gaseous mixture containing carbon dioxide using amine solutions (Astarita *et al.*, 1983; Darton *et al.*, 1988; Doraiswamy and Sharma, 1984). The reaction between H_2S and amines takes place in the instantaneous regime, whereas the reaction between CO_2 and amines usually corresponds to the fast pseudo first-order reaction regime. The selectivity towards H_2S ca be defined as the ratio of the number of overall gas phase mass transfer units for H_2S transfer to that for transfer of CO_2:

$$\text{Sel} = \frac{\text{NTU}_{H_2S}}{\text{NTU}_{CO_2}}.$$

This ratio equals the ratio of the overall (gas-phase) mass transfer coefficients for transfer of H_2S and CO_2; see Darton *et al.* (1988). The overall gas-phase mass transfer coefficient for H_2S is the gas-phase transfer coefficient k_g. The overall gas-phase mass transfer coefficient for CO_2, is $H_{CO_2}RTEk_l$, where E is the enhancement factor for CO_2 transfer. Efficient reactor utilization and improved selectivity are obtained by (i) choosing low values of β, (ii) increasing k_g, and (iii) increasing the ratio k_g/k_l (see Bosch, 1989). Selectivity values Sel have been determined for several modes of gas–liquid contacting by Darton *et al.* (1988), some of which are pictured in Fig. 18. For tray columns, usually used for this selective absorption duty, the value of Sel has been estimated to be 72 for operation at a superficial gas velocity of 1 m/s, and this selectivity value can be increased to 138 by operating at a superficial gas velocity of 2 m/s. The probable explanation for this increase is that by increasing the gas velocity, we shift the flow regime on the tray from the froth regime to the spray regime with consequent decrease of β and increase of k_g. Use of cyclone scrubbers (thin liquid films in contact with high gas velocity stream) yields a selectivity value of 175. Use of a novel co-current upflow swirl tube promises a selectivity value of 1,250; see Darton *et al.* (1988). This exercise shows how a careful study of the factors influencing β, k_g, and k_l can lead to clues on how to achieve improved selectivities by improved contactor configurations. The swirl tube contactor has commercial potential of replacing conventionally used sieve tray absorbers.

Considerations of intrinsic process safety often dictate the choice of β; we often desire to minimize the hold-up of hazardous materials in the reactor.

3. *Gas–Liquid–Solid Systems*

Here we need to choose both the solid particle size d_p and the ratio β. The considerations leading to the choices for these parameters are the

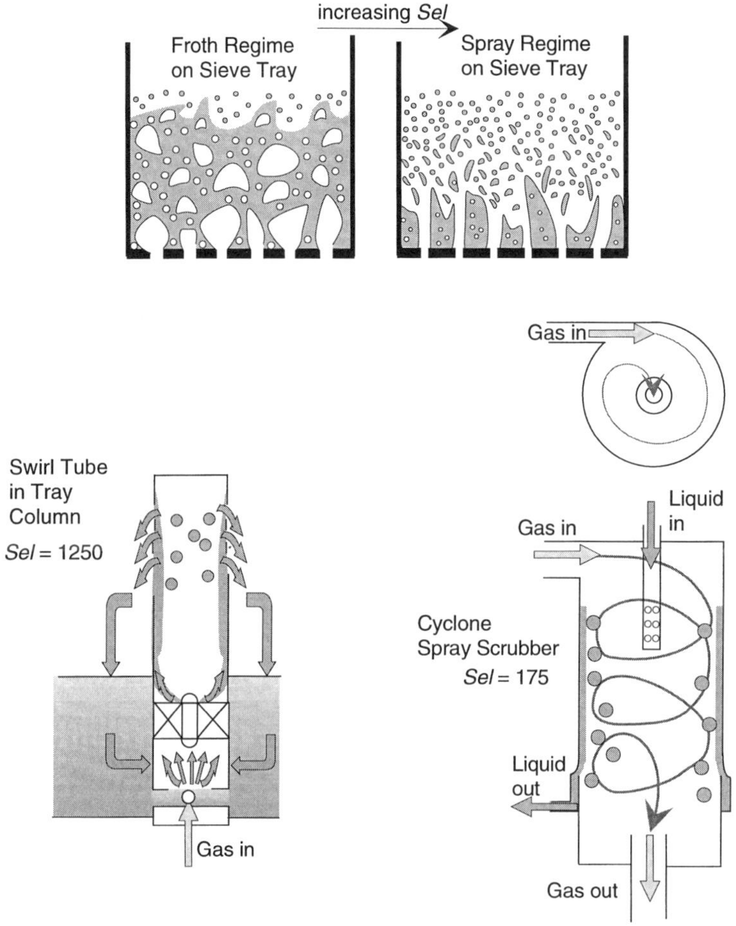

FIG. 18. Some contactors for selective absorption of hydrogen sulfide from carbon dioxide containing gaseous mixtures using amine solutions. Adapted from Darton *et al.* (1988).

same as before. If from a transport-reaction analysis we choose particle sizes smaller than 1 mm, we would need to consider slurry operations. On the other hand, if particle size larger than, say, 2 mm are allowable we have extra flexibility in choosing fixed-bed (e.g., trickle beds) or three-phase fluidized operations. The choice between fixed beds and three-phase fluid-bed operations can be further narrowed down by further analysis in subsets II and III.

4. *Liquid–Liquid Systems*

Let us assume that the reaction takes place in one of the phases say L2. The ideal choice for the parameter $\beta_{L2} \equiv \varepsilon_{L2}/\delta_{L2}a$ is dictated by the same considerations as for gas–liquid systems; *cf*. Fig. 17. To achieve high values of β_{L2} we should disperse phase L1 in the form of drops in the continuous phase L2. Low values of β_{L2} could be achieved by dispersing L2 in the form of drops in the continuous phase L1. Thin liquid film flow, as encountered in gas–liquid systems (*cf*. Fig. 16), though not impossible, is unusual in liquid–liquid systems.

Sometimes practical considerations override the decisions arrived at from a transport-reaction analysis. It is thus advisable to disperse corrosive liquid so as to reduce contact with the reactor walls. Hazardous liquid mixtures are usually dispersed so as to reduce their hold-up, even if this is contrary to conclusions reached from a transport-reaction analysis.

C. Reactor Subset II—Contacting Flow Pattern

This subset involves arriving at decisions on the following aspects of contacting of the individual phases.

(a) The ideal residence time distribution of the individual phases.
(b) For each reactant in the feed to the reactor, we need to evaluate whether it should be introduced at the reactor inlet or whether there is an incentive for progressive, staged addition.
(c) We also need to evaluate the incentives for *in situ* removal of one or more products from the reactor.
(d) The choice has to be made between the three main overall contacting methods: (i) countercurrent, (ii) co-current, and (iii) cross-current.

We consider each of the four items (a)–(d) in turn.

1. *Subset IIa: Ideal RTD of Individual Phases*

From the point of view of choosing the ideal reactor configuration, it is sufficient to decide whether we should aim for plug flow of a given phase or for a perfectly mixed state; this analysis is well covered in standard textbooks such as Levenspiel (1972). For isothermal reaction within a single phase, this decision is often governed by the desire to reduce the reactor volume required for achieving a specified conversion level; see Fig. 19. If we wish to maximize the intermediate A_2 in a consecutive

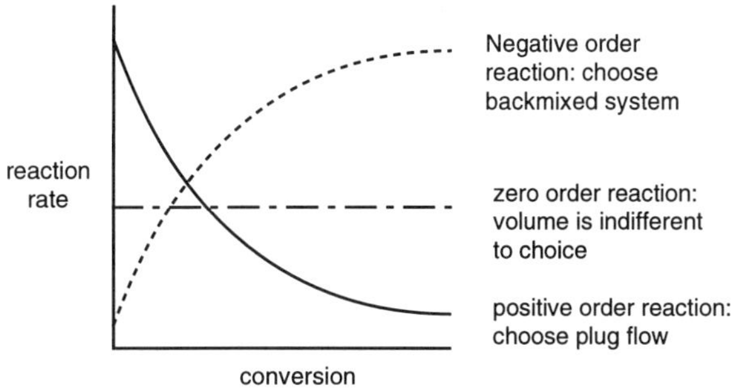

FIG. 19. Choice of residence time distribution for isothermal reactions of positive, zero, and negative order.

reaction scheme $A_1 \rightarrow A_2 \rightarrow A_3$ within a phase, we should aim for plug conditions (minimum axial dispersion); this conclusion is entirely analogous to the avoidance of intra-particle diffusion resistances (see Fig. 14).

For highly exothermic reactions, we usually have the dilemma: To mix or not to mix? From a concentration viewpoint we usually like to approach plug flow conditions, i.e., we do not wish to mix concentrations along the reactor. But from the point of view of temperatures, we would prefer a thermally well-mixed system. Let us consider the specific example of the oxidation of ethene to produce ethene oxide; see Fig. 20. This highly exothermic reaction is conventionally carried out in a cooled multi-tubular packed-bed reactor. Close to the inlet of the reactor we have a temperature peak (hot spot). At increasing temperatures there is loss of selectivity to ethene oxide because of the parallel, parasitic reaction to combustion products. The selectivity profile along the length is shown in Fig. 20; the temperature hot spot clearly leads to a loss of selectivity. Our systems approach leads to the conclusion that we ought to have a system with perfect thermal backmixing (from selectivity considerations) and no concentration backmixing (from the point of view of improved conversions). The question is: Can we achieve both? One solution to this problem is to incorporate a heat pipe on the outside of the tube wall of each packed tube that would help rapid axial thermal equilibration. Such a device has been suggested by Parent *et al.* (1983) for the oxidation of naphthalene to phthalic anhydride. Some of their key results have been summarized in Fig. 21; these show the remarkable improvement in the yield of the desired phthalic anhydride product due to near isothermal operation with heat pipes. Such systems need closer examination and further experimental study. Richardson *et al.* (1988) have incorporated a sodium heat pipe within an (endothermic) reforming reactor with the objective of approaching isothermal operation. This concept has potential application in fixed-

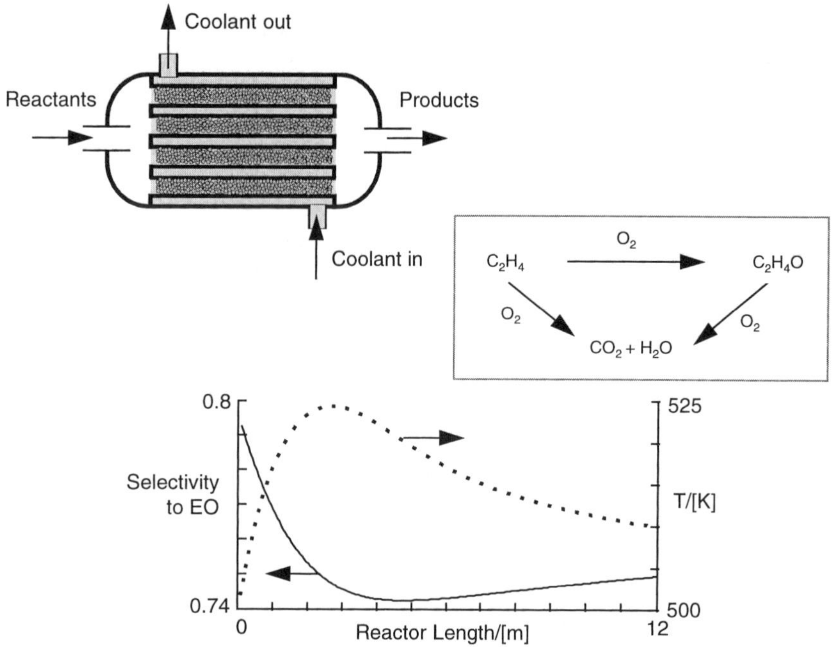

FIG. 20. Temperature and selectivity profiles for the exothermic reaction of oxidation of ethene to ethene oxide in a multi-tubular packed bed reactor. The selectivity to ethene oxide is defined as the number of moles of ethene oxide produced per mole of ethene converted. The simulations for the reactor temperature and selectivity were carried out using the kinetic data of Westerterp and Ptasinski (1984).

bed catalytic reforming where steep temperature gradients are experienced at the reactor inlet because of high endothermicity. Catalyst coking is usually a problem at the entrance to the bed. By using heat pipes to ensure temperature redistribution, we may limit this coking tendency and consequently lengthen cycle times.

Use of cold quench gases or evaporating solvents and recycle of solids are other options to obtain thermal equilibration. In the Du Pont process for production of maleic anhydride by oxidation of butane, a dense phase circulating bed riser reactor is used (Contractor and Sleight, 1988). Solids recycle allows catalyst regeneration and, further, ensures that isothermal conditions are approached. In order to avoid the attrition problems inherent with solids recycle systems, the catalyst may be coated with a thin layer of material such SiC or SiO_2. Circulating bed reactors have tremendous potential for carrying out exothermic gas–solid reactions, especially with deactivating catalysts (see Gianetto *et al.*, 1990); this potential is as yet largely untapped.

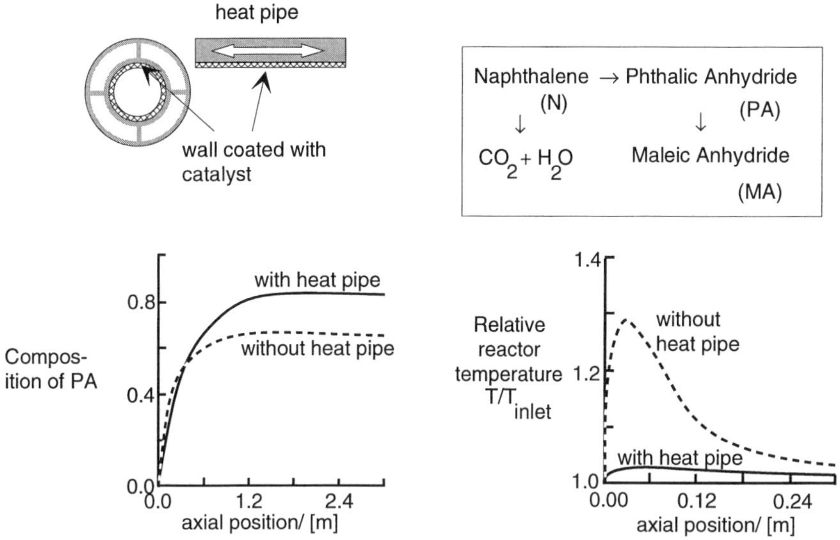

FIG. 21. Composition and temperature profiles in a tube-wall catalytic reactor, with and without heat pipe, for oxidation of napththalene to phthalic anhydride. Adapted from Parent *et al.* (1983).

2. *Subset IIb: Staged (Progressive) Injection of Reactant(s)*

As our first illustration we consider the co-dimerization of propene and butene to produce heptenes (Reaction 1). This reaction is accompanied by two competing, undesirable, reactions: dimerization of propene to hexene (Reaction 2), and dimerization of butene to octene (Reaction 3). The second reaction proceeds extremely rapidly and in order to suppress the formation of hexenes we should have progressive injection of propene into the reactor with all the butenes at the beginning of the operation, as is shown in Fig. 22 (Trambouze *et al.*, 1988).

Consider the process for manufacture of detergent alcohols (ALC) by hydroformylation of liquid olefins in the C_{11}–C_{12} range (OLF) with syngas

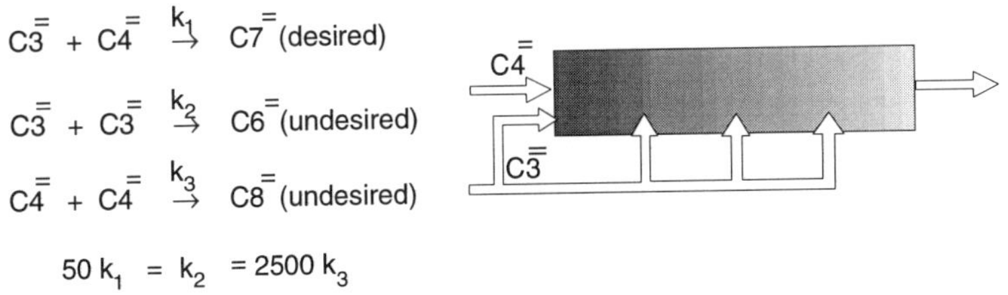

FIG. 22. Co-dimerization of propene and butene. For maximizing selectivity towards heptene we use progressive injection of propene.

(H_2 and CO), using homogeneous liquid-phase cobalt based catalyst. The reaction can be written as

$$\mathrm{OLF} + \mathrm{H_2} + \mathrm{CO} \rightarrow \mathrm{ALD} + \mathrm{H_2} \rightarrow \mathrm{ALC},$$

where ALD is the intermediate aldehyde. Side reactions to produce paraffins (PAR) and dimer alcohols ("heavy ends" = HE) are unavoidable in practice:

$$\mathrm{OLF} + \mathrm{H_2} \rightarrow \mathrm{PAR}; \qquad \mathrm{ALD} \xrightarrow[\text{condensation}]{\text{reaction}} \mathrm{HE}$$

In order to suppress the undesirable side reaction to paraffins, commercial operations employ an H_2/CO ratio lower than the stoichiometric value of 2 : 1. A commercial hydroformylation reactor train, whose configuration is sketched in Fig. 23a, was analyzed with a view to improving the selectivity to detergent alcohols. The systems approach described in this article was used to arrive at the "ideal" reactor configuration. The complete checklist of reactor attributes and subsets was analyzed with the help of a detailed kinetic model. The clue to selectivity improvement was found to lie in the use of staged, progressive addition of hydrogen. The split syngas addition scheme is shown in Fig. 23b. The existing (a) and suggested (b) schemes have the same reactor hardware designs and total feed streams. In the split syngas scheme (b), the first reactor in the train is fed with an $H_2/CO = 1.4$. The balance of hydrogen (to make up for the overall ratio $H_2/CO = 1.9$) is supplied to the subsequent stages 2, 3, 4, and 5, in equal proportions. Figure 23c provides a comparison of the schemes (a) and (b). The higher yield of alcohols in scheme (b) is to be attributed to the suppression of paraffin formation in the first reactor by reduced supply of H_2. The reduced paraffin production is translated into a concomitant increase in alcohol production. For the commercial unit that was studied, the improvement in the product slate had a value of \$2 million per annum. The split syngas injection scheme could be realized quite simply by use of an in-line membrane separator (the Monsanto PRISM separator) for readjustment of syngas composition by selective removal of hydrogen. The payout for the capital investment in the membrane separator was on the order of 6 months.

The hydroformylation case study just discussed underlines the economic incentives for careful examination of existing processes for possible improvements by altering reactor configuration.

We may also consider staged injection of one of the reactants as a method of "quenching" exothermic reactions; cold hydrogen gas quench is used, for example, in hydrocracking of vacuum gas oils.

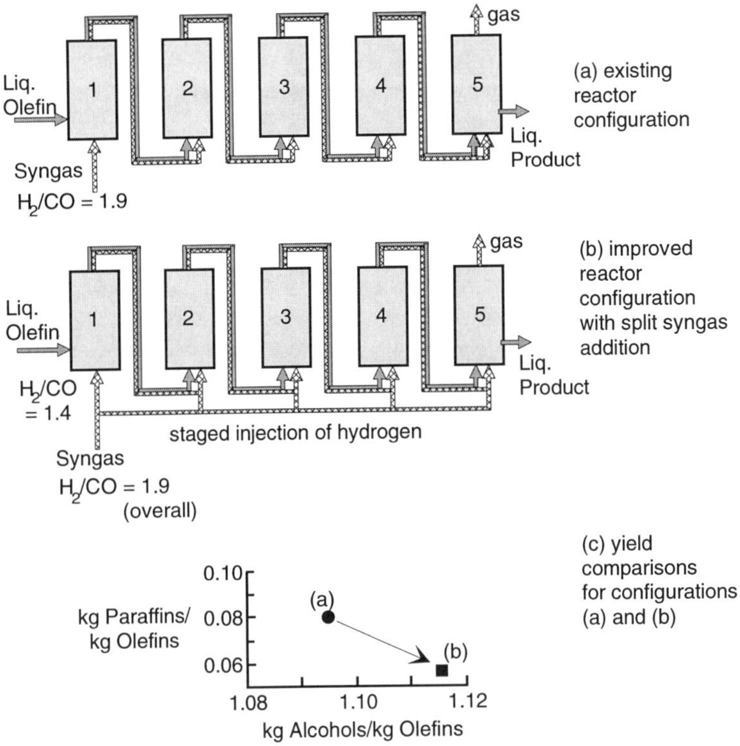

FIG. 23. Hydroformylation of liquid olefins (C_{11}–C_{12}) with syngas (H_2 and CO). (a) Configuration in existing commercial unit consisting of five bubble column reactors in series. (b) Improved configuration arrived at by systems approach, involving staged injection of hydrogen. (c) The yields of alcohols (desired product) and paraffins (undesired product) are compared for configurations (a) and (b).

In the examples just considered, one of the reactants was introduced in a progressive, staged manner. Pursuing this line of attack, we should examine the benefits in keeping the two reactants completely segregated from each other and allowing them to meet only within the pores of the catalyst. The active components of the catalyst could be incorporated within a ceramic membrane with the reactants on either side. Figure 24 shows the schematic diagram of such a catalytic membrane reactor for carrying out the Claus reaction (Sloot *et al.*, 1990):

$$2H_2S + SO_2 \leftrightarrow \tfrac{3}{8}S_8 + 2H_2O.$$

This novel reactor type has specific advantages for chemical processes requiring strict adherence of the feed rates to the reaction stoichiometry. The reaction plane within the catalyst membrane would shift in such a

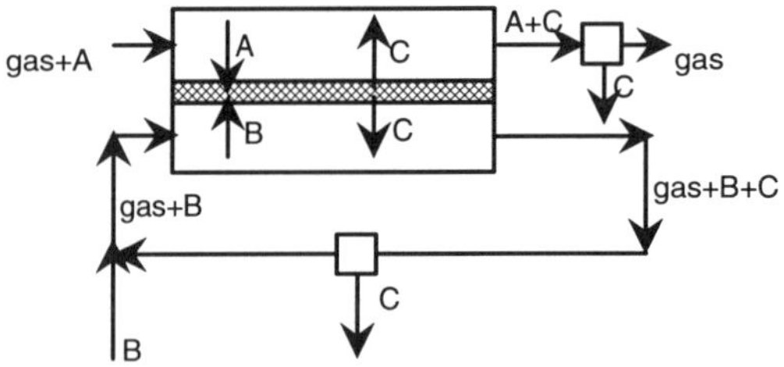

FIG. 24. Catalytic membrane reactor for carrying out the Claus reaction: $2H_2S + SO_2 \leftrightarrow \frac{3}{8}S_8 + 2H_2O$. Adapted from Sloot *et al.* (1990).

manner that the molar fluxes of the reactants across the membrane are always in the stoichiometric ratio; this allows greater flexibility of the reactor to feed rates of hydrogen sulfide and sulfur dioxide. The practical feasibility of this novel concept has been demonstrated by Sloot *et al.* (1990). This concept has also been suggested by Van Swaaij and co-workers (see Sloot, 1991) for catalytic reduction of nitric oxide with ammonia; by keeping the reactants separated and allowing reaction only within the membrane, we will be able to cope with varying ratios of concentration of nitric oxide and ammonia without incurring significant slip of reactants.

Another class of processes where it is advantageous to keep the reactants separated from each other, except within the catalyst pores, is oxidation of light gaseous hydrocarbons (e.g., ethene, propene, butene). Conventionally these processes are carried out in multi-tubular fixed-bed reactors (see, for example, Fig. 20). Flammability considerations usually restrict the feed mixture composition. By adopting the concept of a multi-tubular cooled catalytic membrane reactor (with inclusion of heat pipes?), with reactants kept separate, we should be able to avoid any flammability constraints.

3. *Subset IIc: In Situ Separation of Product(s) from Reactor Zone*

The main reasons for considering *in situ* removal of product(s) from the reaction zone are (i) to enhance conversion in equilibrium limited reactions by shifting the equilibrium towards the right, (ii) to prevent further, undesirable, reaction of products and consequently improve selectivity, and (iii) as a remedy for product-inhibited reactions. The various techniques that can be considered for selective product removal are discussed next.

a. Deliberate Addition of Second Liquid Phase. By deliberate addition of a second liquid phase containing a selective solvent, we may extract the desired product from the reaction zone and prevent further side reactions.

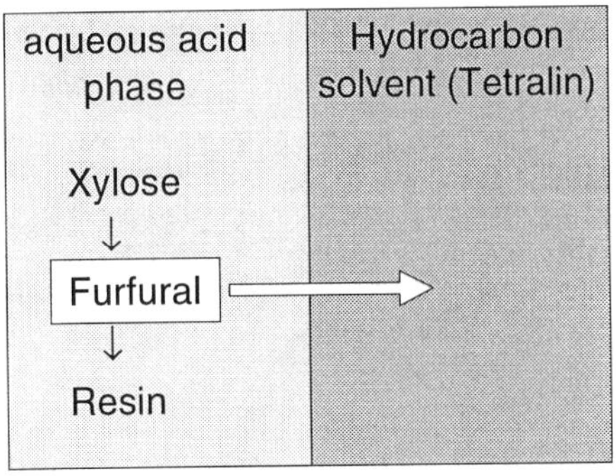

FIG. 25. *In situ* extraction of intermediate furfural (desirable product) by means of hydrocarbon solvent (tetralin).

Figure 25 shows a specific example of extraction of furfural using a hydrocarbon solvent. Sharma (1988) has considered several other examples of reactions which would profit from introduction of an additional phase. Sharma (1988) has also provided several examples of liquid–liquid reactions of industrial interest which could benefit from the addition of substances such as quaternary ammonium and phosphonium salts, crown ethers and trialkyl amines, which function as phase transfer catalysts, significantly enhancing the reaction rates and in some cases improving the reaction selectivity.

b. In Situ Distillation. The technique of reactive distillation is well known for carrying out esterification reactions (Doherty and Buzad, 1992). This concept has gained considerable attention recently for carrying out catalyzed liquid-phase reactions; the catalyst in this case is usually incorporated in the form of a structured packing. Figure 26 shows a schematic diagram of the catalytic distillation concept for the production of tertiary amyl ether (TAME). The rectifying section is packed with catalyst "bales"—a kind of rolled-up structured packing. Another alternative is to incorporate the catalyst in the form of a thin coating on conventionally used structured packing material, e.g., from Sulzer. There is considerable scope for equipment development here. For example, we may envisage suspending the catalyst in the form of "tea bags" within the froth zone of a distillation tray.

In situ product separation by distillation offers applications in esterification (e.g., for ethyl acetate), trans-esterification (e.g., for butyl acetate), hydrolysis (e.g., for ethylene glycol, isopropyl alcohol), metathesis (e.g., for methyl oleate), etherification (e.g., for MTBE, ETBE, TAME), and alkylation reactions (e.g., for cumene).

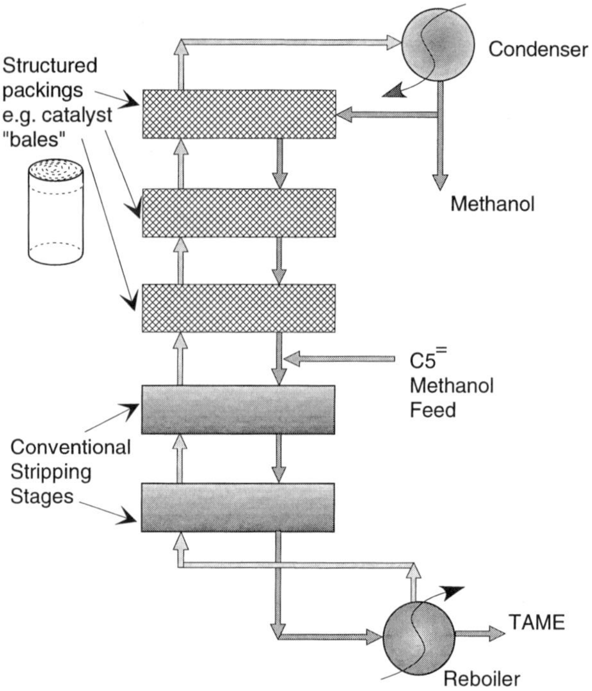

FIG. 26. Catalytic distillation scheme for tertiary amyl ether (TAME) manufacture.

c. In Situ Adsorption. A novel reactor concept suggested by Van Swaaij and Westerterp involves the use of a solid adsorbent, in trickle phase through a packed catalytic reactor, for selective removal of a product; see Fig. 27. This concept has been demonstrated experimentally by Kuczynski (1986) for synthesis of methanol, an equilibrium-limited reaction.

Another possibility for *in situ* adsorption is to fluidize both catalyst and adsorbent phases (i.e., gas–solid–solid fluidized bed or gas–liquid–solid–solid fluidized bed). We may, for example, envisage a *four*-phase methanol synthesis process where the liquid phase, containing an inert hydrocarbon solvent, would serve as a thermal flywheel for this highly exothermic reaction.

d. In Situ Supercritical Extraction. In equilibrium-limited biocatalyzed reactions, removal of the desired products, which are often thermally labile, *in situ* by supercritical extraction with carbon dioxide can lead to substantial benefits. In the lipase-catalyzed interesterification of triglycerides, for example, a high degree of incorporation of required fatty acids into triglyceride cannot be obtained because of its reverse reaction: Tricaprylin

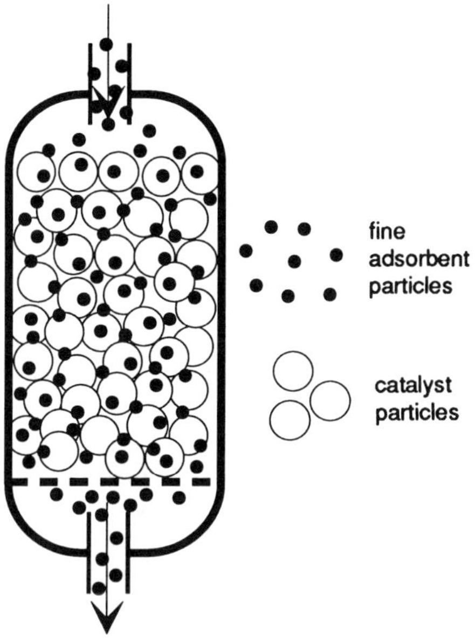

FIG. 27. Gas–solid–solid trickle flow reactor concept for *in situ* adsorption of product.

+ methyl oleate ↔ 1-oleodicaprylin + 1,3-dioleocaprylin + methyl caprylate. Adschiri *et al.* (1992) have applied supercritical carbon dioxide extraction to the removal of products from a liquid-phase reaction system as a means of solving the problem.

e. Membrane Reactor for Selective Removal of Product. A permselective ceramic membrane-walled tubular catalytic reactor can be considered for carrying out dehydrogenation reactions; the membrane serves to selectively remove the hydrogen, thus shifting the equilibrium towards the right. This concept is shown schematically in Fig. 28. An experimental study by Becker *et al.* (1993) has shown that use of this concept for dehydrogenation of ethyl benzene results in a 20% increase conversion over conventional fixed-bed operation. Other reactions where the use of permselective membranes in catalytic reactors can be expected to lead to significant improvements include dehydrogenations of propane, butane, and cyclohexane. A survey of potential applications of inorganic membrane reactors is given by Hsieh (1991).

4. *Subset IId: Counter-, Co-, or Cross-Current Contacting*

The decision whether to adopt counter-, co-, or cross-current contacting (see Fig. 9) is dictated by factors such as equilibrium limitations, flooding,

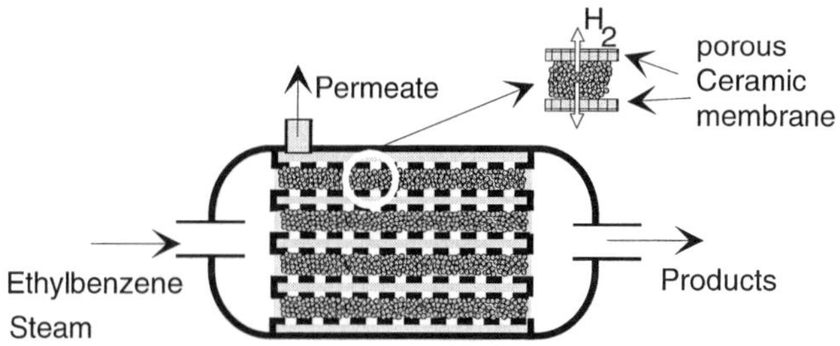

FIG. 28. Permselective membrane reactor concept for dehydrogenation of ethyl benzene to produce styrene.

and pressure drop. For gas–solid moving-bed systems the three possible modes of operation are shown in Fig. 29. Co-current downflow and cross-current moving beds are most commonly used, with the latter configuration (with radial inflow of gas) being preferred in order to reduce the pressure drop. The continuous catalyst regeneration (CCR) technology for reforming of naphtha using Pt-based catalysts uses this cross-current concept. One potential problem which may be encountered during scale-up of such reactors is the pinning of the catalyst particles to the screens; this aspect limits the allowable gas velocities. Also, catalyst attrition may cause problems such as blockage of solids flow and can cause excessive pressure drop.

For gas treatment applications such as absorption of CO_2, H_2S, and COS using amines where high conversion levels are usually desired, it is common to adopt countercurrent operation from considerations of phase and reaction equilibrium.

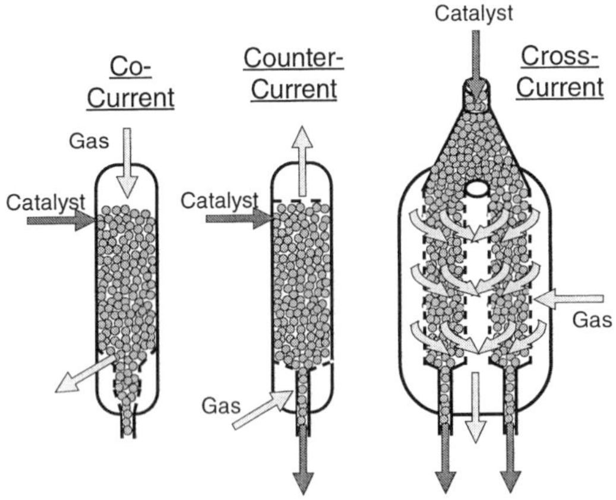

FIG. 29. Co-, counter-, and cross-current contacting for moving-bed gas–solid reactors.

For gas–liquid–solid systems, the commonly used contacting patterns are sketched in Fig. 30. Generally speaking we should anticipate several scale-up problems for three-phase reactors wherein solids are being transported (e.g., for reasons of catalyst deactivation). But the perception of these problems by different development groups could be quite different, resulting in different choices of reactor configurations. This is illustrated quite nicely by the hydrodemetalization (HDM) process. For this application the following widely different configurations are in use, or under development Dautzenberg and De Deken, 1984):

- Fixed trickle beds with co-current down flow of gas and liquid (Fig. 30a)
- Moving beds with co-current down flow of gas and liquid (Shell HYCON process; Fig. 30c)
- Moving beds with co-current up flow of gas and liquid (IFP process; Fig. 30d)
- Three-phase fluidized beds (also called ebullating beds) with particle sizes usually larger than 1.5 mm (Fig. 30g)
- Slurry reactors with fine particles, usually smaller than 1 mm (Fig. 30f).

It is interesting to note the sharp contrast between the options in Fig. 30c and 30d used respectively by Shell and Institut Français du Pétrôle (IFP), respectively. The Shell moving trickle bed technology (HYCON) for HDM was introduced for commercial operation in The Netherlands in 1989; this technology involves co-current downflow of gas, liquid, and catalyst phases. Engineers at IFP have opted for a different solution with upflow of gas and liquid phases. Any fine particles generated by attrition would be fluidized and transported out of the reactor. The two different approaches highlight the different perceptions of Shell and IFP with regard to potential scale-up problems.

In the Shell Middle Distillates Synthesis (SMDS) process starting from natural gas, the reactor configuration chosen for the first commercial unit in Malaysia, successfully commercialized in 1993, is the multi-tubular downflow trickle bed with catalyst inside the tubes (Sie *et al.*, 1991); see Fig. 30e. Because of the enormous exothermicity of the synthesis reaction and the relatively poor heat transfer an extremely large heat transfer area is required. The reactor volume is largely governed by the installable heat transfer area in a vessel of given volume. Use of the multi-tubular three-phase fluidized bed or slurry reactor (see Fig. 30k and 30l) provides much better heat transfer characteristics (an improvement of a factor of five over fixed bed units) and could lead to considerably lower reactor volumes. However, the anticipated scale-up problems with three-phase

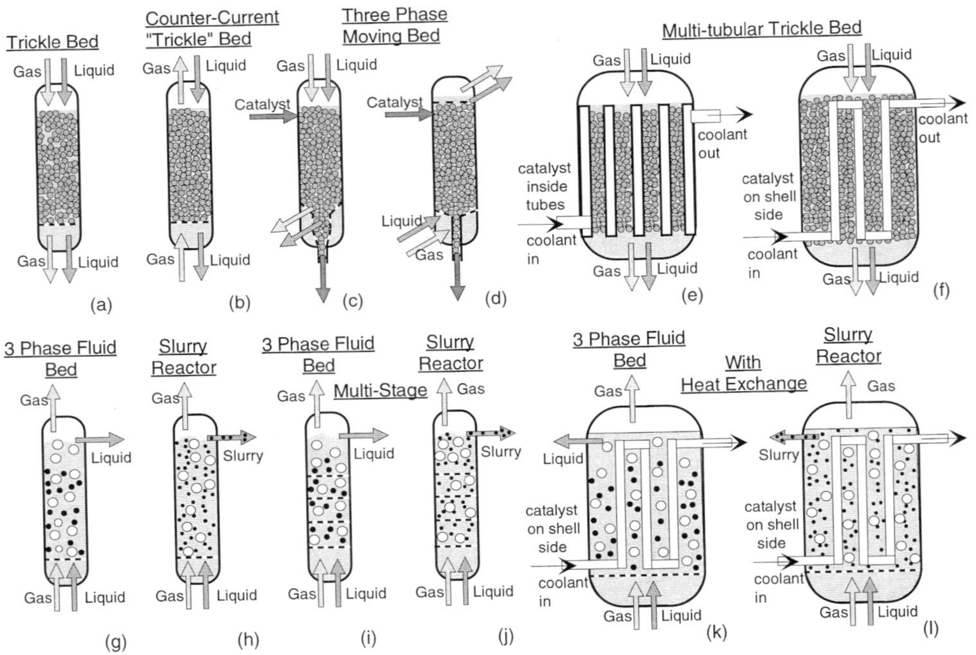

FIG. 30. Contacting patterns and contactor types for gas–liquid–solid reactors. (a) Co-current downflow trickle bed. (b) Countercurrent flow trickle bed. (c) Co-current downflow of gas, liquid, and catalyst. (d) Downflow of catalyst and co-current upflow of gas and liquid. (e) Multi-tubular trickle bed with co-current flow of gas and liquid down tubes with catalyst packed inside them; coolant on shell side. (f) Multi-tubular trickle bed with downflow of gas and liquid; coolant inside the tubes. (g) Three-phase fluidized bed of solids with solids-free freeboard. (h) Three-phase slurry reactor with no solids-free freeboard. (i) Three-phase fluidized beds with horizontally disposed internals to achieve staging. (j) Three-phase slurry reactor with horizontally disposed internals to achieve staging. (k) Three-phase fluidized bed in which cooling tubes have been inserted; coolant inside the tubes. (l) Three-phase slurry reactor in which cooling tubes have been inserted; coolant inside the tubes.

fluidized-bed operation were of overriding concern for Shell, who decided to adopt the fixed-bed technology because of quicker development scenario. The lead time for development of processes in the petroleum and petrochemical industries is usually of the order of a decade, and for first-of-a-kind technology such as the SMDS process there is an incentive to adopt a sure, safe, and quicker process development route.

For aromatic hydrogenations, co-current downflow in fixed trickle beds is normally used, but as pointed out by Trambouze (1990), there are distinct advantages in opting for countercurrent operation because of equilibrium considerations. Hydrocracking of vacuum gas oil is another process traditionally carried out in co-current downflow in fixed beds in trickle flow. Higher conversions are possible with a countercurrent hydrocracking operation. Problems with countercurrent operation, however, are excessive pressure drop and flooding limitations. To overcome these problems we need to consider larger-sized (say, 5 mm) "shaped" catalysts in the form of Raschig rings or Berle saddles (Trambouze, 1990).

D. Reactor Subset III—Choice of Flow Regimes

1. *Gas–Solid Systems*

The various flow regimes for gas–solid systems are shown in Fig. 4. The first major decision is whether to keep the solids fixed (in a packed bed) or to move the solids in a moving bed or fluidized bed (see Fig. 11). This choice is largely dictated by catalyst deactivation kinetics and the time interval between successive regenerations. If this time interval is of the order of one year, fixed-bed operation is usually preferred. If the time interval is of the order of one week we usually opt for swing-type operation using two beds; swing operation is, for example, used in the regenerative naphtha reforming technology. If the time interval between successive regenerations is of the order of a few hours, then moving-bed operations can be considered, such as in the continuous catalytic regeneration (CCR) technology for naphtha reforming. If the time between successive regenerations is of the order of less than one hour, then fluidized-bed operation is appropriate. The decision to transport the solids to and from the reactor is a crucial one because solids motion introduces several complications such as attrition and blockage. If the catalyst is expensive (e.g., Pt-based), it is usually not advisable to fluidize it because of inevitable losses through cyclones.

Other reasons, distinct from catalyst deactivation, for choosing fluidized-bed operation could be the desire to use particles smaller than, say,

1 mm (such particles are usually not allowable in packed- or moving-bed operation because of excessive pressure drop). Sometimes, the desire to have a completely thermally backmixed system (Subset II) would dictate the use of bubbling or circulating fluidized beds. This is the case for combustion of coke from deactivated FCC catalyst. Traditionally, FCC regenerator designs have adopted the bubbling fluid bed regime (R-2 in Fig. 11), because of the good backmixing of the emulsion phase. However, the major disadvantage of bubbling bed regenerator designs is oxygen slip due to poor mass transfer from bubbles; deep beds typically 8 m in height are required even for moderate conversion levels of about 90%. The "fast" fluidization regime, which is the current choice for FCC regenerator operation, has vastly superior gas-to-solid mass transfer characteristics and is the regime currently favored for newer designs. The choice of an "ideal" regime of operation for the FCC regenerator cap be rationalized by an analysis of the gas-to-solid mass transfer characteristics of the regimes R-2, R-4, and R-5 of Fig. 11. For typical operating conditions in the FCC regenerator, the values of the overall volumetric mass transfer coefficient per reactor volume, $k_g a$, have been estimated; these are shown in Fig. 31 along with the pseudo first-order reaction rate constant for reaction of

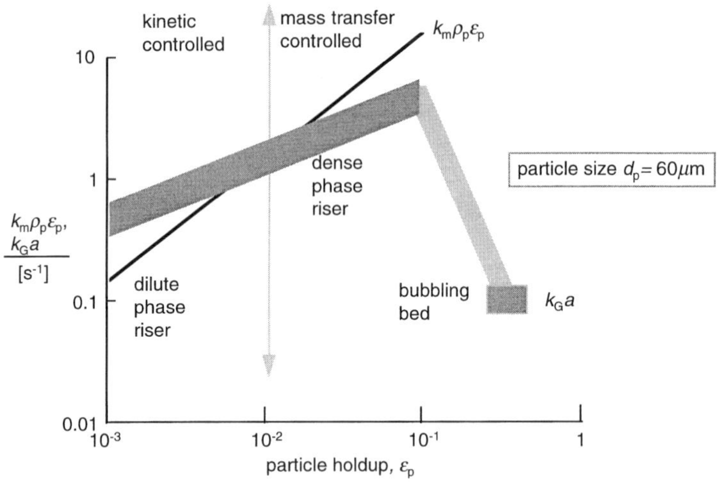

FIG. 31. Gas-to-solid mass transfer characteristics of various regimes of operation for FCC regenerators. R-2, R-4, and R-4 refer to the regimes sketched in Fig. 11. The kinetic data for coke burn off is taken from Hano *et al.* (1975). The gas–solids mass transfer coefficient for riser reactors is estimated from the Van der Ham *et al.* (1993) correlation. The estimation of volumetric mass transfer coefficient in fluid beds is from the model of Krishna (1981). Further details of the calculations presented in this figure can be found in Krishna (1993).

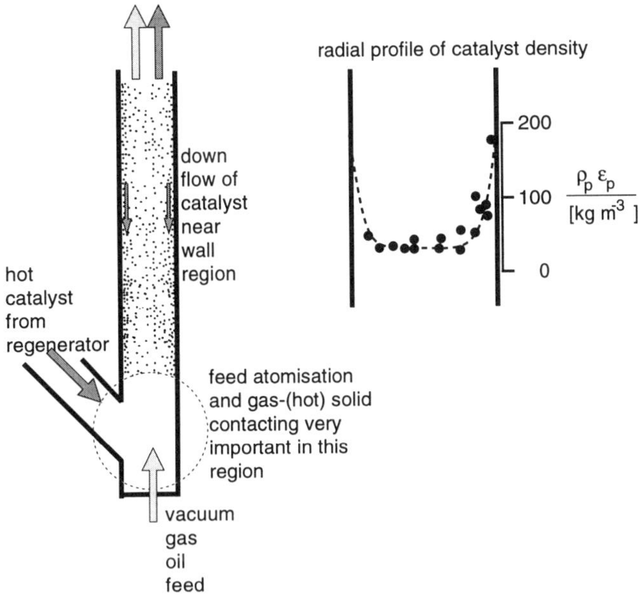

FIG. 32. FCC riser hydrodynamics. The solids concentration near the wall is considerably higher than at the center. Radial catalyst density profile measurements of Schuurmans (1980).

oxygen with coke: $k_m \rho_p \varepsilon_p$. In the bubbling bed regime R-2, the reaction of oxygen with coke is governed by interphase mass transfer, while in dense- and dilute-phase riser transport, regimes R-4 and R-5, respectively, the reaction is kinetically controlled. Despite the large uncertainty in estimation of the $k_g a$ values, it is clear from Fig. 31 that the overall rate of reaction of oxygen is highest at particle hold-ups in the range 0.2–0.3, i.e., in the dense-phase riser transport ("fast" fluidization) regime. This explains the reason why modern regenerators adopt the fast fluidization regime. There is, however, a large degree of uncertainty in the scale-up of circulating dense-phase fluid beds. For the cracking reactor in FCC operations we should aim for pure plug flow of gas and catalyst in order to prevent overcracking of gasoline to light gases. Since backmixing of catallyst is undesirable, the dilute-phase riser transport regime, R-5 of Fig. 11, is normally chosen as the reactor configuration. A closer examination of the riser hydrodynamics (see Fig. 32) reveals that the concentration of solids near the wall of the riser is significantly higher than at the center and there is downflow of catalyst near the wall (Schuurmans, 1980). This higher catalyst concentration in the wall region leads to overcracking. There is a great economic incentive to devise a reactor configuration with a closer approach to plug flow of catalyst. One possible solution is to have co-current downflow of gas and catalyst in the reactor, i.e., a "downer." Other aspects of FCC operation which need attention are better feed atomization and gas–solid contacting at the feed inlet. We may consider pre-fluidization of the hot solids before allowing contact with liquid feed.

2. *Gas–Liquid Systems*

For upflow of gas through liquids, in vertical columns, there is complete correspondence of flow regimes; see Fig. 33. The analogue of the homogeneous fluidization regime is the homogeneous bubbly flow regime. The bubbling fluid bed operation has a complete parallel in the churn turbulent regime in gas–liquid systems (see Krishna, 1993). The choice between the various gas–liquid regimes, therefore, parallels the analysis for gas–solid systems; with increasing reaction rate, our regime choice moves from left to right in Fig. 33. One possible starting point in the choice of the flow regime is consideration of the parameter β, already chosen in Subset I. Regimes to the left of the flow regime map of Fig. 33 correspond to high β (the choice for relatively slow liquid-phase reactions), whereas towards the right we have low β values (a choice for high rates of liquid-phase reactions). To achieve low β values we could, for example, operate in the spray regime in a tray column (see, e.g., Fig. 18). The

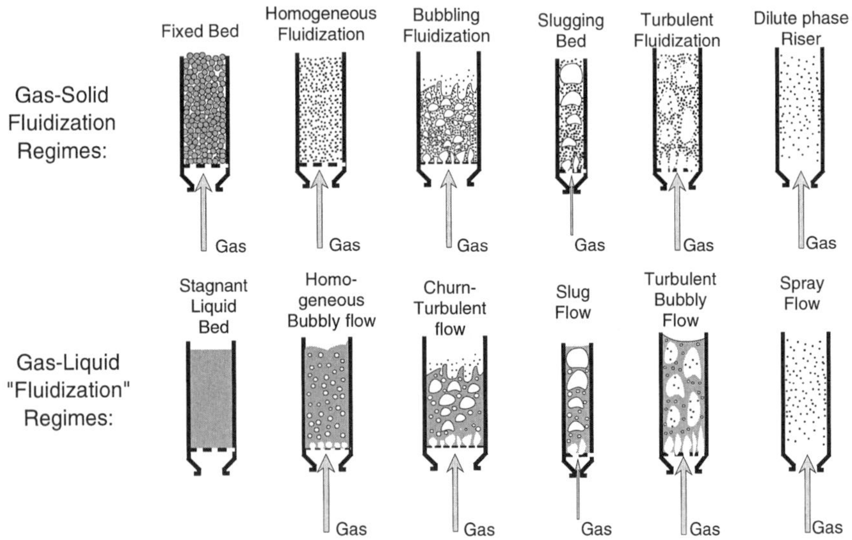

FIG. 33. Gas–solid and gas–liquid flow regimes in vertical columns with upflow of gas.

analogue of the turbulent or "fast" fluidization regime of gas–solids flow is the regime called turbulent bubbly flow in Fig. 33; this is the regime prevalent in air lift fermentors, for example. In air lift fermentors we aim for good gas–liquid mass transfer to prevent oxygen depletion in the liquid phase. Both turbulent, or "fast," fluidization and turbulent bubbly flow regimes are gaining importance for similar reasons: They have superior mass transfer characteristics. A deeper appreciation of the analogies between gas–solid and gas–liquid systems will be helpful in reactor selection and could facilitate scale-up (Krishna, 1993).

While in the foregoing we have stressed the analogies between gas–solid and gas–liquid flow regimes, there are some important practical differences in the hydrodynamics of these systems. The operating window for the homogeneous fluidization regime for gas–solid systems is extremely narrow, and it is normally not possible to design a commercial reactor to operate in a stable manner in this regime. The situation is somewhat different for gas–liquid systems; the homogeneous bubbly flow regime is a common choice for gas–liquid systems because of the much wider operating window with respect to gas velocity. The churn-turbulent flow regime of gas–liquid flow is characterized by the presence of large fast-rising bubbles, typically 50 mm in size, co-existing with small, about 5 mm sized, bubbles (Krishna *et al.*, 1993). These fast-rising bubbles, akin to the bubbles in a gas–solids fluid bed, cause the contents of the reactor to be churned up (i.e., backmixed) and reduce the efficiency of gas–liquid contact. At the regime transition point we should experience a sharp decrease in the reactor performance; this is indeed found to be the case in practice for the Fischer Tropsch synthesis reaction where the liquid phase additionally contains fine catalyst particles (see Fig. 34). The importance of properly selecting the flow regime is demonstrated by this example.

3. *Gas–Liquid–Solid Systems*

Here the solid phase could be a catalyst or an inert packing material. If the solid phase is the catalyst, the first question to answer is whether to transport the solids or not; the considerations leading to this decision are entirely analogous to those for the gas-catalyst system and relate to the time interval between successive regenerations. If it is decided not to transport the solids i.e., to choose fixed beds, we have the following options (see also Fig. 30):

(i) Co-current downflow of gas and liquid,
(ii) Co-current upflow of gas and liquid, and
(iii) Countercurrent flow of gas and liquid.

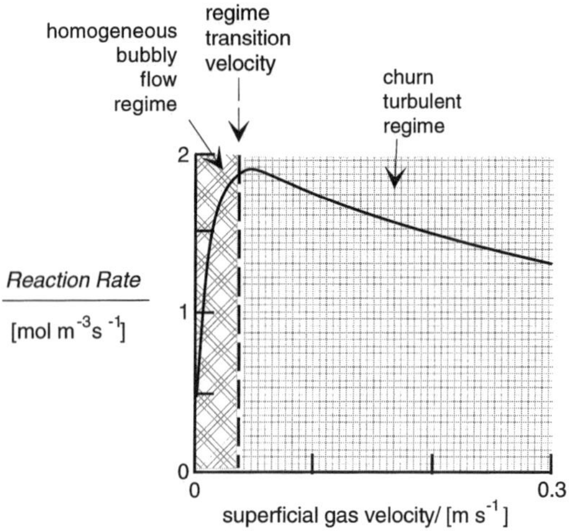

FIG. 34. Rate of reaction of syngas (A = CO + H_2) as a function of superficial gas velocity for Fischer–Tropsch synthesis in the slurry phase. Adapted from Krishna (1993).

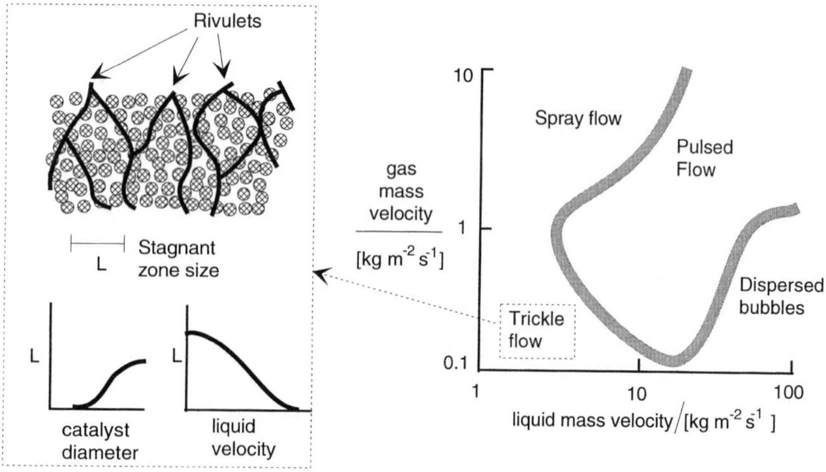

FIG. 35. Flow regime map for co-current downflow of gas and liquid through packed beds.

Let us first consider co-current downflow of gas and liquid (Fig. 30a); for this case the flow regime map is shown in Fig. 35. The most commonly used regime of operation is the trickling flow regime. To achieve good wetting of catalyst, the superficial liquid velocity has to be of the order of 10 mm/s (see Trambouze *et al.*, 1988). Another possible solution to overcome the problem of liquid stagnancy in trickle beds is to increase the gas velocity and operate under pulsing flow conditions. For laboratory columns operating in the pulsing flow regime, it has been shown that the stagnant zones are swept away by the pulses (Blok *et al.*, 1983), resulting in better contacting and mass transfer. It is, however, not certain that commercial units, typically of diameters greater than 2 m, can be made to operate in the pulsing flow regime. Another aspect which needs to be taken into account when choosing the flow regime of operation is the influence of system pressure on flow regime transitions. Increased-pressure operation tends to stabilize the trickle flow regime, and the transition to the pulsing flow regime is "delayed" (Wammes, 1990).

Another strategy to avoid the wetting and stagnancy problems associated with co-current downward trickle flow is to opt for co-current upflow; the various flow regimes are shown in Fig. 36 (Shah, 1979). We normally choose the bubble flow regime. The IFP technology for HDM utilizes this regime of operation.

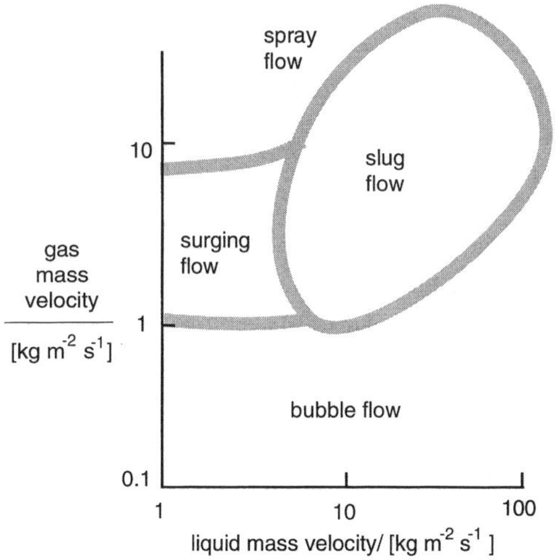

FIG. 36. Flow regimes in co-current upflow of gas and liquid through a packed bed of solids. Adapted from Shah (1979).

The analysis in Subset II may point to the choice of countercurrent operation through a packed bed. The most commonly used regimes here are trickle flow and bubble flow. The possibility of flooding places an important constraint on the choice of the operating gas and liquid flow velocities. The pressure drop is significant for small catalyst particles; this precludes countercurrent operation unless shaped catalyst particles are used.

Three-phase fluidized beds and slurry reactors (see Figs. 30g–l) in which the solid catalyst is suspended in the liquid usually operate under conditions of homogeneous bubbly flow or churn turbulent flow (see regime map in Fig. 33). The presence of solids alters the bubble hydrodynamics to a significant extent. In recent years there has been considerable research effort on the study of the hydrodynamics of such systems (see, e.g., Fan, 1989). However, the scale-up aspects of such reactors are still a mater of some uncertainty, especially for systems with high solids concentration and operations at increased pressures; it is for this reason that the Shell Middle Distillate Synthesis process adopts the multi-tubular trickle bed reactor concept (*cf.* Fig. 30e). The even distribution of liquid to thousands of tubes packed with catalyst, however poses problems of a different engineering nature.

IV. Closing Remarks

In this article we have advocated the use of a systematic, structured approach to reactor selection. The reactor selection exercise is conveniently split into three, separate, sequential decisions on the following subsets, or attributes:

Subset I: Volume-to-surface area of each phase

Subset II: Contacting flow pattern of the phases

Subset III: Multiphase flow regimes.

For each of these subsets we have further provided a checklist of reactor parameters that need to be examined. The choice of each item in the checklist is made on the basis of a wish list, set up right at the beginning of the reactor selection exercise. Figure 37 presents a summary of the reactor attributes and considerations along with a commonly used "wish" list. In the discussions we have stressed the point that a disciplined approach may unravel novel ways of improving reactor performance; this has been demonstrated by means of several examples.

Wish List

- *ease of scale-up*
- *ease of operation*
- *freedom from instabilities and runaways*
- *environmental acceptability*
- *maximum conversion of reactants*
- *maximum selectivity to desired products*
- *low capital and operating costs*
- *intrinsically safe process*
- *minimum hold up of hazardous materials*

Reactor Attributes	Considerations
Reactor Sub Set I: (Volume/Surface area)	- effectiveness factor - influence of intra-particle transport on selectivity - thermal stability - gas-liquid reaction regime (slow, fast pseudo first order or instantaneous)
Reactor Sub Set II Contacting Flow Pattern	
(a) Ideal RTD of each phase	- To mix or not to mix ? thermal stability - selectivity in complex reaction sequence
(b) Staged injection of reactants	- selectivity - thermal quenching - flammability limits
(c) In-situ separation of products from reaction zone	- shift reaction equil-ibrium -selectivity
(d) Counter-, Co- or Cross-current contacting	-reaction equilibrium -pressure drop -flooding - catalyst deactivation and frequency of regeneration
Reactor Sub Set III Choice of Flow Regime - packed/moving bed - homogeneous G-S fluidization = bubbly flow in G-L systems - heterogeneous G-S fluidization = churn turbulent flow in G-L systems - circulating G-S fluid bed = air lift G-L reactor - G-S riser transport = G-L spray system	- realisation of decisions in SubSets I and II - interphase transfer - heat removal capability - backmixing character-istics of individual phases - scale-up know-how - catalyst deactivation rates and frequency of regeneration

FIG. 37. Summary of reactor selection methodology. The "wish" list is used to arrive at various "decisions" on the three reactor subsets. In arriving at the decisions there are several reactor engineering parameters which need to be taken into account; these are listed under "considerations."

The systems approach presented here has been mainly developed for application within the petroleum and petrochemical industries and, therefore, is restricted to continuous "steady-state" processing on a large scale. It is worthwhile examining the extension of these concepts to unsteady-state processing and batch operations. Also, there may be other ways to structure the reactor selection problem to suit one's own work environment and technology culture.

Notation

a	interfacial area per unit reactor volume, m^{-1}
d_p	particle diameter, m
C_A^*	molar concentration of component A which is in equilibrium with the bulk gas phase, mol m^{-3}
C_{Bb}	molar concentration of liquid phase component B, mol m^{-3}
D_{eff}	effective diffusivity within catalyst particle, $m^2\ s^{-1}$
D_l	liquid-phase diffusivity, $m^2\ s^{-1}$
E	enhancement factor for gas–liquid reaction
F	dimensionless parameter $F \equiv (D_{Bl}C_{Bb})/(D_{Al}C_A^*)$
H_{CO_2}	Henry coefficient for CO_2, mol m^{-3} Pa^{-1}
Ha	Hatta number $Ha \equiv \sqrt{k_1 D_l}/k_l$
k_g	gas-phase mass transfer coefficient, ms^{-2}
k_1	pseudo first-order reaction rate constant for homogeneous liquid-phase reaction, s^{-1}
k_l	liquid-phase mass transfer coefficient, ms^{-1}
k_m	pseudo first-order reaction rate constant for catalytic reaction, defined per kilogram of catalyst, $m^3\ kg^{-1}\ s^{-1}$
L	characteristic length of particle, m
NTU	number of overall gas phase mass transfer units
R	gas constant, 8.314 J mol^{-1} K^{-1}
Sel	Selectivity for absorption of hydrogen sulfide from a gaseous mixture in presence of carbon dioxide
S_p	external surface area of particle, m^2
T	temperature, K
ΔT_{max}	maximum temperature rise in catalyst pellet, K
T_o	surface temperature of catalyst pellet, K
V_p	volume of particle, m^3

Greek Letters

β ratio of liquid phase volume to volume of diffusion layer $\beta \equiv \epsilon_l/\delta_l a$
δ_l thickness of diffusion layer of liquid phase $\delta_l \equiv D_l/k_l$, m
ε_l fractional hold-up of liquid phase
ε_p particle hold-up
η effectiveness factor of catalyst particle
ρ_p particle density, kg m^{-3}
τ residence time, s
ϕ Thiele modulus for spherical particle

$$\phi \equiv \frac{d_\mathrm{p}}{2}\sqrt{\frac{k_\mathrm{m}\rho_\mathrm{p}}{D_\mathrm{eff}}}$$

ϕ_gen generalized Thiele modulus

$$\phi_\mathrm{gen} \equiv \frac{V_\mathrm{p}}{S_\mathrm{p}}\sqrt{\frac{k_\mathrm{m}\rho_\mathrm{p}}{D_\mathrm{eff}}}$$

Subscripts

A referring to component A, usually in gas phase
B referring to component B, usually in liquid phase
eff effective parameter
g referring to gas phase
gen generalized parameter
l referring to liquid phase
L1, L2 referring to the two phases in liquid–liquid systems
p referring to particle
1 pseudo first-order parameter

Superscript

$*$ referring to equilibrium value

References

Adschiri, T., Akiya, H., and Chin, L. C., *J. Chem. Engng. Japan* **25**, 104 (1992).
Adaje, J., and Sheintuch, M., *Chem. Engng Sci.* **45**, 1331 (1990).
Astarita, G., Savage, D. W., and Bisio, A., "Gas Treating with Chemical Solvents." Wiley-Interscience, New York, 1983.

Becker, Y. L., Dixon, A. G., Moser, W. R., and Ma, Y. H., *J. Membrane Sci.* **77**, 233 (1993).
Blok, J. R., Varkevisser, J., and Drinkenburg, A. A. H., *Chem. Engng. Sci.* **38**, 687 (1983).
Bosch, H., "Solvents and reactors for acid gas treating." Ph.D. thesis in Chemical Engineering, University of Twente, Enschede, The Netherlands, 1989.
Contractor, R. M., and Sleight, A. W., *Catalysis Today* **3**, 175 (1988).
Darton, R. C., Hoek, P. J., Spaninks, J. A. M., Suenson, M., and Wijn, E. F., *Inst. Chem. Engrs. Symp. Series No. 104*, The Institution of Chemical Engineers, Rugby, U.K., p. A323, 1988.
Dautzenberg, F. M., and De Deken, J. C., *Catal. Rev.—Sci. Eng.* **26**, 421 (1984).
Doherty, M. F., and Buzad, G., *Trans. Inst. Chem. Engrs. Part A* **70**, 448 (1992).
Doraiswamy, L. K., and Sharma, M. M., "Heterogeneous Reactions: Analysis, Examples and Reactor Design," Vol. 2. John Wiley, New York, 1984.
Fan, L. S., "Gas–Liquid–Solid Fluidization Engineering." Butterworths, Boston, 1989.
Gianetto, A., Pagliolico, S., Rovero, G., and Ruggeri, B., *Chem. Engng. Sci.* **45**, 2219 (1990).
Ham, A. G. J., van der, Prins, W., and Swaaij, W. P. M., van, *in* "Fluid–Particle Processes: Fundamentals and Applications" (edited by A. W. Weimer, J. C. Chen, and W. C. Yang), A.I.Ch.E. Symposium Series No. 295, Vol. 89, 1993, 53.
Hano, T., Nakashio, F., and Kusunoki, K., *J. Chem. Eng. Japan* **8**, 127 (1975).
Hsieh, H. P., *Catalysis Reviews—Sci. & Eng.* **33**, 1 (1991).
Krishna, R., "Design and scale-up of gas fluidized bed reactors," *in* "Multiphase Chemical Reactors, Volume II—Design Methods," (edited by A. E. Rodrigues, J. M. Calo, and N. H. Sweed), NATO Advanced Study Institutes Series E: Applied Sciences—No. 52. Sijthoff and Noordhoff, Alphen aan den Rijn, The Netherlands, 1981.
Krishna, R., "Analogies in multiphase reactor hydrodynamics," Chapter 8 in "Encyclopedia of Fluid Mechanics, Supplement 2, Advances in Multiphase Flow" (N. P. Cheremisinoff, editor). Gulf Publishing, Houston, 1993, 239.
Krishna, R., Ellenberger, J., and Hennephof, D. E., *Chem. Engng. J.* **53**, 89 (1993).
Kuczynski, M., "The synthesis of methanol in a gas–solid–solid trickle flow reactor." Ph.D. Thesis in Chemical Engineering, University of Twente, Enschede, The Netherlands, 1986.
Levenspiel, O., "Chemical Reaction Engineering," 2nd Ed. Wiley, New York, 1972.
Levenspiel, O., *Chem. Engng. Sci.* **43**, 1427 (1988).
Parent, Y. O., Caram, H. S., and Coughlin, R. W., *A.I.Ch.E. J.* **29**, 443 (1983).
Poll, I., Krishna, R., Voetter, H., and Van Wechem, H. M. H., "The basis of reactor selection for the Shell shale retorting process," *in* "Recent Trends in Chemical Reaction Engineering" (edited by B. D. Kulkarni, R. A. Mashelkar, and M. M. Sharma), Vol. II. Wiley Eastern Limited, New Delhi, 1987.
Richardson, J. T., Paripatyadar, S. A., and Chen, J. C., *A.I.Ch.E. J.* **34**, 743 (1988).
Schuurmans, H. J. A., *Ind. Eng. Chem. Proc. Des. Dev.* **19**, 267 (1980).
Shah, Y. T., "Gas–Liquid–Solid Reactor Design." McGraw-Hill, New York, 1979.
Sharma, M. M., *Chem. Engng. Sci.* **43**, 1749 (1988).
Sie, S. T., Senden, M. M. G., and Van Wechem, H. M. H., *Catalysis Today* **8**, 371 (1991).
Sloot, H. J., Versteeg, G. F., and van Swaaij, W. P. M., *Chem. Engng. Sci.* **45**, 2415 (1990).
Sloot, H. J., "Development of a non-permselective membrane reactor for catalytic gas phase reactions." Ph.D. thesis in Chemical Engineering, University of Twente, Enschede, The Netherlands, 1991.
Van Swaaij, W. P. M., and Zuiderweg, F. J., "Proceedings of the Fifth European/Second International Symposium on Chemical Reaction Engineering, Amsterdam," pp. B9–B25, pp. C1–C3, 1972.

"Synthetic Fuels Data Handbook" (compiled by G. L. Baughman), 2nd Ed., Cameron Engineers, Inc., 1978; see also: Nowacki, P., "Oil Shale Data Handbook," Energy Technology Review No. 63, Chemical Technology Review No. 182. Noyes Data Corporation, New Jersey, 1981.

Trambouze, P., Van Landeghem, H., and Wauquier, J.-P., "Chemical Reactors. Design, Engineering and Operation." Editions Technip, Paris, 1988.

Trambouze, P., *Chem. Engng. Sci.* **45**, 2269 (1990).

Voge, H. H. and Morgan, C. Z., *Ind. Eng. Chem. Proc. Des. Dev.* **11**, 454 (1972).

Wallman, P. H., Tamm, P. W., and Spars, B. G., "Oil shale retorting kinetics," paper presented at the American Chemical Society Meeting, Division of Fuel Chemistry, San Francisco, California, August 24–29, 1980.

Wammes, W. J. A., "Hydrodynamics in a co-current gas–liquid trickle-bed reactor at elevated pressures." Ph.D. thesis in Chemical Engineering, University of Twente, Enschede, The Netherlands, 1990.

Weisz, P. B., and Hicks, J. S., *Chem. Engng. Sci.* **17**, 265 (1962).

Westerterp, K. R., and Ptasinski, S. A., *Chem. Engng. Sci.* **39**, 245 (1984).

Wilkins, E. S., Nuttall, H. E., and Thakur, D. S., "Oil degradation mechanisms during *in-situ* oil shale retorting—VMIS," Proceedings of the 2nd World Congress on Chemical Engineering, Montreal, Canada, October 4–9, 1981.

POLLUTION PREVENTION: ENGINEERING DESIGN AT MACRO-, MESO-, AND MICROSCALES

David T. Allen

Department of Chemical Engineering
University of California at Los Angeles
Los Angeles, California 90024

I. Introduction

Billions of tons of industrial waste are generated annually in the United States. As shown in Fig. 1, managing and legally disposing of these wastes costs tens to hundreds of billions of dollars each year, and these costs have been increasing rapidly (U.S. Department of Commerce, 1990, 1992). The escalation is likely to continue as emission standards become even more

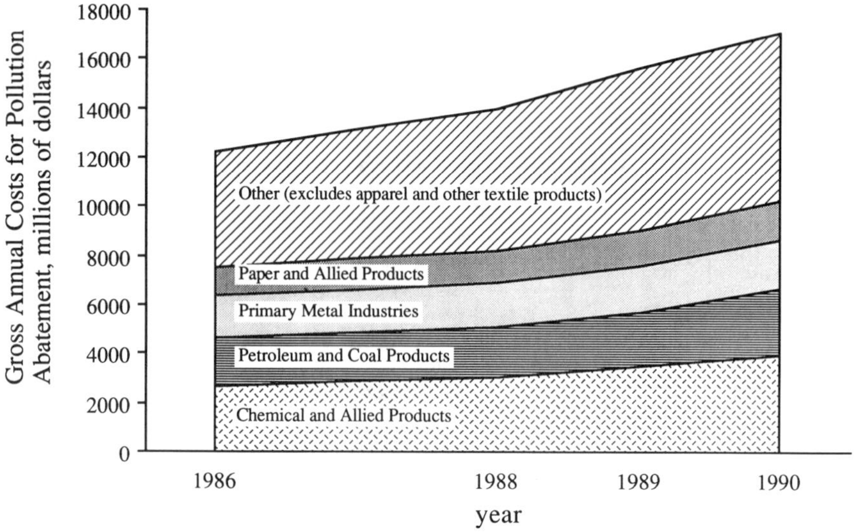

FIG. 1. Pollution abatement costs (U.S. Department of Commerce, 1990, 1992).

stringent. In the face of these rapidly rising costs and rapidly increasing performance standards, traditional end-of-pipe approaches to waste management have become less attractive. The most economical waste management alternatives in many cases have become recycling of the wastes or the redesign of chemical processes and products so that wastes are prevented or put to productive use. These strategies of recycling or reducing waste at the source have collectively come to be known as pollution prevention.

The engineering challenges associated with pollution prevention are substantial. This review will categorize the challenges into three levels. At the most macroscopic level, the flow of materials in our industrial economy, from natural resource extraction to consumer product disposal, can be redesigned. Currently, most of our raw materials are virgin natural resources that are used once, then discarded. Studies in what has come to be called industrial ecology examine the material efficiency of large-scale industrial systems and attempt to improve that efficiency. A second level of engineering challenges is found at the scale of individual industrial facilities, where chemical processes and products can be redesigned so that waste is reduced. Finally, on a molecular level, chemical synthesis pathways, combustion reaction pathways, and other material fabrication procedures can be redesigned to reduce emissions of pollutants and unwanted by-products. All of these design activities, shown in Fig. 2, have the potential to prevent pollution. All involve the tools of engineering, and in particular, chemical engineering.

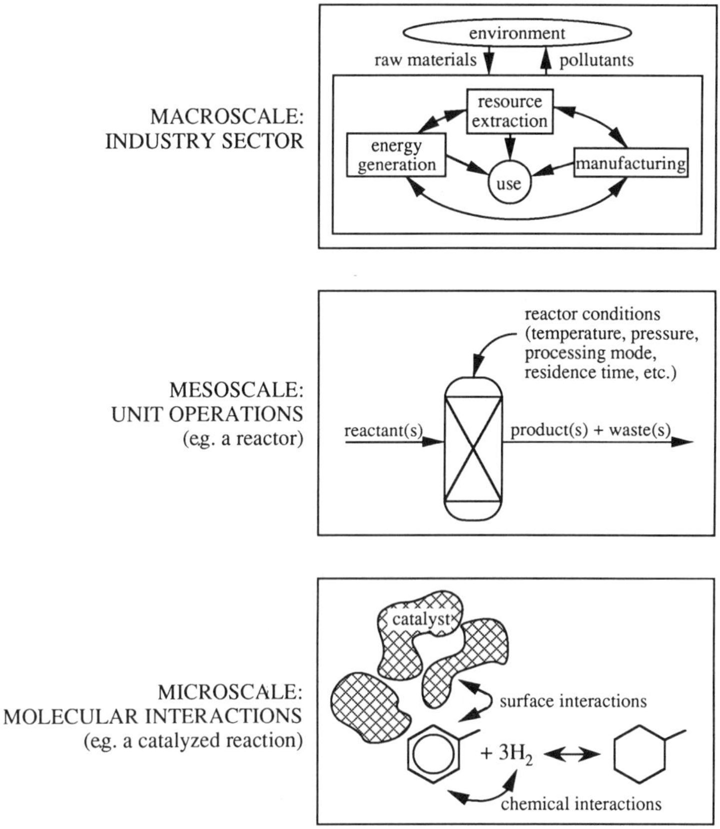

FIG. 2. Pollution prevention can be engineered at macro-, meso-, and microscales (from Friedlander, 1993).

II. Macroscale Pollution Prevention

Following the flow of materials in our industrial economy, from raw material acquisition to product and waste disposal, provides perspective that is essential for pollution prevention. Such studies can help to identify whether materials currently regarded as wastes in one industrial sector could be viewed as raw materials by another sector. These studies also reveal what types of processes and products are responsible for waste generation, and identification of the source of a waste is the first step toward prevention.

This section will examine pollution prevention at the macroscale level from three perspectives. First, an overview of waste generation and management will be presented. This inventory of wastes helps to identify

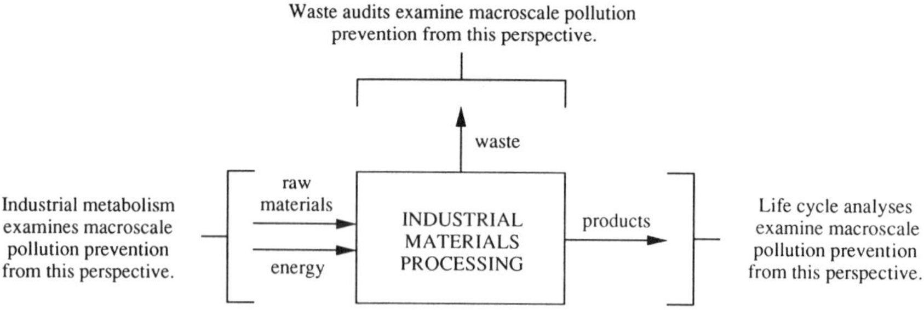

FIG. 3. Macroscale pollution prevention can be studied by examining waste inventories, by examining raw materials (industrial metabolism), or by examining products (life cycle analyses) (U.S. Congress, Office of Technology Assessment, 1992).

processes and products that may benefit from pollution prevention, but a mere listing of wastes and emissions ignores the complex interdependencies of many processes and products. Two related approaches are used to study the complex systems used to convert raw materials to products. One approach, called Industrial Metabolism (Ayers, 1989), involves selecting a particular raw material, for example lead, and following it as it flows through processes and into products. A second approach, called Life Cycle Analysis [Society of Environmental Toxicology and Chemistry (SETAC), 1991], starts with a particular product and identifies all of the precursors that were required for the product's manufacture, use, and disposal. These three elements—waste inventories, industrial metabolism, and life cycle analysis—form the basis of pollution prevention at the macroscale. The relationship of these elements is shown in Fig. 3, and each of the elements will be examined in more detail later.

A. An Overview of Waste Generation and Management in the United States

The best estimates available from national waste generation databases indicate that more than 12 billion tons (wet basis) of industrial waste are generated in the United States annually (Allen and Jain, 1992). To put this rate of waste generation in perspective, consider that the annual output of the top 50 commodity chemicals is only 0.3 billion tons per year (*Chemical and Engineering News*, May 11, 1992) and that the annual rate of generation of municipal solid waste (post-consumer waste) is 0.2 billion tons per year (U.S. Environmental Protection Agency, 1990). Given these massive rates of industrial waste generation, it is clear that waste management and disposal is a problem of staggering magnitude. The problem should not be viewed, however, strictly as a waste treatment and disposal problem. Data to be presented in this section will demonstrate that it may be possible to use the wastes from some industrial processes as feedstocks for other processes. This section will examine the flows of industrial waste streams, their sources and the concentrations of valuable resources in the wastes.

Table I and Fig. 4 identify the sources of the 12 billion tons of industrial waste generated annually in the United States. Over 90% of this waste material is legally classified as nonhazardous under the provisions of the Resource Conservation and Recovery Act (RCRA). As shown in Table I, the major sources of these nonhazardous wastes are mining, petroleum exploration, and electric power generation. In contrast, wastes defined as hazardous under RCRA are generated primarily by chemical manufacturing and petroleum refining. Hazardous wastes constitute less than 10% of the total waste flow, yet the costs associated with treating and disposing of these wastes are a substantial fraction of national waste management expenditures. One of the reasons for the high costs associated with hazardous wastes is the level of treatment required. For example, the hazardous constituents in an organic waste stream must typically be 99%, 99.99%, or 99.9999% destroyed before the waste stream is considered successfully treated—the difference in level of destruction depends on the toxicity of the hazardous constituent. Achieving such high levels of destruction is expensive and typically involves the use of multiple treatment technologies. Figure 5 (Baker *et al.*, 1992) provides a rough mapping of the technologies currently used to treat hazardous wastes in the United States and illustrates the complex interplay of technologies. Consider an organic waste stream requiring incineration. As the waste is incinerated, scrubber wash waters and ash, both defined as hazardous wastes, are generated and must be managed. As noted in Fig. 5, these wastes derived from the treatment of other wastes can be significant (on average, 40 tons of scrubber wash water and ash are generated per ton of hazardous waste incinerated). Management of waste generated in the treatment process can lead to even more wastes. Scrubber wash waters generated by an incinerator might be neutralized, producing a solid waste, which again is defined as hazardous. These cascading treatment technologies can introduce huge costs, providing a strong motivation to recycle or eliminate the waste at its source.

Figure 5 also illustrates the relatively limited range of treatment technologies currently used for hazardous wastes. Only combustion/incineration, a few types of wastewater treatment technologies, land disposal, and a few types of recycling are used to manage virtually all industrial hazardous wastes. Given the diverse nature of the waste streams, this limited range of waste management tools is unlikely to be the optimal manage-

TABLE I
NONHAZARDOUS (RCRA, SUBTITLE D) WASTE GENERATION (USEPA, 1988)

Waste category	Estimated annual generation rate (million tons)
Industrial nonhazardous waste	7600[a, b]
Oil and gas waste[c]	
drilling waste	129–871[d, e]
produced waters	1966–2738[e, f]
Mining waste[c]	> 1400[g]
Municipal waste	158[b]
household hazardous waste	0.002–0.56[b]
Municipal waste combustion ash	3.2–8.1[h]
Utility waste[c]	
ash	69[i]
flue gas desulfurization waste	16[i]
Construction and demolition waste	31.5[j]
Municipal sludge	
wastewater treatment	6.9[b]
water treatment	3.5[b]
Very-small-quantity[k] generator hazardous waste (< 100 kg/month)	0.2[e]
Waste tires	240 million tires[g]
Infectious waste	2.1[e, l]
Agricultural waste	Unknown
Approximate total	> 11,387

[a]Not including industrial waste that is recycled or disposed of off site.
[b]These estimates are derived from 1986 data.
[c]See Science Applications International Corporation (1985).
[d]Converted to tons from barrels: 42 gals = 1 barrel, ~ 17 lbs/gal.
[e]These estimates are derived from 1985 data.
[f]Converted to tons from barrels: 42 gals = 1 barrel, ~ 8 lbs/gal.
[g]These estimates are derived from 1983 data.
[h]This estimate is derived from 1988 data.
[i]These estimates are derived from 1984 data.
[j]This estimate is derived from 1970 data.
[k]Small quantity generators (100–1000 kg/month waste) have been regulated under RCRA, Subtitle C, since October 1986. Before then, approximately 830,000 tons of small-quantity generator hazardous wastes were disposed of in Subtitle D facilities every year.
[l]Includes only infectious *hospital* waste and does not include infectious waste generated by doctors' offices, nursing homes, etc.

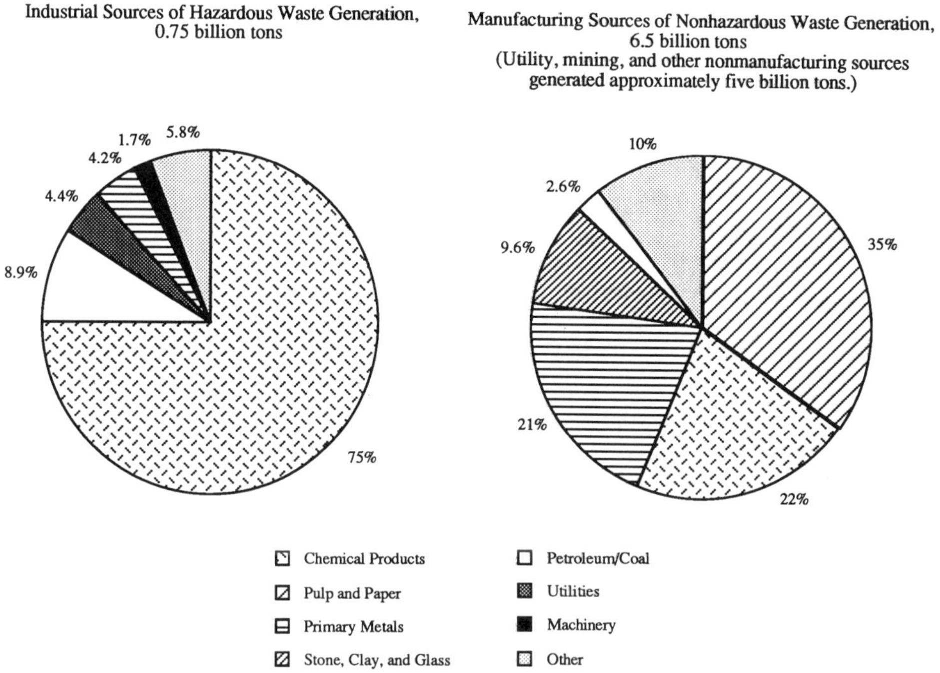

FIG. 4. Industrial waste generation in the United States (U.S. Department of Energy, 1991; Allen and Jain, 1992).

ment solution. The methods used for wastes defined as nonhazardous are even simpler and less varied. As shown in Table II, most nonhazardous wastes are sent directly to landfills or other land disposal operations. Little recycling and treatment are done because the management standards are not as high for nonhazardous waste as they are for hazardous waste.

Identifying which of these industrial waste streams can be prevented is difficult, but as a first step, it is instructive to examine a simpler issue—recyclability. As shown in Fig. 5, a relatively small fraction of waste streams is currently sent to solvent, metal, and other recovery operations. This low rate of recycling might be because waste streams contain few materials worth recovery, or it may be due to legislative, institutional, or technological barriers to recycling of hazardous wastes. To examine whether industrial waste streams have potential value as raw materials, and therefore could be more extensively recycled, consider the Sherwood diagram, shown in Fig. 6 (National Research Council, 1987). The Sherwood diagram demonstrates that the value of a resource scales with the level of dilution at which it is present in the raw material. Resources that are present at

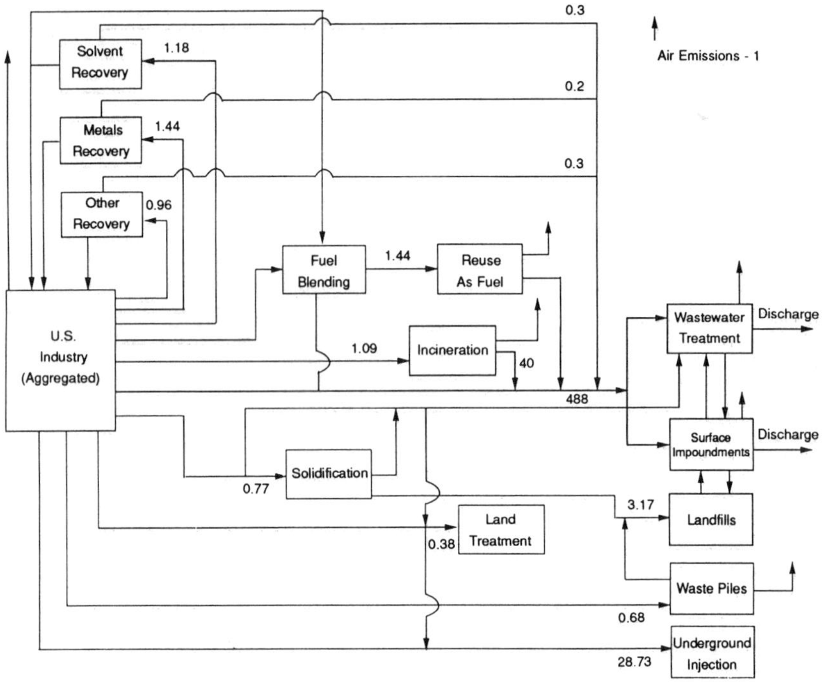

FIG. 5. Flows of hazardous waste in the United States (Baker *et al.*, 1992; data, in million tons per year, are from 1986, USEPA, 1991a).

very low concentration can only be recovered at high cost, while resources present at high concentration can be recovered economically.

Using price and the Sherwood diagram, it is possible to estimate the concentration at which materials can be recovered. As a case study of whether industrial wastes contain materials that are economically recoverable, consider metals. The concentrations of metals in hazardous wastes can be determined using the 1986 National Hazardous Waste Survey [U.S. Environmental Protection Agency (US EPA), 1991a]. Comparing metal prices, minimum economically recoverable concentration (from the Sherwood diagram) and data on the concentration distributions of metals in waste streams, it is possible to estimate what fraction of metals in hazardous waste streams can be recycled (Allen and Behmanesh, 1993). These estimates are reported in Table III and indicate that metals in hazardous wastes are underutilized. This could be because only waste streams with very high metal concentrations are recovered, or because only a small fraction of potential recyclers at all feasible concentration levels recover metals. Figure 7 attempts to differentiate between these two cases. To

TABLE II
INDUSTRIAL NONHAZARDOUS WASTE ON-SITE MANAGEMENT[a]

Industry type (Standard Industrial Classification Code)	Total waste quantity disposed of in all on-site industrial facilities (thousand tons)	Percent of waste disposed of in landfills	Percent of waste disposed of in surface impoundments	Percent of waste disposed of in land application units	Percent of waste disposed of in waste piles
Organic chemicals (2819)	58,864	0.4	96.3	3.1	0.08
Primary iron and steel (3312–3321)	1,300,541	0.3	99.2	< 0.01	0.5
Fertilizer and agricultural chemicals (2873–2879)	165,623	3.5	93.1	0.5	2.9
Electric power generation (4911)	1,092,277	4.9	95.0	0.03	0.08
Plastics and resins manufacturing (2821)	180,510	0.05	98.2	0.02	1.7
Inorganic chemicals (2812–2819)	919,725	0.4	95.1	0.01	4.5
Stone, clay, glass, and concrete (32)	621,974	1.2	97.3	< 0.01	1.5
Pulp and paper (26)	2,251,700	0.3	99.3	0.4	0.07
Primary nonferrous metals (3330–3399)	67,070	2.1	84.3	0.6	13
Food and kindred products (20)	373,517	1.0	78.6	20	0.1
Water treatment (4941)	58,846	0.3	84.5	15	0.1
Petroleum refining (29)	168,632	0.2	99.6	0.2	0.05
Rubber and miscellaneous plastic products (30)	24,198	2.2	97.4	0.2	0.2
Transportation equipment (37)	12,669	1.4	93.1	< 0.01	4.6
Textile manufacturing (22)	253,780	0.03	99.7	0.3	< 0.01
Leather and leather products (31)	3234	0.3	99.4	0	0.3
Selected chemicals and allied products	67,987	0.2	99.1	0.7	0.01
Total	7,616,149	1.1	96.6	1.3	1.0

[a]Percentages (in each row) are rounded and may not total 100%.

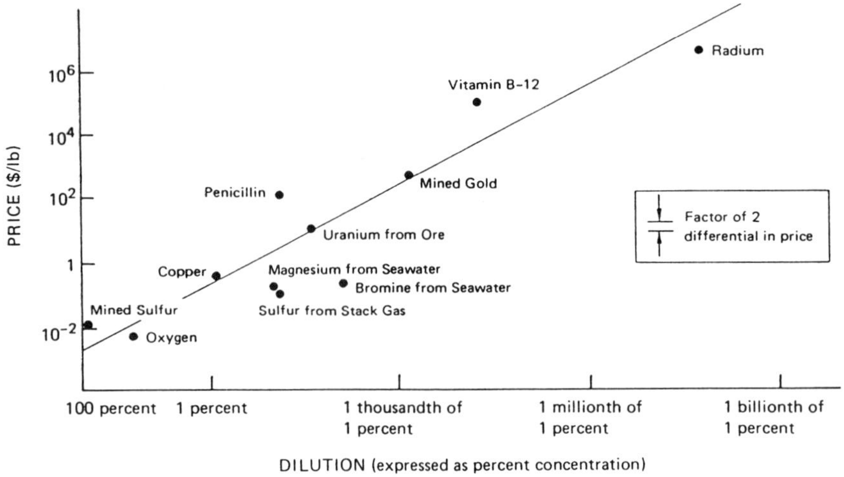

FIG. 6. The Sherwood diagram: the price at which a material can be economically recovered scales with the concentration (National Research Council, 1987).

TABLE III
PERCENTAGE OF METAL LOADINGS IN HAZARDOUS WASTES THAT CAN IN PRINCIPLE BE RECOVERED BASED ON THE PRICE–CONCENTRATION RELATIONSHIP IN THE SHERWOOD DIAGRAM (ALLEN AND BEHMANESH, 1993)

Metal	Minimum concentration recoverable, from Sherwood Plot (mass fraction)	Percent of metal, theoretically recoverable (%)	Percent recycled in 1987 (%)
Sb	0.00405	74–87	32
As	0.00015	98–99	3
Ba	0.0015	95–98	4
Be	0.012	54–84	31
Cd	0.0048	82–97	7
Cr	0.0012	68–89	8
Cu	0.0022	85–92	10
Pb	0.074	84–95	56
Hg	0.00012	99	41
Ni	0.0066	100	0.1
Se	0.0002	93–95	16
Ag	0.000035	99–100	1
Tl	0.00004	97–99	1
V	0.0002	74–98	1
Zn	0.0012	96–98	13

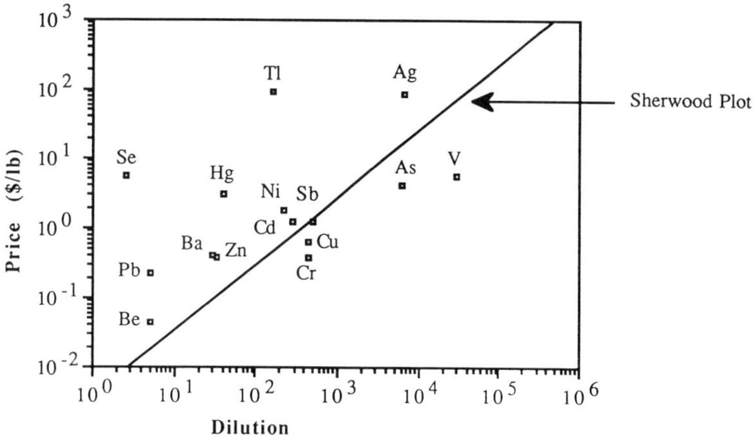

FIG. 7. The Sherwood plot for waste streams: the minimum dilution (1/mass fraction) of metal wastes undergoing recycling is plotted against metal price. The Sherwood plot for virgin materials is provided for comparison. Points lying above the Sherwood plot indicate that the metals in the waste streams are only recycled at very high concentration, i.e., waste streams undergoing disposal are richer than typical virgin materials. Points lying below the Sherwood plot indicate that the waste streams are vigorously recycled.

develop Fig. 7, the concentration distribution of metals in recycled waste streams was examined. The concentration below which only 10% of the metal recycling took place was assumed to be a lower bound for economic metal recovery from the waste. This concentration was then plotted, together with the 1986 metal price (recall that the waste data are from 1986) to generate Fig. 7. Also plotted on Fig. 7 is the Sherwood Diagram for virgin materials. Comparison of the Sherwood plot for virgin materials and the waste concentration data reveals that most metals are only recycled at very high concentrations. A few metals, such as vanadium and nickel, fall close to the Sherwood plot for virgin materials, indicating that some waste generators aggressively recover these metals. Overall, however, these metals remain under-recovered, and only a small fraction of the wastes are recycled.

To summarize, an examination of industrial waste generation reveals the following:

- Billions of tons of industrial waste are generated annually in the United States; tens to hundreds of billions of dollars are spent annually to manage these wastes.
- Only a few technologies (incineration, land disposal, and various forms of wastewater treatment) are used to manage waste streams; there is relatively little use of innovative technologies.

- The waste streams frequently contain valuable materials at concentration levels suitable for recovery; however, relatively little material is reclaimed from wastes.

These conclusions form the foundation for the next section. They indicate that some wastes should be viewed as potential raw materials, but identifying uses for these novel raw materials poses some challenges.

B. Industrial Metabolism

Analysis of waste management data, as presented earlier, represents a first step in performing macroscale studies of pollution prevention. The next step is to integrate waste generation data with production data. These studies, which have been described as Industrial Metabolism (Ayers, 1989), examine the sources and all of the uses of particular materials. By integrating models of the uses of selected materials with data on waste generation for the same materials, it may be possible to identify targets of opportunity for recycling between industrial sectors.

As an example of industrial metabolism, consider lead. Lead is converted into products at a rate of roughly 1.2 million tons per year. The sources of the lead are mining and recycling operations, with recycling supplying approximately 50% of lead use. Most of the 1.3 million tons of lead consumed annually is used in the production of lead storage batteries. Minor uses include metal products, electronics, pigments and additives to glass, ceramics, and plastics. Once converted into products the lead is eventually either recycled or sent for disposal. Recycling is extensive for batteries. According to the US EPA (1989, 1990), 0.9 million tons of lead acid batteries were discarded in municipal solid waste in 1988, of which 0.8 million tons were recycled. Further, approximately 250,000 tons of lead was discarded as industrial waste in 1986, of which 150,000 tons were recycled. Coupling these data with the data on industrial hazardous waste generation and the data on lead production and consumption yields the lead flow diagram shown in Fig. 8. The simplified model of the industrial metabolism of lead can be contrasted with the industrial metabolism of platinum-group metals and iron (Frosch and Gallopoulos, 1989). A simplified model of the industrial ecology of platinum-group metals is shown in Fig. 9. The greatest contrast between the industrial ecology of lead and that of platinum group metals is the fate of materials used in automotive end products. Lead acid batteries from automobiles are recycled at a rate of over 90% (US EPA, 1989, 1990), while metals from catalytic converters are recycled at only a 12% rate. The difference might be attributed to the

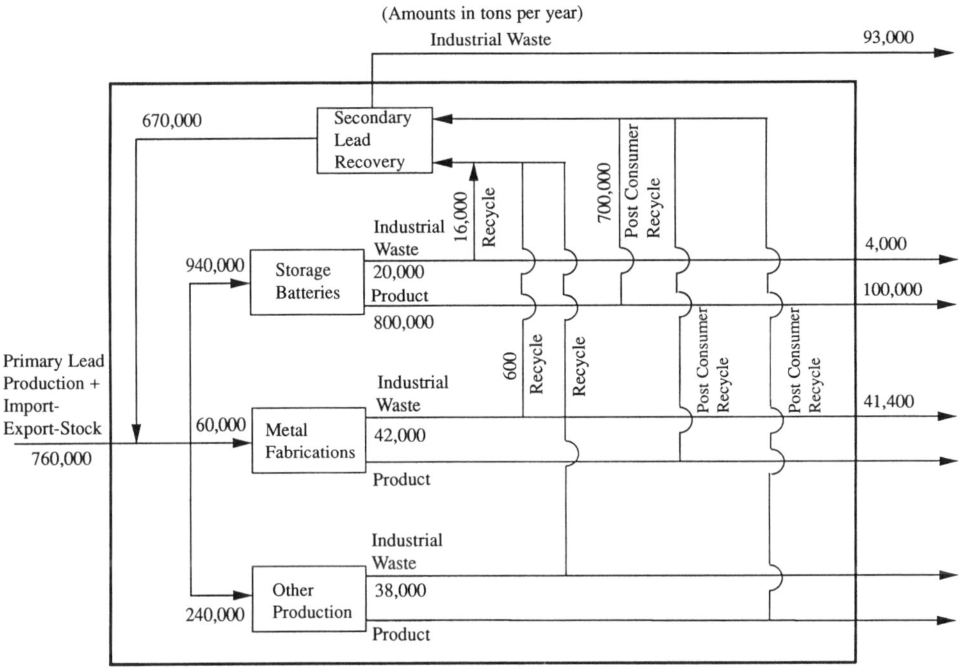

FIG. 8. A simplified model of the industrial ecology of lead (Allen and Behmanesh, 1993).

low concentration of metals in the catalyst, but this argument is not viable when the high recycling rates for industrial catalysts and the low concentrations of metals in virgin ores (several parts per million) are considered. The main reason for low recycling rates for platinum group metals in automotive catalytic converters is the lack of a collection network. Such a network exists for lead acid batteries. Even if a collection network exists, however, technology selection can strongly influence the industrial metabolism of materials. Consider the case of scrap iron. The stockpile of scrap iron awaiting recycling increased from 610 million tons in 1982 to more than 750 million tons in 1987 (Frosch and Gallopoulos, 1989). One of the reasons for this increase in the stockpile of scrap is a technology shift from open hearth to basic oxygen furnaces in steel-making. While open hearth furnaces could accept up to 50% scrap, basic oxygen furnaces accept only 20%. Thus, even when a recycling infrastructure is in place, technology selection can play a key role in encouraging or discouraging recycling.

These simple case studies of the industrial metabolism of metals reveal the importance of infrastructure and technology selection in industrial

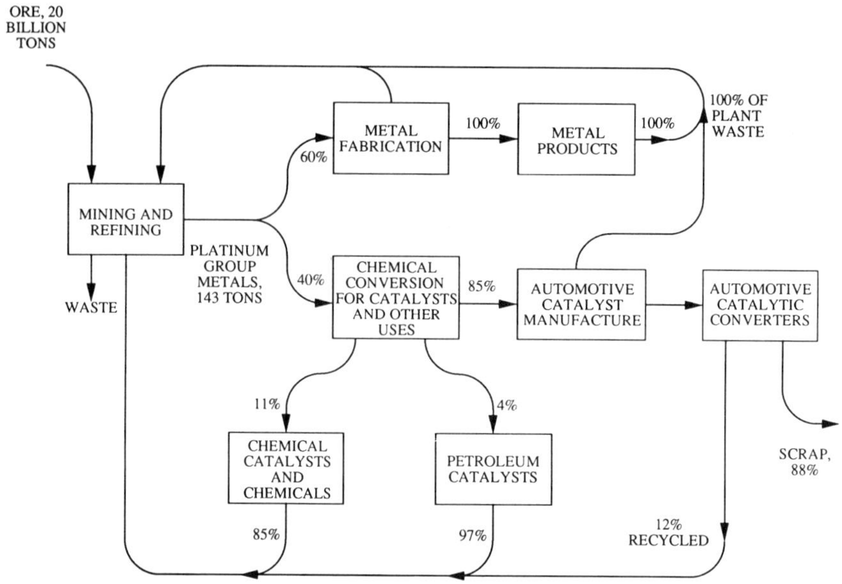

FIG. 9. A simplified model of the industrial ecology of platinum-group metals (Frosch and Gallopoulos, 1989).

metabolism. They also reveal that industrial ecology studies are still relatively elementary. More detailed analysis of potential recovery and recycling opportunities is feasible, however. Detailed chemical characteristics of waste streams could be matched with chemical characteristics of process streams to determine the extent to which an industrial materials processing system can be established which requires minimal input of virgin raw materials. These studies are just beginning, and their ultimate goal is to establish an industrial ecology, similar to natural ecosystems, which requires external sources of energy but completely recycles mass.

Metals are attractive materials for studies in industrial ecology because they are relatively straightforward to follow through chemical processes. Although they may change oxidation state or chemical nature, they are not transmuted into different elements. Performing industrial ecology studies on organics is much more difficult, however. The best framework available for such studies are the models of the chemical process industries developed by Rudd and co-workers (1981). In these structural models of the commodity chemical industry, the flows of raw materials into and products out of approximately 180 types of chemical processes were determined. These processes generate more than 120 different products and form a complex web of material flows that make possible many routes to form chemical products. As a relatively simple case study of the multiple pathways available in chemical synthesis, consider methyl-*tert*-butyl ether (MTBE), an oxygenated additive to gasoline that is being produced in large quantities to satisfy the provisions of the 1990 Clean Air Act Amendments. MTBE is produced by reacting methanol with isobutylene using one of two processes. In addition to having two processes to choose from in the MTBE synthesis, there are options in the synthesis of the raw materials. The methanol fed to the MTBE process can be made from methane, via carbon monoxide or via fermentation. The isobutylene can be made by cracking petroleum, by isomerizing butenes, or by dehydrogenating butanes. These different processes allow more than a dozen routes from raw materials to MTBE. Each route will have different energy requirements and rates of waste generation. Selecting the cleanest and most economical route is a difficult proposition. It is made even more difficult when we realize that our selection of a particular process may influence the rates of waste generation in the rest of the chemical industry. For example, if we choose to produce methanol via carbon monoxide, we may be able to generate the carbon monoxide through partial oxidation of a material that is currently wasted. On the other hand, to convert the carbon monoxide into methanol requires hydrogen, which is an energy-intensive material.

Only a few comprehensive analyses of the technological structure of the chemical industry have been performed, and most of these studies were motivated by the energy crises of the 1970s. Their focus therefore tended to be on the role technology selection could play in improving the energy efficiency of the chemical industry. Wastes and emissions were not explicitly considered. One of the few studies available on the impact that technology selection can have on the environmental performance of the chemical industry was published in 1985 by a group at UCLA (Fathi-Afshar and Yang, 1985). This study examined the mix of technologies that would result in the minimum cost of production for 124 chemical products and would also result in the lowest gross toxicity of the chemical intermediates used in the synthesis. The results are summarized in Fig. 10. The point labeled A on Fig. 10 corresponds to the cost of production of the 124 chemicals if the sole criterion for process selection is the toxicity of the intermediates required. Point C corresponds to the total cost of chemical production if cost is the only criterion used in selecting technologies. The line connecting points A and C is the collection of possible technology mixes. The ideal point is B, which represents the lowest possible cost and the lowest possible toxicity of intermediates, but which is not obtainable using current technologies. Clearly, a mix of technologies located somewhere near point D represents the best compromise between economics

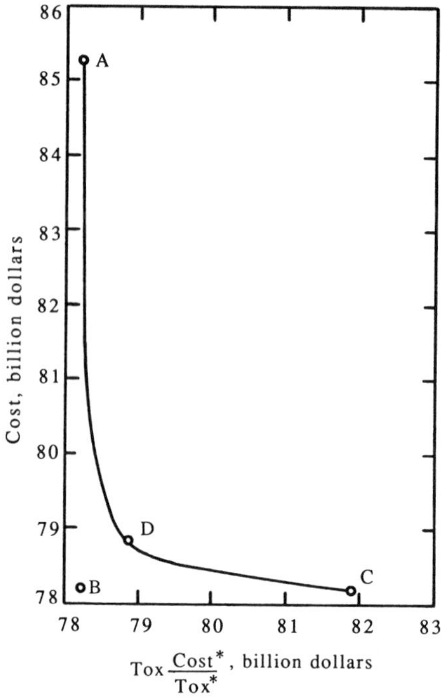

FIG. 10. Trade-offs between cost and the use of toxic intermediates in the chemical industry. Point A is the lowest-toxicity route currently feasible, but it comes at a greater cost than the most economical approach (Point C). Point B (low cost, low toxicity) is not currently technologically feasible. Point D is the closest feasible technology mix to Point B (Fathi-Afshar and Yang, 1985).

and the environmental objective of lowest toxicity of intermediates. In addition to selecting desirable mixes of technologies, this type of analysis can help to identify critical areas for technology improvement. If, for example, we were to select a mix of technologies that resulted in the lowest total cost of chemical production, we could then identify the chemical intermediates that contribute to toxicity. Such an analysis is presented in Fig. 11 and reveals that just a few chemical intermediates dominate the toxicity of the entire system. In this example, toluene diisocyanate, phosgene, and methylene diphenylene dominate. Finding technological alternatives to these intermediates could dramatically reduce overall toxicity.

The example just described demonstrates the utility of structural analyses of the chemical industry. Similar studies could be done, examining the trade-offs between economics, energy consumption, and waste generation, if process-specific waste generation data were available. Unfortunately,

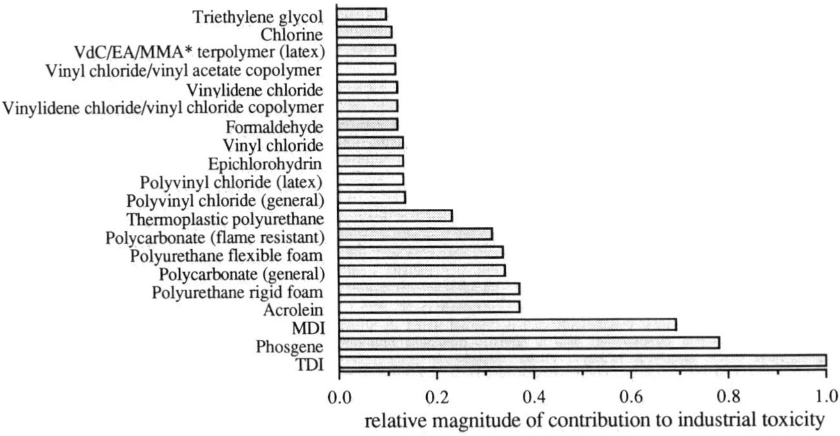

*VdC/EA/MMA: Vinylidene chloride/ethyl acrylate/methyl methacrylate

FIG. 11. Major contributors to the total toxicity of the chemical intermediates industry (Fathi-Afshar and Yang, 1985).

few such sources of data are available (Allen and Jain, 1992), and the quality and timeliness of the data are questionable. Thus, studies of the industrial ecology of organics remain at a rather rudimentary level.

C. LIFE CYCLE ANALYSES

The previous section described how the flows of individual materials can be tracked from their initial acquisition to their final disposition in a product or a waste stream. Even relatively simple materials generally have a multitude of uses, which creates interesting opportunities for recycling. While the identification of such pollution prevention opportunities is most readily done by tracking individual materials, an alternative approach that is gaining considerable popularity considers an individual product and maps the flows of energy and raw materials that were required to create the product. These studies, commonly referred to as life cycles analyses, follow a basic framework, which is summarized in Fig. 12.

Figure 12 shows the basic framework for compiling an inventory of wastes, emissions, and energy use associated with the manufacture, use, and disposal of a product (SETAC, 1991). Compiling an inventory is just the first step in a life cycle analysis, however. After the inventory is compiled, the impacts of raw material use, waste generation, and emission generation must be assessed. Finally, after the life cycle impacts are assessed, mechanisms for reducing adverse environmental impacts can be

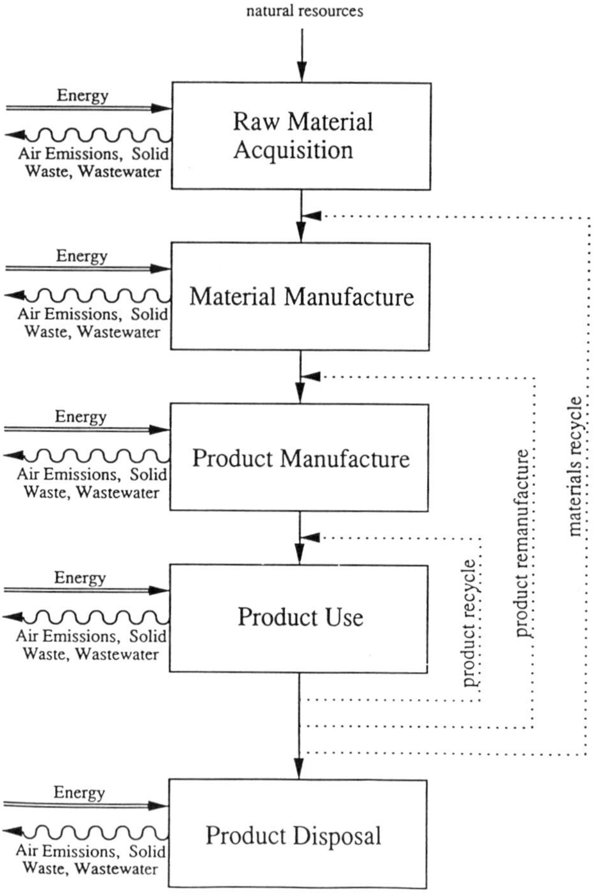

FIG. 12. Life cycle analysis framework.

sought. Thus, a life cycle analysis consists of three components: an inventory, an impacts assessment, and an improvement analysis (SETAC, 1991). Methodologies have been developed and demonstrated for performing life cycle inventories. In contrast, methods for performing life cycle impacts are currently in their infancy. Finally, improvement analyses can be done in an elementary way, but until tools are developed for evaluating life cycle impacts, only limited analysis can be performed.

Table IV summarizes some well known life cycle inventories that have been conducted in the United States. As shown in Table IV, life cycle inventories have been most frequently used to compare different products—for example, cloth and disposable diapers. Such comparisons are generally ambiguous, however, providing no clear answer about which

TABLE IV
A SAMPLING OF LIFE CYCLE ASSESSMENTS[a]

Client (reference)	Practitioner	Product	Year
USEPA (1974)	MRI	Beverage containers	1974
SPI (MIR 1974)	MRI	Plastics	1974
Unknown (Hunt and Franklin, 1975)	MRI	Beer containers	1974
EPA (Koch and Kuta, 1991)	MRI	Milk containers	1978
P & G (USEPA 1978)	Franklin	Laundry detergent packaging	1988
P & G (Kock and Kuda, 1991)	Franklin	Surfactants	1989
Unknown (Franklin Associates, 1989)	Franklin	Soft drink delivery systems	1989
P & G (Little, 1990)	A. D. Little	Cloth and disposable diapers	1990
Council for SW Solutions (Franklin Associates, 1990a)	Franklin	Foamed polystyrene and bleached paperboard	1990
American Paper Institute (Franklin Associates, 1990b)	Franklin	Cloth and disposable diapers	1990
Council for Solid Waste Solutions (Franklin Associates, 1990c)	Franklin	Grocery sacks	1990
Vinyl Institute (ChemSystems, 1991)	ChemSystems	Vinyl packaging	1991
Council of State Governments (Tellus Institute, 1991a)	Tellus	Packaging	1991

[a]Derived from Freeman *et al.*, 1992.

product is "greener." Consider a classic example of this ambiguity, the case of paper and plastic grocery sacks.

1. *Paper or Plastic: A Life Cycle Case Study*

At the supermarket checkstand, consumers are asked to choose whether their purchases should be placed in unbleached paper grocery sacks or in polyethylene grocery sacks. Many consumers make their choice based on their perception of the relative environmental impacts of these two products. Using the mass balance approach of a life cycle inventory, it is possible to quantitatively examine the relative environmental impacts of paper and plastic grocery sacks. Figures 13 and 14 give graphic representation to the life cycle stages of grocery sacks. For paper sacks, there are steps involving timber harvesting, pulping, paper making, product use, and waste disposal. For polyethylene sacks there are steps involving petroleum extraction, ethylene manufacture, ethylene polymerization, polymer processing, product use, and waste disposal. In most of these steps, energy is required and wastes are generated. Comparing Fig. 12, the general frame-

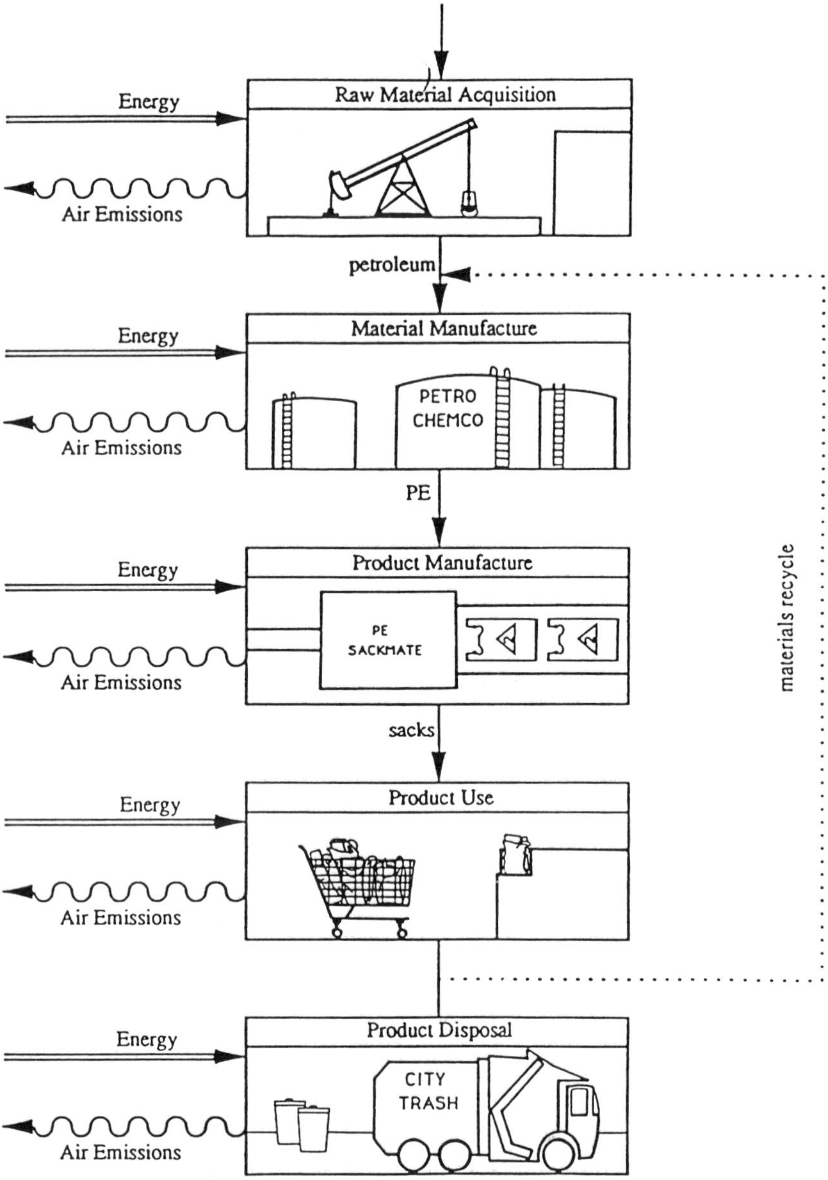

FIG. 13. Life cycle analysis framework for plastic grocery sacks.

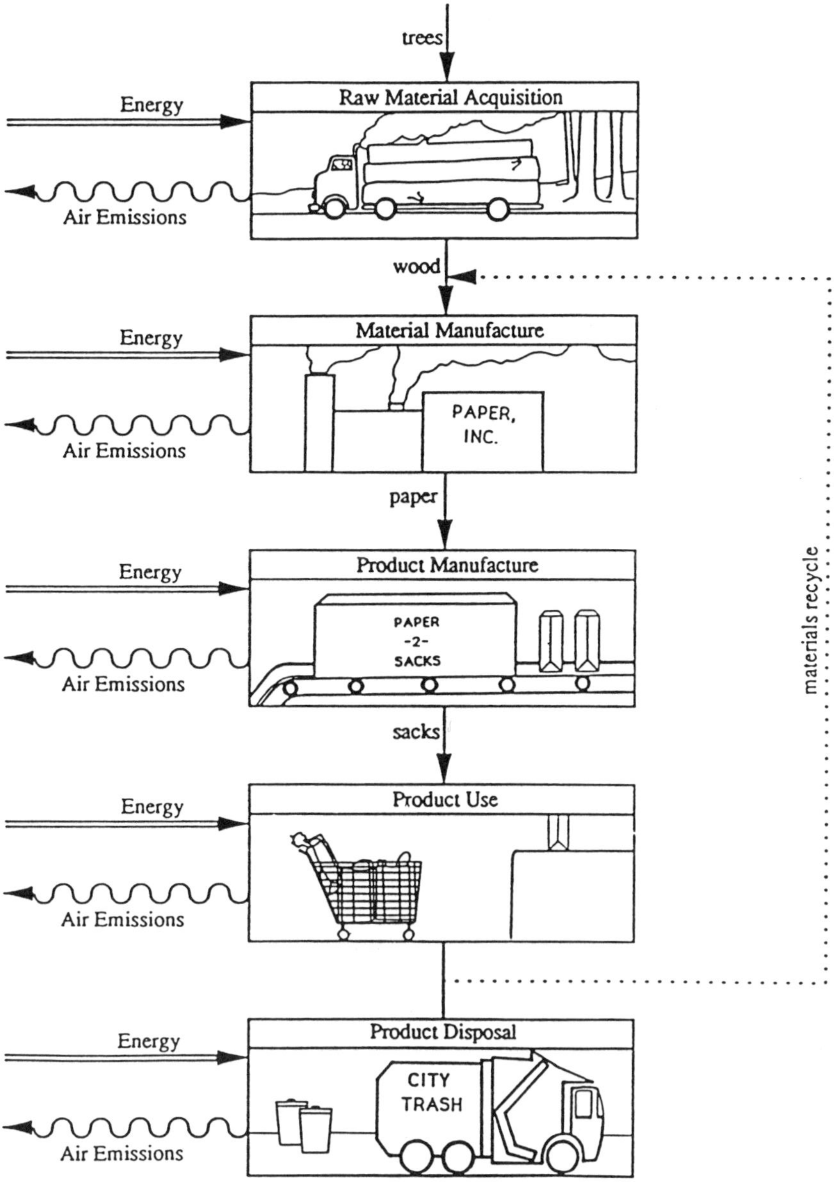

FIG. 14. Life cycle analysis framework for paper grocery sacks.

work for life cycle inventories, and Figs. 13 and 14 reveals some small differences. Most notably, the product reuse and product remanufacture loops present in Fig. 12 are missing in Figs. 13 and 14. They are ignored because almost all recycled grocery sacks are returned to the material manufacture stage rather than product remanufacture or consumer grocery sack reuse. Also, note that the only wastes considered in this example are air emissions, so solid waste and wastewater do not appear in Figs. 13 and 14.

Now, consider the use of the inventory in comparing paper and plastic grocery sacks. Life cycle waste and emission inventories of paper and polyethylene grocery sacks have resulted in the data given in Table V, and these data serve as a basis for comparing these two products. Before a quantitative comparison between the two products can be made, however, differences in product use must be considered. Although both types of sacks are designed to have a capacity of $\frac{1}{6}$ barrel, fewer groceries are generally placed in polyethylene sacks than in paper sacks, even if the practice of double-bagging paper sacks (one sack inside the other), used in some stores, is taken into account. There is no general agreement on the number of polyethylene grocery sacks needed to hold the volume of groceries usually held by a paper sack. Reported values range from 1.2 to 3; for the calculation presented here a value of 2.0 polyethylene grocery sacks required to replace a paper grocery sack was used.

Using the data in Table V, it is possible to determine the amount of energy required and the quantity of air pollutants released per 1000 lb of production of polyethylene sacks. The results are shown in Fig. 15. At 0% recycle, polyethylene sacks (on an equal use basis, 2 polyethylene sacks per paper sack) require approximately 20% less energy than paper sacks. However, as the recycle rate increases, this difference in energy requirement decreases linearly. At recycle rates above 80% there appears to be no significant difference in energy requirements for polyethylene and

TABLE V
AIR EMISSIONS AND ENERGY REQUIREMENTS FOR POLYETHYLENE AND PAPER GROCERY SACKS (FRANKLIN ASSOCIATES, 1990C)

Life cycle stages	Air emissions, oz/sack		Energy required, btu/sack	
	Paper	Polyethylene	Paper	Polyethylene
Materials manufacture plus product manufacture plus product use	0.0516	0.0146	905	464
Raw materials acquisition plus product disposal	0.0510	0.0045	724	185

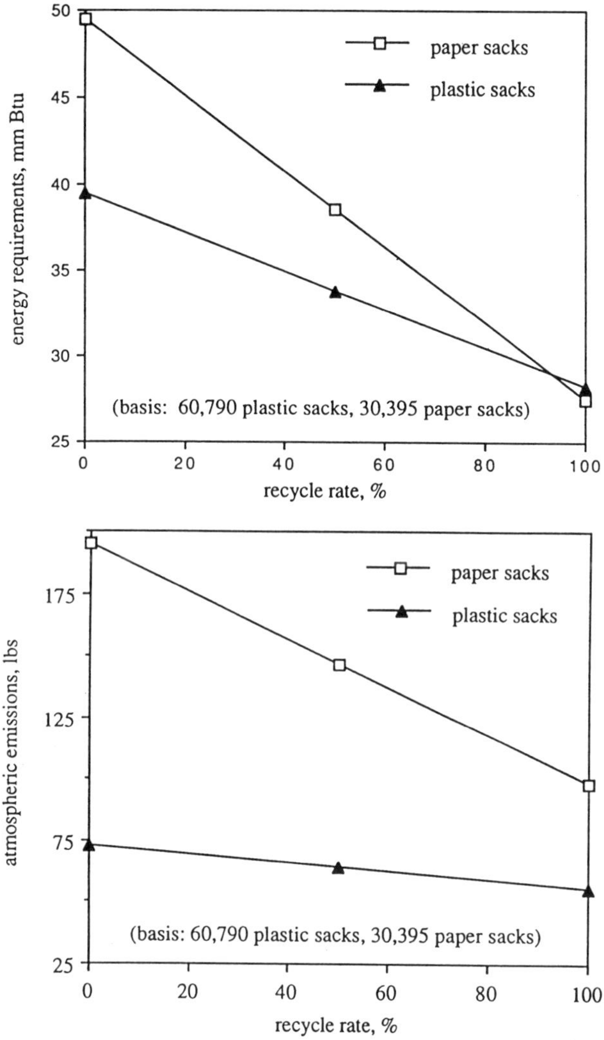

FIG. 15. Energy requirements and atmospheric emissions for paper and plastic grocery sacks, as a function of recycle rate (Franklin Associates, 1990c).

paper sacks. Therefore, on the basis of energy alone, paper sacks would be considered competitive with polyethylene sacks at high (> 80%) recycle rates. The plot for total atmospheric emissions shows a similar declining difference between the products with increasing recycle rates. At 0% recycle, total atmospheric emissions are 60–70% lower for polyethylene sacks; this difference gradually declines to 40% at 100% recycle.

TABLE VI
PROFILE OF ATMOSPHERIC EMISSIONS FOR PAPER AND PLASTIC GROCERY SACKS (FRANKLIN ASSOCIATES, 1990C)

	Atmospheric emissions per 10,000 sacks (lb)			
	Polyethylene sacks		Paper sacks	
Pollutant category	0% Recycling	100% Recycling	0% Recycling	100% Recycling
Particulates	0.8	0.8	24.6	2.8
Nitrogen oxides	2.1	1.7	9.2	8.0
Hydrocarbons	5.8	3.2	4.9	3.9
Sulfur oxides	2.6	2.7	13.6	10.6
Carbon monoxide	0.7	0.6	7.0	6.5
Aldehydes	0.0	0.0	0.1	0.1
Other organics	0.0	0.0	0.3	0.2
Odorous sulfur	—	—	4.5	0.0
Ammonia	0.0	0.0	0.0	0.0
Hydrogen fluoride	—	—	—	—
Lead	0.0	0.0	0.0	0.0
Mercury	—	—	—	—
Chlorine	—	—	—	—

In making these comparisons, it is important to recognize the uncertainties inherent in the analysis. One glaring uncertainty apparent in the calculations of this example is the issue of how many plastic sacks must be used to match the function of one paper sack. In this problem, two plastic sacks were assumed to be equivalent to one paper sack. If a value of 1 or 3 were used, the comparison would be quite different. Further, while polyethylene sacks generate lower amounts of atmospheric emissions than paper sacks at all recycle rates, there are qualitative differences between the emissions. Table VI shows the differences in the types of emissions assigned to polyethylene and paper. In the case of paper sacks, the amount of particulates, nitrogen oxides, and sulfur oxides is higher than for polyethylene. As might be expected, higher levels of hydrocarbon emission are assigned to polyethylene sacks. These hydrocarbons are also very likely to be qualitatively different from the hydrocarbon emissions generated by paper sack production. It would be difficult to assess the respective environmental impacts of the hydrocarbon emissions without a much more detailed description of the emissions. Also, lack of emission data from other sources within the life cycle (i.e., incineration and emissions from landfills) makes the comparison of polyethylene and paper sacks incomplete and any comprehensive comparison difficult.

This example has demonstrated that life cycle analyses do not generally result in the identification of an environmentally superior product. In the case of paper and plastic grocery sacks, the plastic sack appears to require less energy and result in less atmospheric emissions than a paper sack. On the other hand, plastic sacks require the use of petroleum, a nonrenewable resource, while paper sacks are based on forest resources which are generally regarded as renewable. Besides the problem of providing ambiguous results, environmentalists frequently argue that life cycle inventories comparing products do not really ask the right question. For example, in the case of grocery sacks, it could be argued that "paper or plastic?" is not the correct question. Why not ask customers whether they prefer a reusable or a disposable sack?

Thus, there are significant controversies associated with life cycle inventories directed at product comparisons. The situation becomes even more contentious as the life cycle analysis moves past inventories, into the assessment of impacts. Despite these controversies, life cycle inventories and analyses can have productive uses. Life cycle inventories can be used without great controversy to identify, for a single product, where the greatest environmental improvements for that product can be made. For example, while it may not be clear whether a paper or plastic sack is environmentally preferable, it is clear that most of the energy requirements and air emissions for plastic sacks are due to manufacturing steps (see Table V). So if improvements in energy efficiency and decreases in atmospheric emissions are sought for this product, the logical place to focus attention is the manufacturing step. A number of companies, such as Procter & Gamble, have successfully used life cycle information in this way. It is also clear that while life cycle analyses are in their infancy, they are developing rapidly. Interested readers should follow closely the publications of the Life Cycle Analysis Advisory Group of the Society for Environmental Toxicology and Chemistry (SETAC) (e.g., SETAC, 1991, 1993), and the Life Cycle Analysis group at the EPA (e.g., US EPA 1991b, 1993a, b). These publications will outline accepted procedures for performing life cycle assessments, as they develop.

D. Conclusion

This section has examined macroscale pollution prevention from three perspectives: the wastes generated by industrial processes, the raw materials required by industrial processes, and the products resulting from industrial processes. Each perspective provides unique insights, and all serve as methodologies for identifying targets of opportunity for pollution prevention. The main goal of the section has been to describe the benefits and limitations of each of the analysis methods. A complete listing of potential prevention targets is beyond the scope of this manuscript;

however, the interested reader can study some of the material available in the literature (Allen and Jain, 1992; Allen and Behmanesh, 1993; Frosch and Gallopoulos, 1989). Moving beyond identifying opportunities for pollution prevention will require product redesign, raw material substitutions, and process modification. These methods for pollution prevention, which are generally focused on the manufacturing step of the product life cycle, will be the topic of the remainder of this review.

III. Mesoscale Pollution Prevention

Macroscale studies of pollution prevention, outlined in the previous sections, are useful in identifying research needs and targets of opportunity for pollution prevention. Once the targets have been identified, then the design of cleaner chemical processes and products can begin. Over the past decade, a variety of approaches have emerged. Some of these strategies are simply good housekeeping, maintenance, and operating practices. Frequently characterized as "low-hanging fruit," such methods have been extensively exploited in many manufacturing operations. A second tier of strategies involves relatively simple process modifications, employing currently available technology. Many of these approaches to waste reduction are still underutilized; some process modifications for reducing waste require technological innovation and are just beginning to be explored. Finally, product reformulation and raw material substitution have occasionally been used to reduce wastes. The U.S. Department of Energy's Office of Industrial Technologies (1991) has summarized these approaches in the matrix of Table VII.

In this section we will examine generic methods and specific examples of each of these strategies for reducing wastes. The focus will be on the chemical process industries: chemical manufacturing and petroleum refining. Focusing on a particular industrial sector will allow a fairly comprehensive treatment of waste reduction methods. In addition, an emphasis on chemical manufacturing and petroleum refining is relevant because these industries are responsible for over half of all hazardous wastes generated in the United States (Allen and Jain, 1992; Chemical Manufacturer's Association, 1990); they are also the source of approximately half of the releases of chemicals reported through the Toxic Release Inventory (US EPA, 1991c), and they are a significant source of wastes legally classified as nonhazardous (see Table I and Fig. 4). The presentation of pollution prevention methods will be divided into two broad categories: process modifications and product design/raw material substitution. To

TABLE VII
STRATEGIES FOR CLEANER TECHNOLOGIES (U.S. DEPARTMENT OF ENERGY, 1991)

Strategies	Housekeeping measures	In-process recycling	Process redesign	Input substitution	Product changes
Timing of impacts	Near-term	Near- and midterm	Mid- and long-term	Near- and midterm	Long-term
Capital cost	Low	Varies	High	Low	Moderate to high
Operating cost	Low	Low to moderate	Low	Moderate to high	Varies
Industry incentives	High	Moderate	Low	Moderate	Low
Energy-saving potential	Moderate	Moderate	High	Varies	High
Characteristics of industries where application is possible	All industries	All industries except those with very stringent or high quality demands	Frequently changing, high-tech industrial products; some commodity goods; consumer goods; manufacturers	Frequently changing, high-tech industrial products; job shops for industrial processes; some commodity goods; consumer goods manufacturers	Large-scale manufacturers of consumer goods
Industry examples	Rubber, electroplating, textiles, chemicals	Electronic components, chemicals, appliances	Steelmaking, medical, chemicals equipment, automobiles	Electronic components, foundries, printing, paints, chemicals	Consumer electronics, chemicals

TABLE VIII
EXAMPLES OF PROCESS MODIFICATIONS FOR WASTE REDUCTION

	Changes in operating practices	Currently feasible modifications	Process modifications requiring technology development
Storage vessels	Use of mixers to reduce sludge formation	Floating roof tanks, high-pressure tanks, insulated tanks	Process specific changes to eliminate the need for storage, particularly intermediates
Pipes and valves	Leak detection and repair programs for fugitive emissions	"Leakless" components	Process designs requiring the minimum number of valves and other components
Heat exchangers	Use of anti-foulants; innovative cleaning devices for heat exchanger tubes	Staged heat exchangers and use of adiabatic expanders to reduce heat exchanger temperatures	Heat exchanger networks to lower total process energy demand
Reactors	Higher selectivity through better mixing of reactants, elimination of hot and cold spots	Catalyst modifications to enhance selectivity or to prevent catalyst deactivation and attrition; recycle reactors for catalyst recycling	Changes in process chemistry; integration of reaction and separation units
Separators	Reduce wastes for reboilers	Improvements in separation efficiencies	New separation devices, efficient for very dilute species

give the presentation on process modifications a logical structure, we will group the waste reduction methods using a unit operations approach. This approach recognizes that most chemical processes consist of a common sequence of steps or unit operations—raw material storage, reaction, separation and purification of products, heating and cooling of process streams, product storage—with similar design procedures and pollution prevention approaches. We will group waste reduction methods according to the unit operation to which they apply. Thus, this section will develop a matrix of approaches to waste reduction in the chemical process industries (Table VIII). The rows of the matrix are common unit operations such as storage, pipes and valves, reactors, heat exchangers, and separation equipment. The columns of the matrix separate the methods into changes in operating practices, currently feasible changes in process technologies, and process changes requiring technology breakthroughs.

A. Process Modification for Waste Reduction

1. Waste Reduction Methods for Storage Vessels

Methods for reducing tank bottom wastes, fugitive emissions from tanks, residuals in shipping containers, and even the shipping containers themselves are abundant, and many are relatively simple. Tank bottoms, which are solids or sludges that accumulate at the bottom of large storage vessels, are typically composed of rusts, soil contaminants, and heavy feedstock constituents. If the tank bottoms are composed primarily of heavy feedstock constituents (e.g., sludges from heavy oils), then mechanical mixers can often be used effectively (American Petroleum Institute, 1991). Mechanical mixing is not the only option available for solubilizing tank bottoms. Emulsifying agents have been used in the oil industry to solubilize tank bottoms, but care must be exercised in making sure that the emulsifier is compatible with downstream processing.

Fugitive emissions from tanks can also be reduced using fairly simple technologies. Floating roofs, insulated walls to prevent temperature and pressure swings, walls designed to withstand higher pressure (which reduce the need to vent), and vapor condensation and recovery systems can all be employed. Many of these technologies are expensive, however, and the amount of material that is saved by the tank design change will not always cover all of the capital costs.

In addition to the waste reduction strategies outlined for tanks, there are a number of simple approaches for reducing the wastes associated with the containers used to ship reactants and products (rail cars, drums and other packages). Proper location of drainage valves can often reduce the amount of residual material in storage vessels. Storage drums dedicated to a specific use can reduce clean-out wastes, and product storage containers compatible with the end use of the product, e.g., water-soluble, biodegradable packages for water-soluble pesticides, can reduce packaging wastes. As an example of reducing container waste, consider a case study reported by Chevron (in Cairncross, 1992), which produced 10,000 oil samples each month, each contained in a glass vial. The used vials were considered hazardous waste and were landfilled until Chevron developed a recycling operation for both the glass and the traces of oil left in the vials. The cost of the recycling system was recouped in less than a year.

More sophisticated solutions to reducing storage wastes generally involve designing out the need for storage. For example, the release of methyl isocyanate (MIC) that killed thousands in Bhopal was from a storage vessel. The MIC, which is a chemical intermediate in the manufacture of an agricultural chemical, is now no longer stored. The MIC is created on-demand in the chemical reactor that consumes the MIC, thus eliminating the need for storage.

2. *Waste Reduction Methods for Piping and Valves*

The most significant environmental problem associated with valves, pumps, compressors, flanges, and other pipe fittings is fugitive emissions. Fugitive emissions are the uncontrolled releases from the thousands of process components in a chemical manufacturing process. Typically, the vast majority of fugitive emissions from a chemical manufacturing operation are associated with a small percentage of process components that are actively leaking. If these leaking components are detected and repaired or replaced, then fugitive emissions can be dramatically reduced. The potential effectiveness of such Leak Detection and Repair (LDAR) programs can be assessed using average data compiled for the Synthetic Organic Chemical Manufacturing Industries by the US EPA (1985). These emissions data indicate that between 500 and 1500 pounds of material are lost due to fugitive emissions per million pounds of chemical production (Berglund and Hansen, 1990). In contrast, for chemical manufacturing operations that have aggressive LDAR programs (often due to the toxicity or other hazardous properties of the chemicals involved), rates of losses due to fugitive emissions can be substantially lower. In 1,3-butadiene manufacturing, loss rates are estimated at 450 lb per million lb of product; for ethylene oxide, the rate is 35; for acrolein, the rate is 0.5, and for phosgene the rate is 0.1 (Berglund and Hansen, 1990). The exceptional leak-free performance of ethylene oxide, acrolein, and phosgene manufacturing is mainly due to aggressive leak detection and repair, careful equipment installation practices, critical evaluation of equipment vendors, and the design of process units for rapid start-up and shutdown (many leaks occur during the rapid changes in process operation that occur during start-up and shutdown). Expensive leakless equipment is used only sparingly.

While simple, the reduction of fugitive emissions is not inexpensive. In a case study involving ethylene oxide manufacturing, \$1.5 million was spent over 2 years, with 55% spent on materials, 30% spent on labor, and 15% spent on a study of equipment leak rates. Just the labor involved in regular monitoring of the status of the thousands to tens of thousands of pieces of equipment typically found in an oil refinery or chemical manufacturing facility can be expensive. Added to that are the costs of replacement and repair, and if appropriate, expensive leakless components. In a fugitive emission reduction project for a moderately sized petroleum refinery (Klee, 1992), an LDAR program was estimated to have an annual cost of \$150,000, largely due to labor. The project was projected to reduce emissions by 705 tons per year, yielding a cost per ton recovered of \$213.

A long-term solution to fugitive emissions is the design of processes with a minimum number of pumps, valves, flanges, and other components. While minimizing the number of components is attractive for reducing fugitive emissions, safety concerns dictate that some redundancy be designed into chemical manufacturing systems.

3. *Waste Reduction Methods for Reactors*

Reactors are a key element in any chemical manufacturing process and are particularly important in waste generation. The reactor is, after all, the unit in which most of the undesired by-products that will eventually make up the waste streams are created. In examining reactor designs for waste reduction potential, there are five levels of analysis that need to be considered. The first level of analysis considers selectivity, i.e., whether the reactor is producing the maximum amount of product and the minimum amount of by-product (which may become waste) per unit mass of feed material. The tools for optimizing selectivity are well known to chemical reaction engineers and have been continuously incorporated into chemical reactor designs for several decades. High levels of selectivity are already achieved in chemical manufacturing operations, but some room for improvement is available, as shown in Table IX. In some rare cases waste reduction may require different reaction conditions than those that maximize selectivity, but in general the only changes in reactor design that are likely to result in waste reduction involve recycle reactors. Three possible configurations are shown in Fig. 16. Configuration A shows a typical recycle reactor where unconverted reactants are recycled to a single process reactor. Conventional recycle reactors can be very effective in reducing wastes if undesired by-products are produced in a reversible reaction that reaches equilibrium. In this case, recycling the by-product inhibits the net formation of waste in the reactor. Configurations B (Hagh and Allen, 1990; Kalnes and James, 1988) and C (from Nelson, 1990) offer opportunities for reducing wastes because the optimal conditions for converting recycle streams into products are generally different than for converting feed streams into products.

TABLE IX
REPRESENTATIVE PRODUCTION AND YIELD DATA FOR COMMODITY CHEMICAL MANUFACTURING (ADAPTED FROM ALLEN, 1992)

Chemical and production process	Annual production (1,000 tons)	Yield (%) calculated[a]
Acrylonitrile	2182	
1. Ammoxidation of propylene		65
2. Cyanation/oxidation of ethylene		76
Maleic anhydride	359	
1. Oxidation of benzene		39
2. Oxidation of *n*-butane		48
Phthalic anhydride	863	
1. Oxidation of *o*-xylene		77
2. Oxidation of naphthalene		69
Vinyl chloride	8439	
1. Chlorination and oxychlorination of ethylene		96
2. Dehydrochlorination of ethylene dichloride		98

[a]Calculated using data reported in Rudd *et al.* (1981).

A second level of analysis for waste reduction in chemical reactors considers the fact that hazards associated with many wastes are due to trace contaminants. For example, if a reactor produces a by-product stream that is considered a waste only because it contains a trace of a chlorinated dibenzodioxin, then eliminating the trace level of dioxin may allow the by-product stream to be used productively. Eliminating the production of very hazardous trace-level components may involve far different reactor designs than those used for maximizing selectivity. These types of improvements are still in their infancy and will require significant fundamental research to become practical. They are discussed in more detail in Section IV.

A third level of analysis involves reconsidering reaction chemistry, which may mean the use of different precursors or the use of a different catalyst. Consider the example of propylene polymerization. Throughout the late 1970s the manufacturing of linear polypropylene generated non-linear polypropylene waste amounting to 7–10% of the total product. The nonlinear polypropylene was generally landfilled or used as an auxiliary fuel. In 1980 the total quantity of the nonlinear polypropylene generated was 200 million pounds. Process research into the chemistry of propylene polymerization, after a number of years, led to a new catalyst which reduced rates of nonlinear polypropylene (waste) generation by 90% (U.S. Department of Energy, 1991). This case study illustrates the potential for

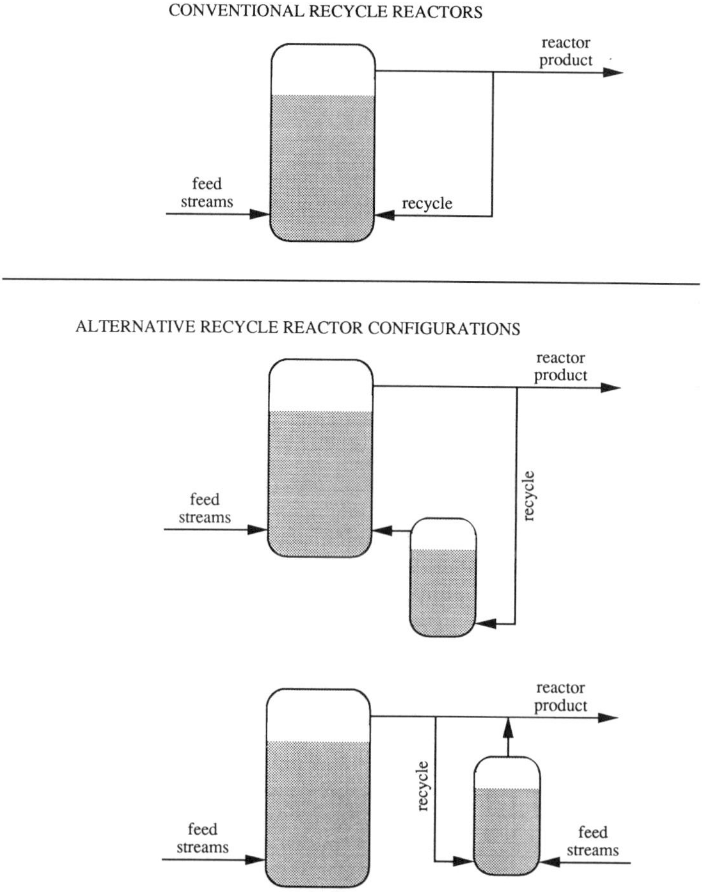

FIG. 16. Recycle reactor configurations.

new catalytic technologies in reducing waste. Other examples include the following (Cusumano 1992; see also Allen, 1992):

- *"Elimination of toxic reagents and intermediates [via novel catalysis]:* ... Anhydrous hydrofluoric and fuming sulfuric acids are used as catalysts throughout the chemical and petroleum industry. Replacing these materials with safe, solid catalysts could have a profound positive impact on industry.
- *"Elimination of toxic streams and by-products [via new catalytic technologies]:* One example is the development of a catalyst system to retrofit current acetaldehyde technology. This technology produces significant amounts of chloro-organic by-products. This requires col-

lection and disposal of aqueous and volatile chloro-organics. A catalyst system has been developed that can be retrofitted into existing technology. This technology reduces by more than 100-fold the chloro-organics formed, thereby making this a much safer process.
- "*Elimination of toxic emissions [using new catalysts]:* An example is the catalytic combustion of hydrocarbons such as methane to obviate the formation of NO_x. By developing catalytic systems capable of reducing the flame temperature from 1800°C to 1300°C, it is possible to reduce the NO_x level from 200 ppm to less than 1 ppm, an amount which will meet all anticipated future regulations."

A fourth method for waste reduction in reactors focuses on spent catalyst wastes where recycling, controlling attrition, and limiting deactivation may reduce wastes. Consider the case of hydroprocessing catalyst wastes, which are extensively recycled to recover cobalt, molybdenum, nickel, vanadium, and alumina (*Chemical and Engineering News*, October 26, 1992, p. 20). More than a third of the domestic demand for vanadium is met via these recovery processes (*Chemical and Engineering News*, November 23, 1992, p. 2).

Finally, integrating chemical reaction and separation in a single vessel offers opportunities for waste reduction. As an example of this strategy, consider the synthesis of methyl-*tert*-butyl ether (MTBE). Two processes are in common industrial use in the synthesis of MTBE from methanol and isobutylene. In one process, a series of fixed-bed catalytic reactors send a mix of product, unreacted methanol, and unreacted isobutylene to a series of separation devices. In an alternative process configuration, the feed materials are sent to a distillation column that contains a series of catalytic beds. The processes are contrasted in Fig. 17. There are several advantages to the catalytic distillation configuration:

> Because the less volatile MTBE product moves down the distillation column, away from the reaction zones as it is produced, thermodynamic limitations to conversion are reduced. The simpler catalytic distillation design involves fewer valves, flanges, and components that can be a source of fugitive emissions; it requires fewer heat exchangers which can generate wastes (see below), and capital costs are lower.

Catalytic distillation and other process configurations that combine reaction and separation in a single vessel are relatively new. Currently, only a few commodity chemicals are manufactured using catalytic distillation. This is not due to a lack of versatility of this design concept. Rather it is a reflection of the timing of process selection. The choice between process configurations that are as different as fixed bed reactors and catalytic

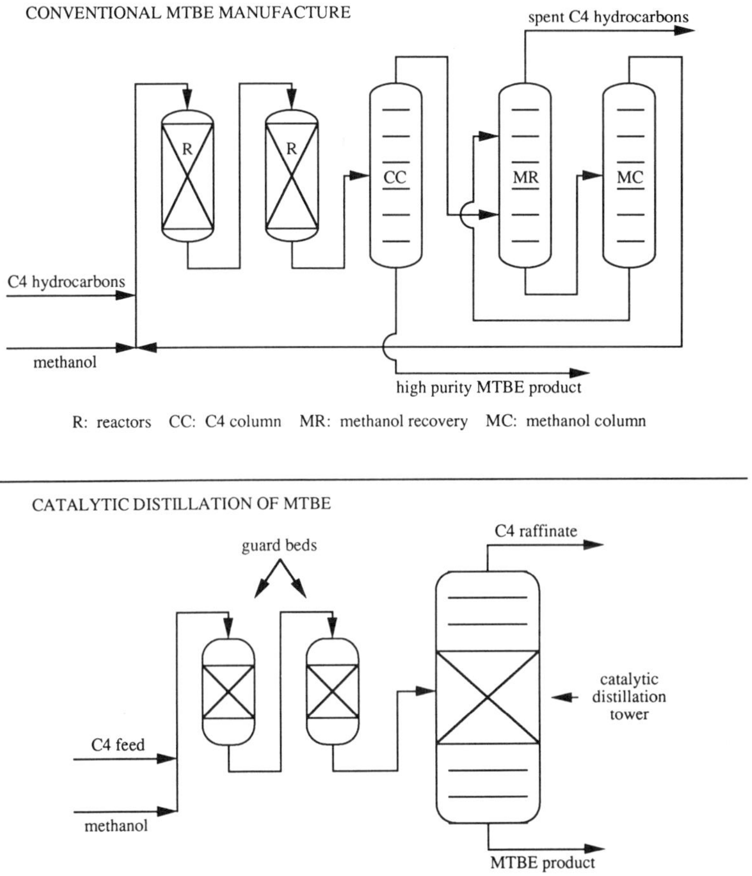

FIG. 17. Integration of reaction and separation (e.g., catalytic distillation) in a single vessel can reduce waste; shown are the conventional and catalytic distillation processes for manufacturing methyl-*tert*-butyl ether.

distillation is generally made when a plant is initially built; retrofitting existing plants this drastically is not generally feasible.

4. Waste Reduction Methods for Heat Exchangers

Heat exchangers can be a source of waste when high temperatures in the exchangers cause the fluids to form sludges. These sludges reduce the effectiveness of the exchanger and therefore must be periodically removed. Methods for reducing wastes from heat exchanger cleaning fall into two major categories. One approach is to alter the cleaning process, which is often blasting with high-pressure steam, a method that generates significant quantities of wastewater. Alternatives include sandblasting with recyclable sand and blasting with dry ice. Another approach attempts to reduce the generation of sludges by injecting anti-foulants or by reducing the temperatures used in the heat exchangers. Most of these approaches are relatively simple, with the exception of the use of temperature reductions. To understand how temperature reductions in heat exchangers are accomplished, consider how a heat exchanger is designed. In order to accomplish a given amount of heat exchange, a process designer attempts a compromise between the temperature driving force for heat exchange and the area available for the heat transfer. For example, the designer could choose a relatively low temperature difference between process fluids, then contact those fluids over a large surface. The same amount of energy transfer could also be achieved by imposing a large temperature difference over a much smaller area. The low temperature difference/high area alternative will generate less heat exchanger waste, but in general has been avoided for two reasons. The first is capital costs. A large-surface area exchanger costs more than a smaller area exchanger. The second reason for avoiding the low temperature difference/high surface area alternative is more subtle. In many large chemical process facilities, heat is supplied by steam, which generally is available at a set of fixed temperatures. The designer confronted with heating a process fluid from 200 to 350°F may be forced to choose between steam at 275°F (30 psig) and high-pressure steam at 400°F (235 psig). Clearly the low-pressure steam is inadequate to do the job, but the high-pressure steam may generate significant sludges. An alternative to choosing only the low- or high-pressure steam is the adiabatic expander shown in Fig. 18. This low-cost device can mix the low- and high-pressure steam to achieve the optimal heat transfer temperature (Nelson, 1990).

5. *Waste Reduction Methods for Separation Equipment*

Separation equipment can be regarded as both generators and minimizers of waste. An effective separation technology can be used to recycle materials within a chemical process. For example, solvent emissions are a significant problem in some sectors of the chemical industry (e.g., pharmaceuticals) Cost-effective condensers to separate evaporating solvent from an air stream can be used to economically recycle these emissions (see case study of Brayton-Cycle Solvent Recovery, U.S. Department of Energy, 1991). On the other hand, separation devices can be a significant source of waste. Since separation units are designed to generate pure

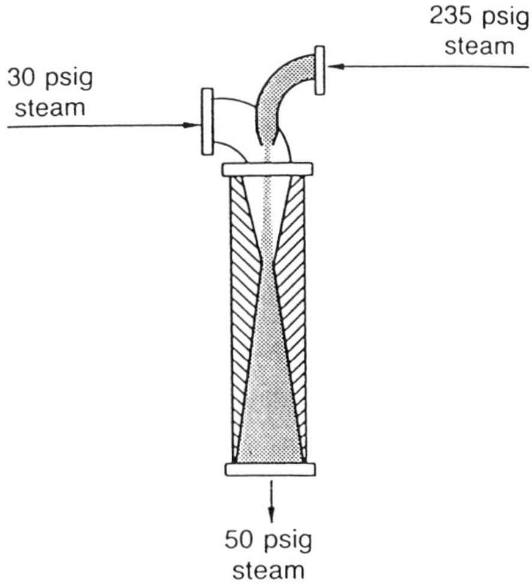

FIG. 18. Use of an adiabatic expander can allow the designer to precisely control the temperature of steam used in a heat exchanger; if lower temperatures can be used, wastes can often be reduced (Nelson, 1990).

products and isolate contaminants, they are by nature waste-generating. The amount of waste generated can be minimized by performing clean separations, i.e., leaving the smallest possible amount of product in the separated contaminants. For some separation devices, such as distillation columns, this can be accomplished by varying the operating conditions of the separation unit (e.g., the reflux ratio), but such improvements are difficult to generalize about. To examine the complexity of the issue, consider the acetone recovery system shown in Fig. 19. Acetone in a gas stream is removed by scrubbing with water; the water is sent to a second separation column where pure acetone and water are recovered. The water in the second column contains some acetone, and some fraction of this water may become waste. The other potential waste stream for this process is acetone in the air which exits the scrubber. A complex optimization of the design parameters for these columns reveals (Ciric and Jia, 1992)

- it is not economical to generate any wastewater, and
- the cost of the acetone recovery is a highly nonlinear function of the amount of acetone in the gas escaping as waste (see Fig. 19).

So, in this case study one of the waste streams can be completely eliminated economically. The other waste streams may be reduced economically (from point a to point b in Fig. 19), but complete elimination is

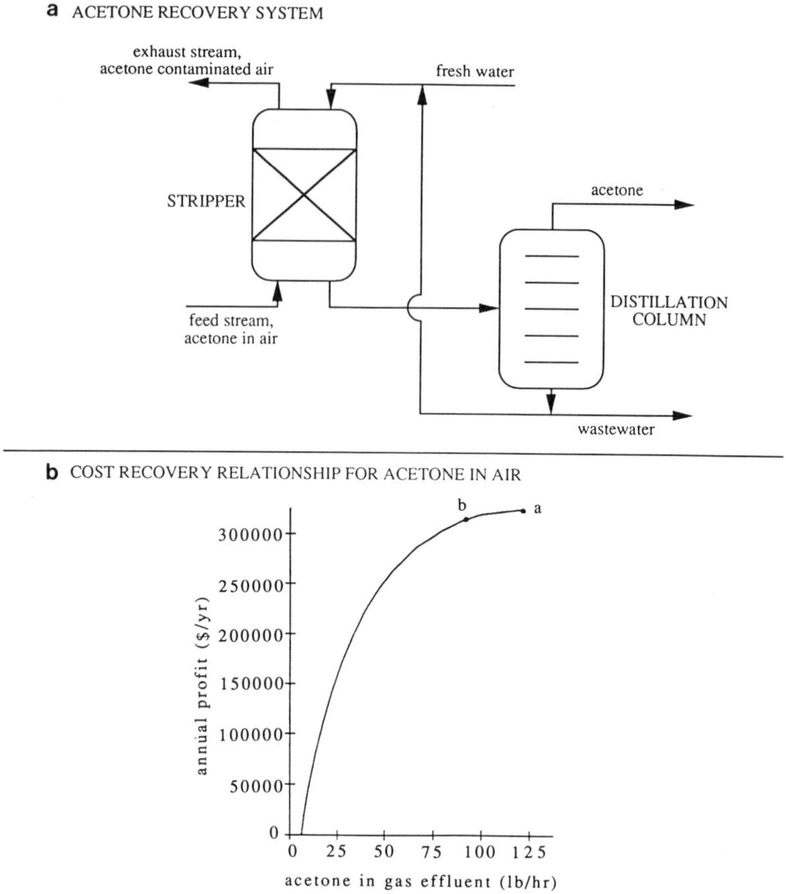

FIG. 19. Acetone recovery system. (a) flow diagram of the system; note there are two waste streams: wastewater and air contaminated with acetone. Complete recycle is possible and economical for the wastewater, but not for the air stream. (b) costs for recovering acetone from the air stream increase dramatically as the percent recovery increases (Ciric and Jia, 1992).

not economically feasible. This case study is not unusual and illustrates the fact that for some waste streams from separation units, complete elimination is possible; for other streams, some reduction, but not complete elimination, is possible.

A more straightforward way to minimize wastes from separation devices is to focus on the heat exchange equipment associated with the units. Methods such as those described earlier for heat exchangers can also be effective for reboilers and condensers.

B. Product Redesign and Raw Material Substitution for Waste Reduction

It is far more difficult to describe generic methods for raw material substitution and product redesign than it is to identify process modifications to reduce waste. However, some chemical manufacturers have developed aggressive and systematic efforts to identify productive uses for waste streams. For example, Du Pont found a market in the pharmaceuticals and coating industry for hexamethyleneimine, a by-product of nylon manufacturing. The market is now so strong that demand exceeds supply and in 1989, Du Pont had to find a way to intentionally manufacture what had formerly been a waste. A Chevron subsidiary sends caustic to nearby pulp and paper manufacturers, and Dow has set up a formal program to find uses for by-product streams (from Cairncross, 1992). Waste exchanges to facilitate these transfers are emerging across the country.

C. Process Synthesis and Flowsheet Restructuring for Waste Reduction

The analysis presented in the previous sections focused on reducing wastes from individual unit operations. This approach implicitly assumes that a process with an established sequence of unit operations exists. Another set of methods for waste reduction involves synthesizing or restructuring the process flowsheet. Identifying flowsheet structures that minimize waste is a challenging task; however, a number of design tools have recently emerged that allow the problem to be approached systematically. This section will describe two of these methods: the hierarchical design procedures of Douglas (1992), and the Mass Exchange Network (MEN) synthesis methods developed by Manousiouthakis and co-workers (El-Halwagi and Manousiouthakis, 1989, 1990).

1. Hierarchical Design Procedures

The design of a chemical process involves many decisions. Choices of raw materials, catalyst, reactor design, separator design, and level of energy integration can lead to a large number of possible flowsheets. Since in a typical process, 10^4–10^9 flowsheet configurations may be possible (Douglas, 1988), not all of the flowsheeting alternatives can be fully evaluated on the basis of waste generation, or any other criterion. To systematically address flowsheet decision making, Douglas (1988) has developed a hierarchical approach. Flowsheeting decisions are made se-

TABLE X
HIERARCHICAL DECISION LEVELS FOR PROCESS SYNTHESIS
(DOUGLAS, 1992)

Level 1.	Input information: type of problem	
Level 2.	Input–output structure of the flowsheet	
Level 3.	Recycle structure of the flowsheet	
Level 4.	Specification of the separation system	
	Level 4a.	General structure: phase splits
	Level 4b.	Vapor recovery system
	Level 4c.	Liquid recovery system
	Level 4d.	Solid recovery system
Level 5.	Energy integration	
Level 6.	Evaluation of alternatives	
Level 7.	Flexibility and control	
Level 8.	Safety	

quentially at a variety of levels, as shown in Table X. The number of possible flowsheets is reduced as the designer proceeds to higher and higher levels. This hierarchical design procedure allows the systematic incorporation of waste reduction alternatives at all levels of design decision making. Shown in Table XI are a number of waste reduction opportunities that could be considered at various design levels. This framework (Douglas, 1992) offers a systematic approach to constructing a flowsheet that generates a minimum of wastes. The advantage of the method is that it explicitly recognizes that waste reduction cannot be relegated to the end of the design process; rather, it must be integrated into all decision levels. At present, the method is somewhat qualitative; a more quantitative approach is described in the next several sections.

2. *Mass Exchange Network Synthesis: Introduction*

The construction of a flowsheet that produces the minimum possible quantity of waste is a design problem that is somewhat analogous to the problem of constructing a flowsheet that consumes the minimum amount of energy. In one case, we are striving for energy efficiency; in the other case, we are striving for mass efficiency. While this simple analogy has some flaws, we will utilize it to develop the concept of MEN synthesis. Heat exchange network synthesis is one of the most powerful flowsheeting tools available for maximizing the energy efficiency of a flowsheet. Simply stated, heat exchange network synthesis systematically examines all of the heating and cooling requirements called for in a flowsheet and determines the extent to which streams that need to have their temperature raised can be heated by streams that need to be cooled. As a very simple example,

TABLE XI
POSSIBLE WASTE REDUCTION STRATEGIES TO BE EVALUATED AT EACH DESIGN LEVEL (DOUGLAS, 1992)

Level 2. Input–output structure of the flowsheet
- a. Problems caused by the reaction chemistry: change the chemistry
- b. Problems caused by air oxidation to NO_x: change to O_2 in recycle CO_2 oxidations
- c. Problems caused by spent catalysts: regenerate the catalyst

Level 3. Recycle structure of the flowsheet
- a. Problems caused by adding reactor diluents to shift the product distribution or to shift the equilibrium conversion: change the diluent
- b. Problems caused by adding heat carriers: change the heat carrier
- c. Problems caused by adding reactor solvents: change the solvent

Level 4. Specification of the separation system

Level 4a. General structure: phase splits

Level 4b. Vapor recovery system
- a. Problems caused by absorber solvents: change the solvent
- b. Problems caused by regeneration of adsorption beds: change the bed stripping agent
- c. Problems with removing spent adsorbents: change to absorption or condensation
- d. Problems caused by the use of reactive absorbers to remove toxic materials

Level 4c. Liquid recovery system
- a. Problems caused by stripping agents: change the agent
- b. Problems caused by extraction solvents: change the solvent
- c. Problems caused by crystallizer (recycle and) purge streams (almost pure water): reuse the purge water elsewhere in the process
- d. Problems caused by crystallizer (not almost pure water): remove the contaminants and recycle the water or look for a different separation system
- e. Problems caused by reactive crystallization by-products: look for a different separation technique
- f. Problems caused by spent adsorbents: regenerate the adsorbent

Level 4d. Solid recovery system
- a. Problems caused by cake washing: same as for crystallizer; filter mother liquor streams

consider Fig. 20. In this example a process stream at 50°C is to be heated to 200°C and a process stream at 200°C is to be cooled to 90°C. Rather than exclusively using utilities to accomplish this heating and cooling, the two process streams can be contacted as shown in Fig. 21, reducing energy requirements. The relative heat capacities and flow rates of the two streams place additional constraints on the amount of energy that can be transferred between the two streams. In this example, there are no thermodynamic limitations at the high-temperature end of this heat transfer problem. In principle the hot stream might be used to heat the cold stream to 200°C. In practice, however, an infinitesimally small temperature

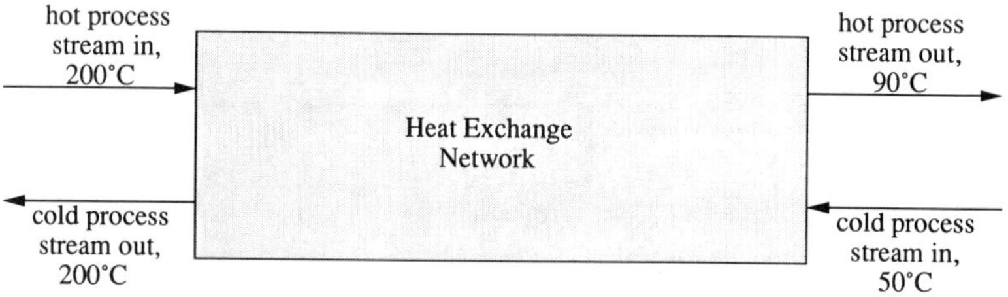

FIG. 20. A simple heat exchange network synthesis problem: stream H needs to be cooled from 200°C to 90°C; stream C needs to be heated from 50°C to 200°C.

difference between hot and cold streams would require infinite heat transfer area. Thus, consideration of the minimum temperature differences required by heat transfer equipment imposes additional constraints on heat exchange network design. Details and more complete treatments of heat exchange network synthesis can be found in modern chemical process design texts (e.g., Douglas, 1988). Our goal here is not to fully develop the concepts of heat exchange networks, but to remind readers of the basic principles to illustrate the analogy between heat and mass exchange networks. Mass exchange network synthesis has been developed by Manousiouthakis and co-workers (El-Halwagi and Manousiouthakis, 1989, 1990). The synthesis considers thermodynamic and concentration difference constraints which are analogous to the simpler temperature and thermodynamic constraints used in heat exchange network synthesis. A brief introduction to mass exchange constraints is given next.

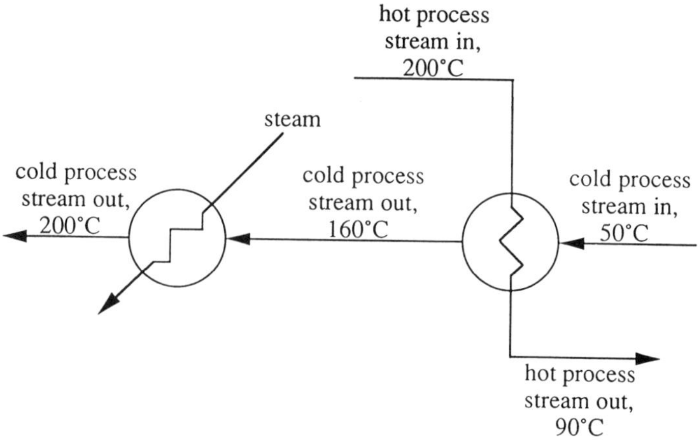

FIG. 21. Heat exchange network for the hot and cold streams of Fig. 20.

3. Thermodynamic and Mass Balance Constraints

In a mass exchanger, the amount of solute that can be transferred from a rich stream to a lean stream is limited by mass balance constraints and concentration driving force constraints, as follows: (i) the total mass transferred by the rich stream must be equal to that received by the lean stream, and (ii) mass transfer is possible only if a positive driving force ε exists for all rich stream/lean stream matches.

The equation describing the first constraint is found by performing a material balance on the solute to be transferred from rich stream i to lean stream j (Fig. 22), which results in

$$R_i\left(y_{ki}^{\text{in}} - y_{ki}^{\text{out}}\right) = L_j\left(x_{kj}^{\text{out}} - x_{kj}^{\text{in}}\right), \tag{1}$$

where R_i is the flow rate of rich stream i, L_j is the flow rate of lean stream j, y_{ki} is the mass fraction of solute k in rich stream i, and x_{kj} is the mass fraction of the solute k in lean stream j. For the analysis in this section, the flow rates of the streams are assumed to be constant. While this is not strictly the case, it is a good approximation if the concentration of solute in the streams is low and little transfer of material other than solute occurs. Equation (1) represents the operating line for the mass transfer of solute from the rich stream to the lean stream. An operating line for contact between a single rich and a single lean stream is plotted in Fig. 23. Note that the slope of the operating line is equal to L/R.

Equilibrium between a rich and a lean stream can be represented by an equation of the form

$$y_{ki} = m_{kj}x_{kj}^{*} + b_{kj}, \tag{2}$$

where x_{kj}^{*} is the mass fraction of component k in stream j that is in equilibrium with the mass fraction y_{ki} in stream i. The constants of Eq. (2) are thermodynamic properties and may be obtained through experimental data. A plot of an equilibrium line is shown in Fig. 23. The positive driving force constraint for mass transfer is satisfied when the equilibrium line lies to the right of the operating line.

FIG. 22. A mass exchanger.

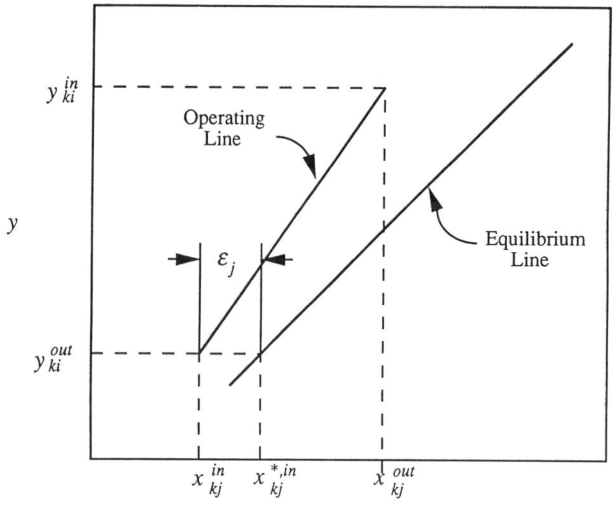

FIG. 23. Equilibrium and mass conservation constraints on mass exchanger design.

4. Composition Interval Diagrams and Load Lines

The operating and equilibrium lines of the previous section are familiar tools for separator design. However, in MEN synthesis, the design of individual separators is not considered. Instead, the streams to be contacted and the extent of transfer possible is determined. Equilibrium and operating lines are not sufficient for this task. The tools of MEN synthesis are composition interval diagrams and load lines. A composition interval diagram (CID) depicts the lean and rich streams under consideration in MEN synthesis. CIDs for the rich and lean streams of Table XII are shown in Fig. 24. Inspection of this figure reveals that for each rich stream, an arrow is drawn with its tail at the entering mass fraction and its head at the exiting mass fraction. Similar arrows are drawn for lean streams.

In the CID of Fig. 24, the compositions of the rich and lean streams are on separate axes. These axes can be combined through the equilibrium relationship. If the equilibrium relationship in the region of interest for

TABLE XII
STREAM DATA FOR A SCENARIO WITH TWO RICH STREAMS AND ONE LEAN STREAM

Rich streams				Lean stream			
Stream	Flow rate, kg/s	y^{in}	y^{out}	Stream	Flow rate, kg/s	x^{in}	x^{out}
R_1	5	0.10	0.03	L	15	0.00	0.05
R_2	10	0.07	0.03				

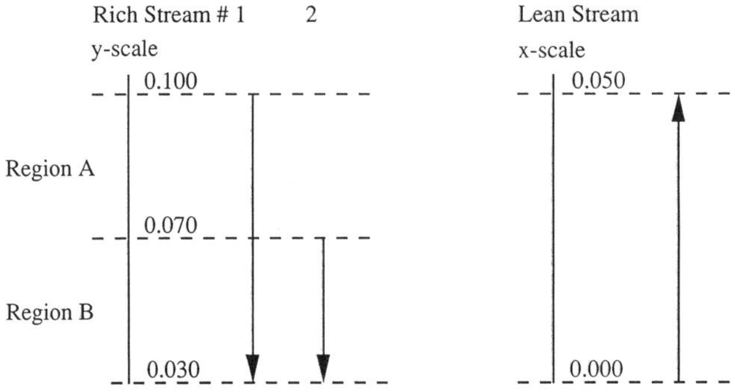

FIG. 24. Composition interval diagram (CID) for the streams of Table XII.

the species considered in this problem is given by

$$y = 0.67x^*, \tag{3}$$

then a mass fraction of $y = 0.1$ in the rich stream is in equilibrium with a mass fraction of $x^* = 0.15$ in the lean stream. By converting the lean stream compositions of Fig. 24 to the rich stream compositions with which they are in equilibrium, and vice versa, a combined CID with shared axes as shown in Fig. 25 can be constructed.

Load lines depict the flow rate of solute transferred as a function of stream composition. Take, for example, R_1 of Table XII. At its inlet, this stream has not begun exchange of solute, so one end point of its load line is $y^{in} = 0.10$, mass exchanged = 0 kg/s. At its outlet, this stream has exchanged −0.35 kg/s or [5 kg/s (0.03–0.10)], so the coordinates of the other end point are (0.07, −0.35 kg/s). This load line and load lines for each of the streams in Table XII are shown in Fig. 26. Note that the rich

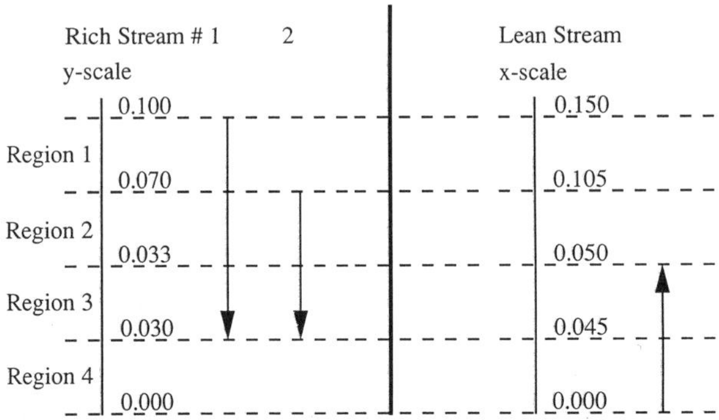

FIG. 25. Combined composition interval diagram (CID) for the streams of Table XII. The equilibrium relationship is used to scale rich and lean stream axes.

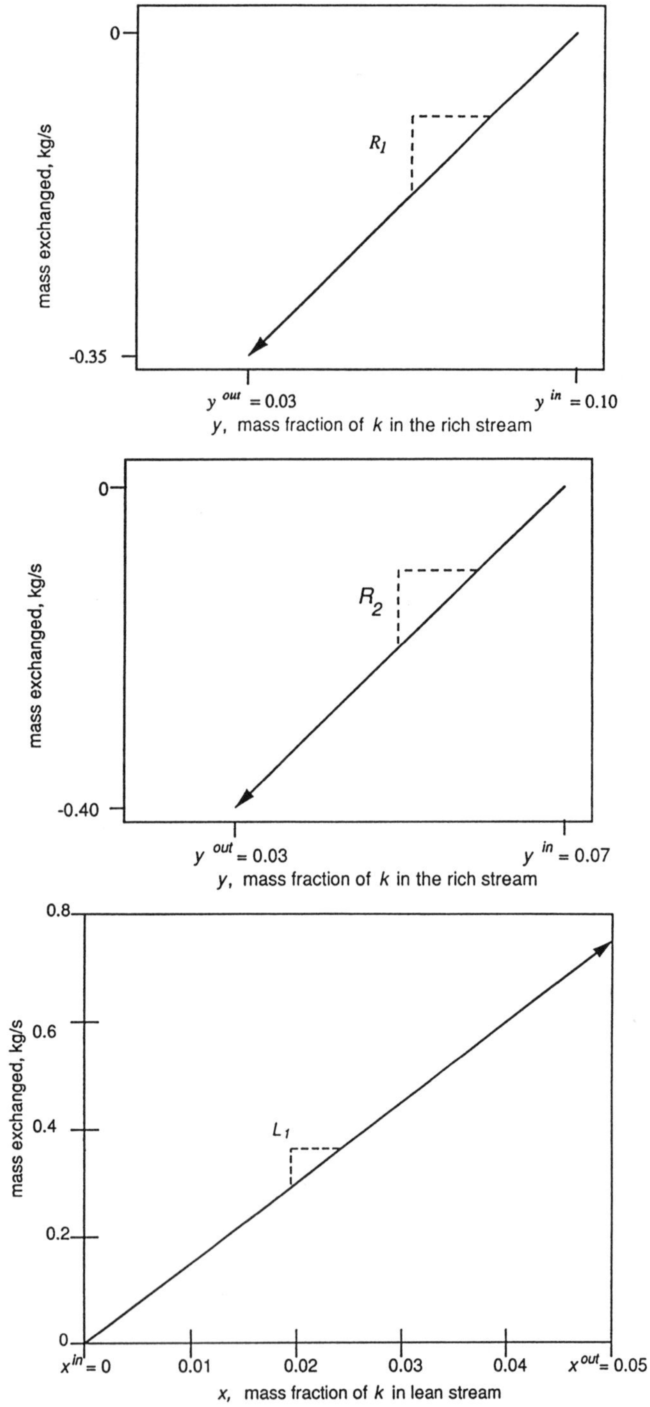

FIG. 26. Load lines for the streams of Table XII. Mass fraction is plotted versus mass exchanged for each stream. The slope of the line equals the flow rate of the stream.

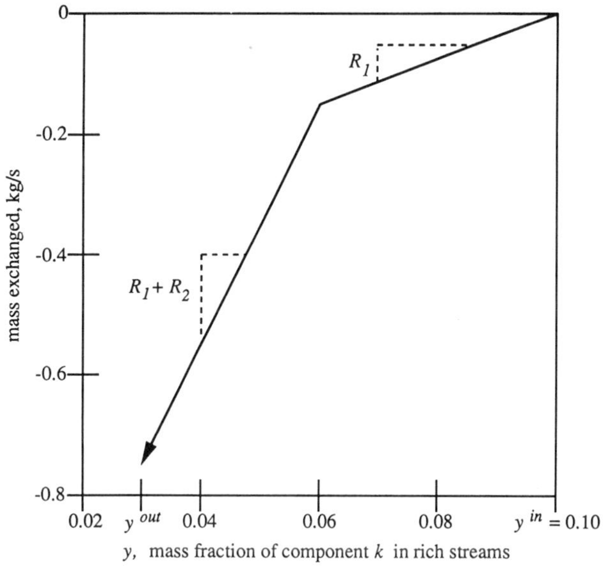

FIG. 27. Composite load line for the two rich streams of Table XII.

stream vectors point down and to the left, while the lean stream vectors point up to indicate the direction of transfer.

The load lines shown in Fig. 26 were for single rich and lean streams. When there is more than one rich stream or more than one lean stream to consider, a line representative of the multiple streams must be constructed. This line, called a composite load line, is the sum of the individual load lines and is developed with the aid of a CID. As an illustration, the composite load line for the rich streams of Fig. 26 is plotted in Fig. 27. This composite line is the sum of the individual rich stream load lines. It consists of two segments, corresponding to the regions shown in the CID of Fig. 24. In region A are the rich streams with mass fractions less than 0.1 and greater than 0.07 ($0.1 \leq y \leq 0.07$). Only R_1 falls into this category, so the total flow rate of the rich streams in this composition range is 5 kg/s. The starting point for the load line is $y = 0.1$ and 0.0 kg/s transferred. Recall that the mass transferred in each CID region is equal to the mass fraction exiting the region minus the mass fraction entering the region, multiplied by the sum of the flow rates in the region. Therefore, at $y = 0.07$, -0.15 kg/s [5 kg/s (0.07–0.1)] have been transferred, and the end point of the load line in this region is (0.07, -0.15 kg/s). As before, the slope of the load line equals the mass flow rate of the stream. In region B are the rich streams with mole fractions less than 0.07 and greater than 0.03. Both rich streams fall into this region. When the load line is plotted, it has a slope equal to the sum of the flow rates of all streams in this region. The starting point for this segment of the load line is the termination point of the previous segment.

The next step in constructing load line diagrams is to plot the composite lean and rich streams on the same axes. As with combined CIDs, load line diagrams can be combined by making use of the equilibrium relation, which for this case is

$$y = 0.67x^*$$

in the region of interest. A combined figure can be made following several different conventions, each of which gives the same final results. The convention used here for constructing the combined figure is to first plot the load line of the lean stream. The rich stream composite load line is added to the figure after converting the rich stream mass fractions into the lean stream mass fractions with which they are in equilibrium. These conversions were made in order to construct the CID of Fig. 25. The rich stream composite load line is free to move vertically; its placement determines the contact between the lean and rich streams. The rich stream load line has this freedom to move vertically because the values for mass exchanged on the y-axis are not absolute: they are useful only in relative terms, i.e., in terms of the differences in mass transferred between points. Therefore, the composite rich stream load line begins at a value x^*, which represents the lean stream mass fraction with which the rich stream is in equilibrium. In the example of Fig. 27 the rich stream load lines begin at mass fraction x^* of 0.15 (0.10/0.67) and continue downward and to the left with a slope of $0.67R_1$. The next point falls at $x^* = 0.10$, where the slope changes to $0.67(R_1 + R_2)$. The load line ends where $x^* = 0.045(0.03/0.67)$. The load lines for the lean and rich streams of Table XII are plotted together in Fig. 28. As stated before, the composite rich stream load line could have been located in any number of different vertical positions.

In Fig. 28, the lean stream load line has been drawn to the left of the composite rich stream load line at every point. This indicates that the desired mass exchange is thermodynamically feasible, and that the transfer could be accomplished using exchangers of finite size. In Fig. 29, the lean stream load line lies to the left of the rich stream load line, except at a point, called the pinch point, where the lines meet. Mass exchange in a case such as this is thermodynamically feasible, but would require an infinitely large mass exchanger (an infinite number of trays or stages, for example). Therefore, there is a practical requirement that conditions be manipulated so that a positive horizontal ε exists between the load lines. This ε is the driving force for mass transfer. If at any point the lean stream

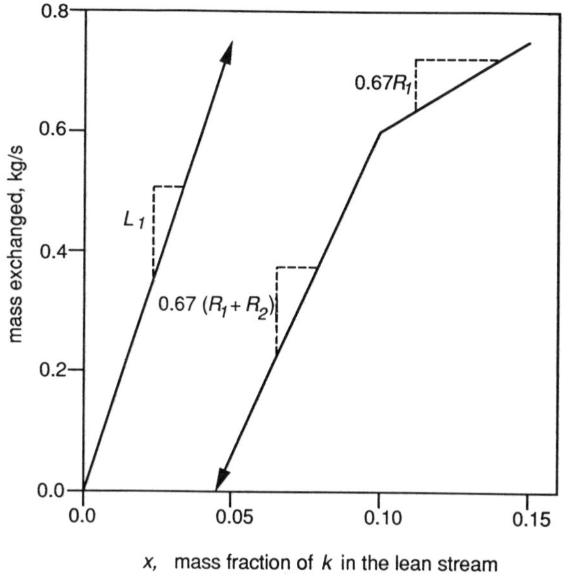

FIG. 28. Composite rich and lean stream load lines for the example of Table XII. Note that the rich stream mass fraction is plotted as an equivalent lean stream mass fraction using the equilibrium relationship.

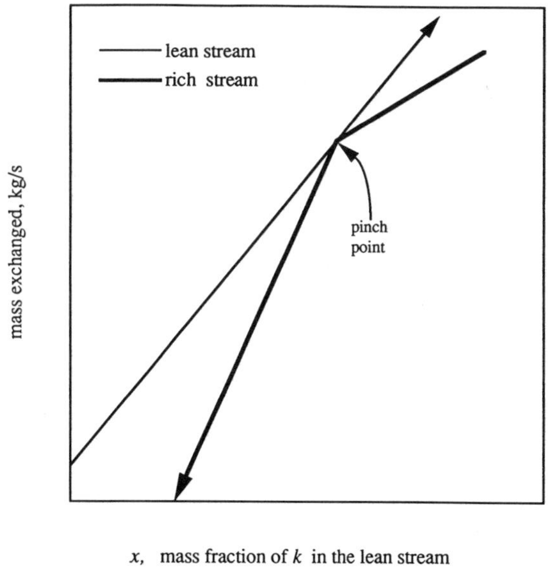

FIG. 29. Pinch point in a load line diagram.

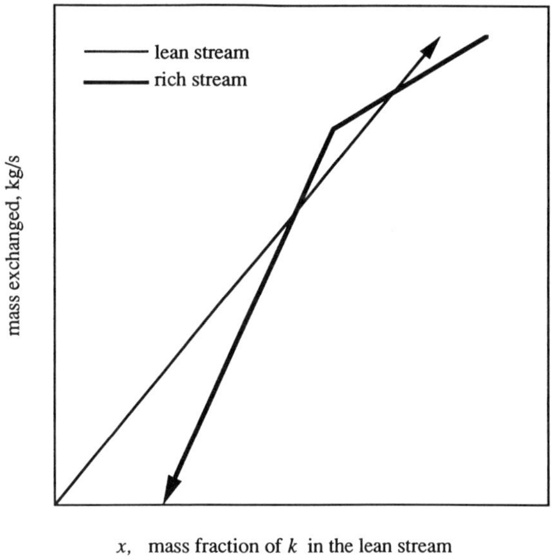

FIG. 30. Load line diagram illustrating thermodynamic infeasibility.

load line lies to the right of the rich stream load line, as shown in Fig. 30, mass exchange in the desired direction is not thermodynamically feasible. In fact, if streams with such characteristics are contacted, mass exchange from the lean stream to the rich stream occurs. This infeasible situation could be made feasible by moving the rich stream load line down, but there is a utility cost associated with moving the rich stream down in a case such as this.

Diagrams that combine the rich and lean stream load lines not only determine the thermodynamic feasibility of mass exchange, but also show the amount of excess mass transfer capacity available from the lean stream and the amount of excess mass transfer capacity available from the rich stream. These regions were deliberately, if unrealistically, omitted in Fig. 29 for the sake of illustrating thermodynamic feasibility. In Fig. 31 three regions labeled I, II, and III are clearly identified. In region I, the lean stream has the capacity to exchange more mass and become richer, but there is a "shortage" of rich stream. The lean stream must be brought up to its specified concentration in a manner other than through mass exchange with the rich stream. For instance, solute k may be added to it. In region II, mass exchange can occur through contact between the rich and lean streams. In region III, the rich stream is capable of mass exchange, but there is a "shortage" of lean stream. An external lean stream mass separating agent is required to achieve the rich stream's

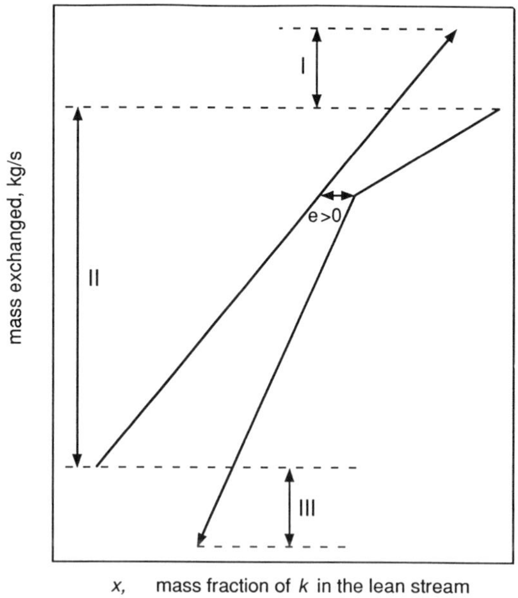

FIG. 31. The three regions of a mass exchange network. Region I represents unused lean stream capacity. There is a net shortage of the solute for the lean streams. Region II represents process mass exchange. Region III represents excess rich stream load.

target concentration. For example, an adsorbent such as activated carbon might be used to take up the excess solute, which is a pollutant in the rich stream. For the lean and rich streams depicted in Fig. 31, the least amount of k and external lean stream or mass separating agent is required when the rich stream load line is manipulated to form a pinch point ($\varepsilon = 0$). As ε increases, operating costs (the cost of k and the cost of the mass separating agent) increase and capital costs (the cost of the network) decrease. As ε decreases, operating costs decrease and capital costs increase. It is possible to find the ε at which total annualized costs are minimized.

5. *Case Study*

The practical application of MEN synthesis can be made clearer through examination of a solved problem, drawn from pesticide formulation.

The active ingredients in pesticides are generally too potent to be used or marketed in pure form. To formulate pesticides, the active ingredients are sometimes diluted with water or a solvent; in other cases they may be mixed with a solid such as sand or clay. One product at a large pesticide formulation plant is created by mixing a liquid active ingredient with sand in a ratio of 9 g active ingredient per kilogram sand. Between runs, the mixer is generally cleaned with sand that becomes final product, but when the mixer requires maintenance it must be cleaned with high-pressure steam. Steam cleaning generates 20,000 liters a year of wastewater with an active ingredient concentration of 3 g/L. This wastewater stream is currently mixed with wastewater streams containing other active ingredients and treated, generating solid waste with high disposal costs. The objective in this case study is to determine if wastewater from steam-cleaning the mixers could be purified to the extent desired by contacting it with sand in a continuous crosscurrent adsorber. The sand from the adsorber would become final product, eliminating waste due to steam-cleaning the mixers.

The equilibrium between wastewater and the sand is described by the Freundlich equation,

$$S = bC^m,$$

where S is the concentration of the adsorbate loading on the solid and C is the concentration of the adsorbate in the liquid. Assume that 9 g/kg is the loading for the active ingredient on sand in equilibrium with the pure adsorbate, which has a density of 1000 g/L. Another approximation is to set the exponent m equal to 0.7, which is its value for Aldicarb in sand. Aldicarb is a pesticide known for its high mobility through soil. These approximations result in the equilibrium expression

$$S = 0.07C^{0.7},$$

where S is in g/kg and C is in g/L. Since this equation probably represents a less favorable relationship than actually exists between the active ingredient of this example and sand, it is suitable for a preliminary analysis.

The combined composition interval diagram is pictured in Fig. 32. In this case, the flow rate of the lean stream is unknown, so the rich stream load line is plotted first on the load line diagram. Because of the nonlinear equilibrium expression, the solution is best obtained by plotting the rich stream load line against the lean stream equilibrium concentrations, so that the lean stream load line is linear. The lowest possible slope for the lean stream load line (minimum flow rate of sand) is obtained when the lean stream load line begins at the left end of the rich stream load line, and ends at a pinch where the rich stream load line begins. The combined load line diagram is given in Fig. 33. It can be seen from the slope

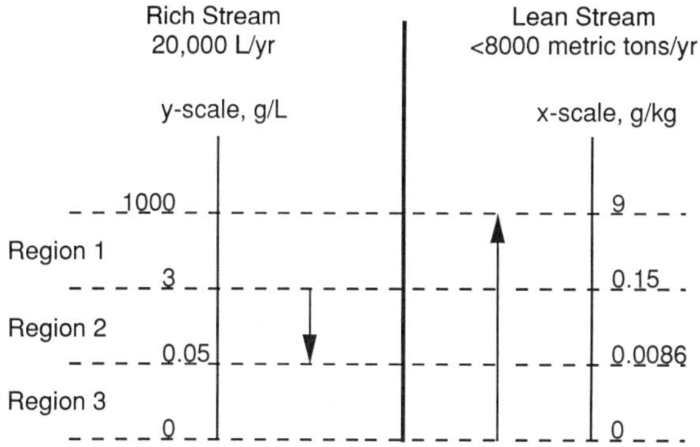

FIG. 32. Combined composition interval diagram for pesticide-contaminated wastewater.

of the lean stream load line that the minimum flow rate of sand required to purify the wastewater to the extent desired is 400 tons/yr (−59,000 g/yr)/(0.15 g/kg) which is more than an order of magnitude less than the sand used to formulate this particular pesticide. The next step in this analysis would be to determine the economic viability of such an adsorber.

A number of additional case studies have been published by Manousiouthakis and co-workers (El-Halwagi and Manousiouthakis, 1989, 1990) to determine the theoretical limits for recycling in a number of chemical processes. As this field continues to mature in a manner analogous to heat exchange network synthesis, more varied and complex case studies will become available.

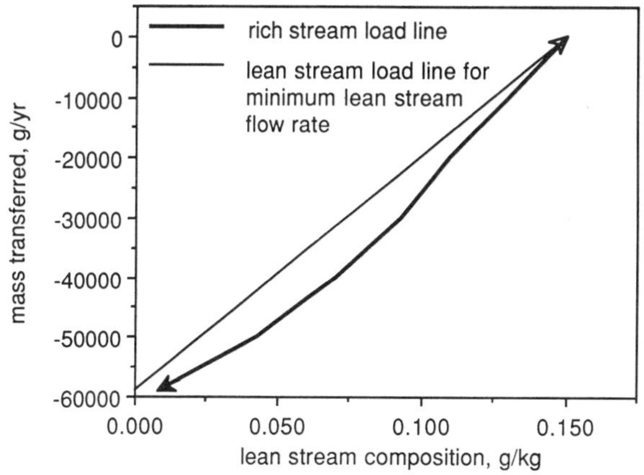

FIG. 33. Load line diagram for pesticide-contaminated wastewater.

D. Adoption of Cleaner Technologies

The waste reduction measures described in the previous sections, in many cases, appear to be relatively simple and easy to implement. Have they been broadly implemented by the chemical industry? The answer is not entirely straightforward. Consider the evidence.

Releases and off-site transfers of the 320 "core" chemicals that have been listed every year in the Toxic Release Inventory (TRI) have been reduced by 47% from 1987 to 1990 (Chemical Manufacturers' Association, 1992). A number of large companies such as Dow, Du Pont, 3M, and Monsanto have widely publicized waste reduction programs that describe successes in making chemical manufacturing technologies cleaner. Yet, this self-reporting of the adoption of cleaner technology by the chemical industry creates much skepticism. Critics of the industry contend and often successfully document that many of the TRI reductions are the result of changes in emission estimation procedures or are the result of actions such as plant closing (see *Chemical and Engineering News*, December 14, 1992, p. 16). Further, the documentation of isolated success stories does not provide an industry-wide audit of the extent of adoption of waste reduction technologies. The only study available that truly approximates an independent audit of the chemical industry's adoption of clean technologies is documented in a pair of reports issued by INFORM (Dorfman *et al.*, 1985; 1992), focused on 29 chemical manufacturing facilities in California, Ohio, and New Jersey. "The plants were selected to be broadly representative of the wide diversity of facilities across the organic chemical industry," and "thus, the plants vary in size . . . , in age . . . , in the types of products they produce and in the types of process they use (batch or continuous)" (Dorfman *et al.*, 1992). By examining the use of source reduction in these facilities in both 1985 and 1992, INFORM has effectively measured, albeit for a relatively small sample of facilities, a measure of the adoption of clean technologies by the chemical industry. Among the conclusions reached by the INFORM team were:

> . . . The organic chemical plants INFORM studied have dramatically decreased their releases of toxic and hazardous wastes, saved money, and increased product yields through source reduction.
>
> Source reduction offers waste generating facilities continuing opportunities to significantly reduce the amounts of toxic and hazardous waste they generate and subsequently release into the air, land, or water or transfer to treatment or disposal facilities. Large reductions continue to be achieved even at plants that have been implementing source reduction for many years.

The cost of implementing many source reduction activities is low (no capital investment was required for one-quarter of the source reduction activities in INFORM's study for which capital cost data were provided, and investments of under $100,000 were required for just under half of the source reduction activities).

Companies can recoup their initial investments rapidly (in 6 months or less for two-thirds of the source reduction activities in INFORM's study for which information on payback periods was reported).

Implementation times, including research and development, are short (6 months or less for nearly two-thirds of the source reduction activities for which plants reported implementation time to INFORM, and 6 months to 3 years for another 30%).

Product yields increase (for 97% of the source reduction activities in INFORM's study for which information on changes in product yield was provided).

Process changes, operations changes, and equipment changes accounted for 87% of the source reduction activities reported to INFORM. Such efficiency-oriented opportunities continued to be found by plants that had previously achieved significant reductions in waste generation.

Product changes and chemical substitutions accounted for only 13% of the source reduction activities in INFORM's study.

Clearly, the impression left from an examination of INFORM's study is that the chemical industry is successfully adopting cleaner technology. A complex set of calculations leads to the conclusion that the source reduction measures at these facilities led to a 33% reduction in the releases and off-site transfer of TRI chemicals (Dorfman *et al.*, 1992, p. 89). The INFORM authors also conclude that "managers of waste generating facilities can continually find many low-technology, efficiency oriented source reduction opportunities when they look for them." INFORM President Joanna Underwood is quoted in *Chemical and Engineering News* (November 16, 1992) as stating that "source reduction is an essential key to economic competitiveness as well as an environmentally sound future." However, as noted by Dennis Redington, Monsanto's director for regulatory management, this view is not entirely shared by the industry. "I would like to be able to say that we knew how to get financial payback, but we have not worked out how to make this all a positive return on investment... some of the individual projects will be cost effective, but in the aggregate, it is going to be hard, if not impossible, to achieve [pollution prevention]... with projects that yield enough savings to make the whole program [economically] positive." (*Chemical and Engineering News*, November 16, 1992.)

Thus, the chemical industry is implementing cleaner technologies and substantially lowering emissions. Are these technologies economical? Certainly some individual projects will be, but when viewed in the aggregate, is a chemical manufacturing operation employing cleaner technologies more economically efficient than its competitors? Alternatively, is cleaner process technology a more competitive way to address strict environmental regulations than conventional clean-up technologies? There are no universal answers to these questions, and in fact, there are relatively few comprehensive case studies that address this issue. The next section will discuss these issues in more depth.

E. Costs and Benefits of Cleaner Technologies

The economic analysis of cleaner chemical manufacturing technologies is a complex issue, largely because of uncertainties in the quantitative evaluation of the benefits of clean technologies. This section will describe some of the economic benefits associated with clean technologies and will outline some of the barriers that companies have encountered in attempting to evaluate these benefits. Finally, the semi-quantitative approach taken by most companies in evaluating clean technologies will be outlined, and the results of a detailed case study will be presented in summary form.

A number of studies have outlined accounting methods for evaluating the economic benefits of clean technologies (for a comprehensive review, see Tellus Institute, 1991b). Most of these methods include the same basic features. They divide costs and benefits into a number of categories, ranging from the readily quantifiable to the inestimable. The most readily quantified costs are those associated with equipment, labor, and material expenses required for the new technology. Readily quantified benefits can include reduced raw material costs and avoided waste treatment and disposal costs. If these are the only costs and benefits considered in the economic analysis of clean technologies, then relatively few will have a positive rate of return. There are, however, other potential, quantifiable benefits associated with cleaner technologies that can be categorized under the general heading of "hidden costs." Tables XIII and XIV list just a few of the "hidden" costs associated with the generation of wastes. To the extent that clean technologies avoid the generation of wastes, they reduce these costs. Cleaner technologies can also reduce costs associated with permits, fees, and licenses. All told, these "hidden" costs can be quite significant, but they can be quite difficult or burdensome to evaluate.

Another type of benefit associated with clean technology is the avoidance of long-term remediation liability. Stated simply, if no wastes are being sent to landfills, then no additional remediation liability is being incurred. While clear in principle, accurately quantifying the reduced

TABLE XIII
HIDDEN LABOR COSTS ASSOCIATED WITH POLLUTION TREATMENT: CLEAN TECHNOLOGIES AVOID SOME OF THESE COSTS[a]

Time to fill drums or storage tanks with waste
Time to properly label waste drums
Time to move waste drums within the plant
Time to load waste drums for shipment
Time to pump out drums or empty a storage tank
Time to schedule waste transportation
Time to fill out waste manifests
Time to mail manifests
Time to file and record manifests
Time to cut checks for waste disposal and transportation firms
Time for waste information training
Time to approve waste disposal invoices
Time to supervise personnel engaged in waste-related activities
Time to select disposal facilities, transporters, consultants, laboratories, etc.
Time to inspect disposal rate site or sites
Time to obtain waste samples
Time for learning regulatory compliance requirements
Time for other waste-related activities

[a]Source: Waste Advantage (1988).

liability benefits of clean technology is difficult. No responsible company plans to create a Superfund site. Instead, these sites are created by the failure of disposal technologies, and the rate of these failures can only be estimated probabilistically. Thus, the potential benefits can only be expressed as a highly uncertain expected value, based on an assumed rate of disposal site failure. A final set of benefits associated with clean technologies is even less quantifiable. They include company image with customers, stockholders, and employees, and achieving targets associated with voluntary emission reduction programs.

In the face of these quantifiable, semi-quantifiable, and inestimable costs and benefits, how do companies determine whether or not to proceed with a particular clean technology project? The most common procedure involves a semi-quantitative estimate of a set of clean technology benefits. One such set, taken from a study by Amoco Oil Corporation, is given in Table XV. The project evaluation criteria are grouped into three major categories: risk reduction, technical factors, and cost factors. In a joint study with the U.S. EPA, Amoco evaluated over a dozen clean technology options for its Yorktown, Virginia, refinery and ranked them based on these criteria (Klee, 1992). The highest-rated projects tended to score well in all of the areas. The implementation costs ranged from under $150,000 to over $30 million. Only a few of the projects generated a

TABLE XIV
HIDDEN COMPLIANCE COSTS:
CLEAN TECHNOLOGIES MAY AVOID SOME OF THESE COSTS
(50 TYPICAL ENVIRONMENTAL COMPLIANCE ACTIVITIES)[a]

1.	Title III—Emergency planning	26.	Scheduling waste shipments
2.	Title III—Emergency notification	27.	Handling rejected waste shipments
3.	Title III—Community right-to-know reporting	28.	Air quality permits
4.	Title III—Toxic chemical release reporting	29.	Approve invoices
5.	Waste generator biennial reports	30.	Hire consultants
6.	Apply for construction permits	31.	County reporting requirements
7.	Apply for operating permits	32.	D.O.L. waste handling requirements
8.	Compliance scheduling	33.	D.O.T. waste shipping requirements
9.	Conduct testing and monitoring	34.	Annual reports for exporting waste
10.	Underground tank requirements	35.	Report waste information to management
11.	Self-monitoring requirements	36.	Mailing waste manifests
12.	Waste generator surveys	37.	Modeling requirements
13.	Recordkeeping requirements	38.	Selection of laboratory(s) for waste analysis
14.	Contingency plan	39.	Waste sampling
15.	Episode plan	40.	NPDWR permit
16.	Pollution incident prevention plan	41.	NPDES permit
17.	Employee waste training programs	42.	Read and understand new regulations
18.	Federal inspections	43.	Attend regulatory seminars
19.	State inspections	44.	CERCLA activities
20.	Non-compliance reporting	45.	Inspect waste disposal facilities
21.	Fire Marshal inspections	46.	Inspect waste transporters
22.	Completing waste manifests	47.	Inspect laboratories
23.	Disposal facility(s) selection	48.	Evaluate bids and proposals
24.	Waste transporter(s) selection	49.	Manifest exception reporting
25.	Waste container labeling	50.	Supervise waste-related activities

[a]Source: Waste Advantage (1988).

positive rate of return; however, the source reduction projects were generally more economical than treatment and disposal options. The source reduction options had an average cost of $650/ton of pollutant recovered, while the other options (largely treatment and disposal) had an average cost of $3200/ton, nearly five times higher. Details are available in Klee (1992).

To summarize, companies are proceeding with the implementation of clean technologies based on a number of quantifiable and semi-quantifiable costs. In the limited number of comprehensive analyses available, relatively few of the possible clean technology projects can be economically justified based only on the value of recovered materials. Source reduction options seem to be more economical than treatment and disposal based on the Amoco case study. To justify many source reduction projects, however, "hidden" costs must be exposed and subjective issues

TABLE XV

CRITERIA USED IN EVALUATING CLEAN PROCESS TECHNOLOGIES (KLEE, 1992)

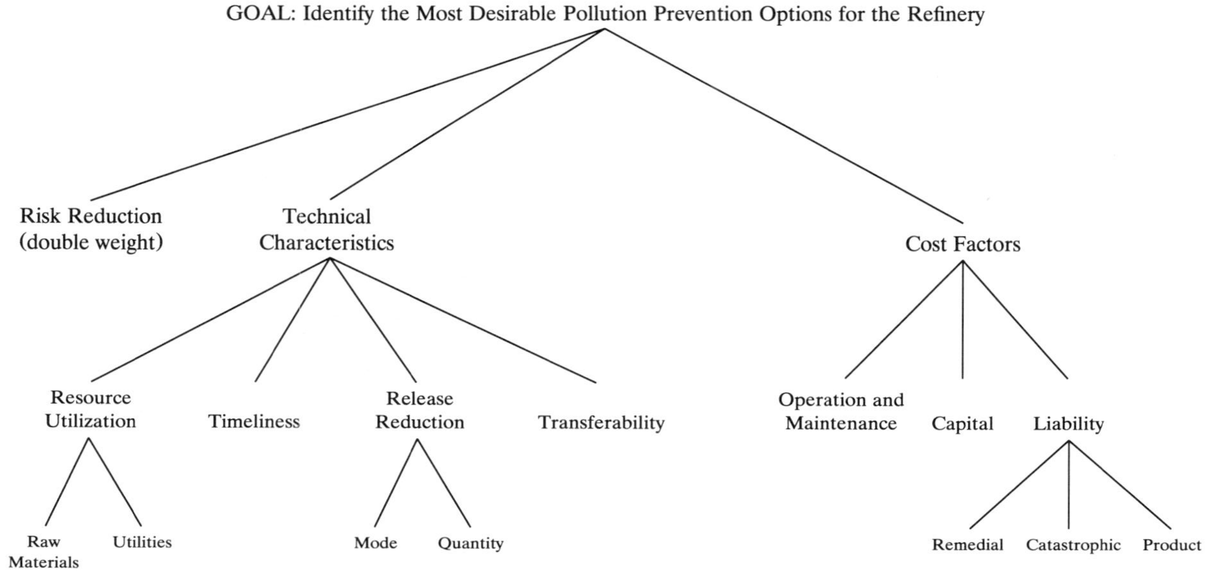

such as avoided liability costs and the value of corporate image must be addressed.

F. Conclusion

This section has provided an overview of some of the design methods available for preventing pollution in chemical processes. Many of the ideas are elementary and focus on isolated unit operations. One of the primary reasons for the simplicity of these pollution prevention methods is that they consider waste streams largely as bulk materials, ignoring their molecular composition and ignoring the molecular processes that generate the wastes. A molecular-level understanding of waste composition and waste generation can reveal entirely new design opportunities for pollution prevention. These design tools, some of which are summarized in the next section, encompass almost all of the sciences that form the basis of chemical engineering.

IV. Microscale Pollution Prevention

The previous sections have outlined pollution prevention strategies at the process level and on the scale of entire industry sectors. While these process changes have been characterized in this review as macro- or mesoscale, many of the approaches that have been described rely upon a molecular-level understanding of chemical and physical processes. For example, the synthesis of new catalysts, which results in higher reaction yields and less wastes, relies on an understanding of surface chemistry. The design of highly selective separation technologies relies on an understanding of adsorption and other phenomena. The minimization of particulate pollutants relies on an understanding of aerosol physics and chemistry. These and a large number of other general engineering principles are employed in pollution prevention. A detailed discussion of all of these principles is beyond the scope of this review. So instead of attempting to be comprehensive, just a few select examples of molecular-level design for pollution prevention based on the author's own experiences will be presented. These case studies of solvent substitution and reaction pathway synthesis illustrate how general engineering principles are used as a foundation upon which pollution prevention approaches are built.

A. Solvent Substitutions

1. CFC Replacements

The case of chlorofluorocarbons (CFCs) provides an interesting illustration of the general problem of finding substitutes for targeted pollutants and the variety of engineering approaches that can be employed in solving the problem. CFCs were first synthesized in the 1930s as a refrigeration fluid and have been used in a variety of other applications because of their chemical stability and low toxicity. In the early 1970s, it was suggested (Molina and Rowland, 1974) that chlorine released by CFC degradation in the stratosphere could cause depletion of stratospheric ozone. These findings led to a 1978 ban by some countries (including the United States) on the use of CFCs in non-essential applications such as aerosol propellants. With the discovery of polar ozone holes, beginning in 1985 (Farman *et al.*, 1985), a movement to ban all uses of CFCs began, resulting in an international agreement on the production and use of CFCs known as the Montreal Protocol [United Nations Environment Program (UNEP), 1987]. With the ratification of the Montreal Protocol, an intense search for CFC substitutes began, and some of the engineering methods employed in these searches will be the focus of this section.

CFCs have many industrial uses, but in this section the focus will be on the use of CFCs as solvents and the search for potential solvent substitutes. CFCs are used extensively in the electronics and aerospace industries to clean metal parts. Their chemical inertness insures against damage to the surfaces to be cleaned, and their relatively high vapor pressure makes drying the surface after cleaning simple. In the early 1970s, CFCs were used extensively, frequently as replacements for other chlorinated solvents that had been identified as either potential health hazards or as potential precursors in the formation of photochemical smog. In fact, between 1974 and 1985, use of CFCs as solvents tripled (Glas, 1989), largely because of environmental concerns about other solvents. The most common method for finding CFC substitutes has been to simply compare the desired properties of the CFCs to the properties of lists of potential substitutes. When CFCs are used as solvents, particularly for solubilizing hydrocarbon greases adsorbed onto metal substrates, the target properties are solubility parameters compatible with long-chain hydrocarbons, low flammability, and a boiling point slightly above room temperature. Other properties that must be considered are toxicity, potential for the depletion of stratospheric ozone, the smog formation potential, and the global warming potential of the material. Databases containing these and other properties for hundreds of potential CFC substitutes have been compiled

(Hughes Aircraft Company, 1991). These lists include rather conventional substitutes such as 1,1,1-trichloroethane, unusual substitutes such as terpene extracts from orange rinds, and solvents as simple as lemon juice and soapy water. Unfortunately, ranking potential CFC replacements from a finite list of solvents will not lead to the best replacement if the best replacement is not on the list. A more systematic approach to engineering a solvent replacement is afforded by thermodynamic group contribution methods.

2. *Group Contribution Approaches*

The basic premise of group contribution methods is that a molecule can be considered as a collection of functional groups, which each contribute in a well-defined manner to the properties of the molecule. Consider estimating solubility parameters. Potential solvent replacements for CFCs can be found by matching solubility parameters (Joback, 1989), which characterize the intermolecular forces that determine solvation ability. Several different types of solubility parameters are available, which characterize the dispersive, polar, and hydrogen-bonding forces that influence solubility. Each can be estimated using a group contribution approach, using Eqs. (4)–(6):

$$\delta_d = 13.29 + \Sigma\Delta_{1,\delta_d}, \tag{4}$$

$$\delta_p = 5.07 + \Sigma\Delta_{1,\delta_p}, \tag{5}$$

$$\delta_h = 7.23 + \Sigma\Delta_{1,\delta_h}, \tag{6}$$

where δ_d is the solubility parameter describing dispersive forces, δ_p is the solubility parameter describing polar forces, δ_h is the solubility parameter describing hydrogen bonding, and Δ_i are the contributions of group i to the dispersive, polar, and hydrogen-bonding parameters. The summations in Eqs. (4)–(6) are taken over all functional groups in the molecule. To illustrate the use of these group contribution approaches, the solubility parameters for ethyl alcohol will be estimated. Ethyl alcohol contains one methyl ($-CH_3$) group, a $-CH_2-$ group, and a hydroxyl group ($-OH$). The contributions of each of these groups to the various solubility parameters are shown in Table XVI; the application of Eqs. (4)–(6) then results in values of the solubility parameters of 13.3, 9.4, and 16.2. The challenge now is to systematize this procedure so that all feasible solvents with the desired solubility parameters can be identified. For simplicity of illustration, we will consider only the polar and hydrogen-bonding solubility parameters. Our goal is to find a material with parameters within a target

TABLE XVI
SELECTED GROUP CONTRIBUTIONS FOR SOLUBILITY PARAMETERS
(JOBACK, 1992)

Group	δ_d	δ_h	δ_p
$-CH_3$	0.34	−0.85	−0.59
−Cl	−0.15	0.26	3.11
−Br	2.23	−0.69	1.61
−OH	−0.65	10.63	5.55
$-CH_2-$	0.34	−0.85	−0.59
> C=O	−1.14	4.85	4.67

distance of the parameters for the material to be replaced. This target area for replacement of toluene as a solvent is shown as the circle in Fig. 34 (Joback, 1992). The search is begun at point (5.07, 7.23), which is the value of the solubility parameters from Eqs. (5) and (6) if no groups are present. Each group added to a potential replacement molecule can be represented as a vector in Fig. 34. For example, the hydroxyl group (–OH), which has group contributions of 5.55 and 10.63, can be represented by the vector shown in Fig. 35. As groups are added to the molecule, group vectors are added, head to tail, to update the value of the molecule's solubility parameter. As shown in Fig. 34, groups can be added until the value of the property is in the target range. Groups must be

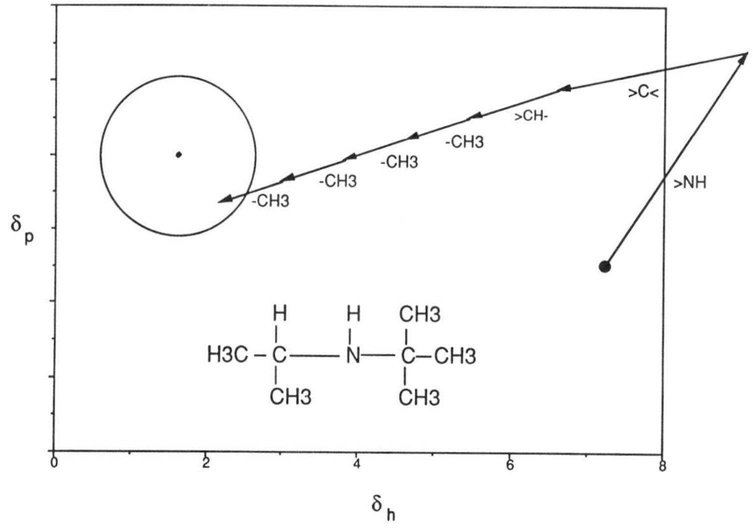

FIG. 34. Property targets for a solvent replacement. The replacement molecule is constructed by adding functional group property vectors until the target area is reached (Joback, 1992).

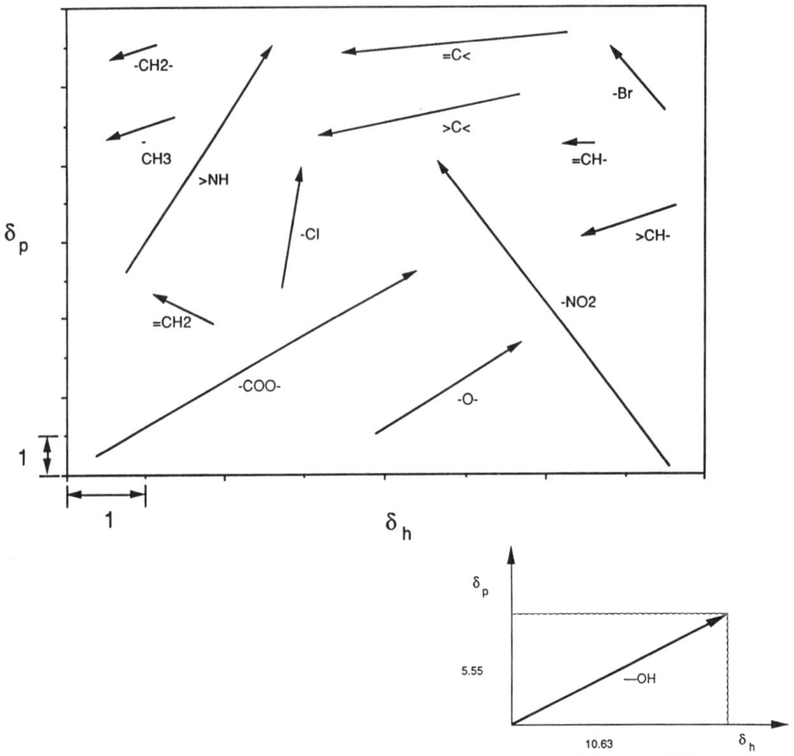

FIG. 35. Typical functional group property vectors (Joback, 1992).

chosen such that a feasible molecule is constructed (for example, the choice of three methyl groups and no other functionalities is not a feasible molecule), but otherwise the approach is quite general. Using the approach, it is possible to design molecules that will contain a distribution of functional groups that result in the target properties.

While this simple example of molecular design for specified physical properties has focused on only two parameters, the polar and hydrogen-bonding solubility parameters, there is no limitation in principle to the number of physical properties that could be considered in the optimization. The most serious limitations of this approach are the following:

- The optimization may lead to structures that, while feasible, are difficult to synthesize.
- The optimization may not be able to consider molecules containing functional groups for which no group contributions are available.

- The group contributions are based on regressions from data on a limited set of compounds; these group contributions may not be accurate for structures generated by the optimization. For example, the group contribution of a hydroxyl group to a property such as vapor pressure in an alcohol can be quite different than in a molecule such as glycol. Thus, care must be taken in applying group contribution methods to new structures.
- Group contribution methods may not be available for all relevant properties.

Each of these difficulties could be addressed in the optimization; as an example, consider the problem of estimating the potential for stratospheric ozone depletion in a new material. Stratospheric ozone depletion potentials have only been calculated for a few compounds, and simple group contribution methods for estimating this property are not yet available. Nevertheless, it is clear that the property depends strongly on two parameters: atmospheric lifetime, and the number of chlorine and bromine atoms in the molecule. Both of these parameters can be estimated using a group contribution approach (see Allen *et al.*, 1992, and references cited therein), and so it should be possible to include at least a crude estimate of stratospheric ozone depletion potential, as well as other properties relevant to the environmental impact of the material, into the design. The group contribution approach to the molecular design of chemical products is already in widespread use in applications such as pharmaceutical design. The development of group contribution or molecularly based approaches to estimating properties of environmental interest is the major impediment to the use of these methods for pollution prevention.

While group contribution methods have great potential, they could ignore revolutionary design innovations. For example, in the selection of replacement solvents, the use of supercritical fluids or eliminating the need for the solvent entirely might be overlooked. Further, our experience with CFCs suggests caution in labeling any material as totally environmentally benign. Recall that CFCs were initially regarded as environmentally beneficial, and 40 years were required after their invention to identify their severe environmental impacts.

B. Reaction Pathway Synthesis

The selection of chemical synthesis pathways that minimize the formation of undesired by-products is a central concept in pollution prevention.

A number of detailed case studies have been presented which describe how, once the reaction pathways are known, reaction conditions can be selected to minimize pollutants. For example, Hopper *et al.* (1992) examined the production of acrylonitrile and allyl chloride. Senkan used a detailed chemical kinetic model to describe the high-temperature oxidation and pyrolysis of C_2HCl_3, a prototypical chlorinated hydrocarbon (Senkan, 1992; Chang and Senkan, 1988, 1989). The high-temperature reactions of chlorinated hydrocarbons are of interest both in the production of commodity chemicals such as ethylene dichloride and vinyl chloride, and in the formation of undesired by-products, such as chlorinated dibenzodioxins and dibenzofurans. A group of approximately 150 elementary reactions was used in this case study to follow the formation of by-products such as phosgene and carbon tetrachloride in the oxidation of C_2HCl_3, revealing major formation pathways and reaction conditions that minimize the formation of the by-products. A number of additional examples of reaction pathway synthesis for pollution prevention are available. Chapman and Tsou (1993) have proposed a synthesis of styrene that avoids the use of benzene; Gladfelter (1993) has proposed a route to isocyanates that avoids phosgene. Generalizing these successes in reaction pathway synthesis is a substantial challenge, however. A number of tools are available for predicting equilibrium product distributions (see, for example, Govind, 1985), but general methods for predicting pathways and rates are in their infancy.

While the challenges of predicting by-product formation in chemical manufacturing are substantial, additional challenges are posed when the reactions of complex natural products such as petroleum are considered. Petroleum fractions are mixtures of thousands of molecular species. As these mixtures are processed into fuels and petrochemicals, each of the molecular species can undergo hundreds of reactions. For the past several decades, the engineering models of the processing of these extraordinarily complex materials have been simplified by the nature of the products derived from the processes. In the case of fuels derived from petroleum, only bulk properties such as volatility, viscosity, and octane number were important, and the detailed molecular composition was relatively unimportant. In the case of chemical feedstocks, such as ethylene derived from petroleum naphthas, only the target product and a few select by-products were typically monitored. Thus, since detailed molecular information about the problems was not required, molecular-level models of the processes were not necessary. Lumped models (see, for example, Weekman, 1979), which grouped many similar compounds into pseudo-components, were sufficient. Now, however, new regulations, such as those limiting the levels of benzene allowed in gasoline, are driving petrochemical manufacturers toward a molecular understanding of their products. Molecular-level modeling of petroleum is difficult because a typical process stream may contain 10^4 different chemical species, each of which can undergo 10^2 elementary reactions. This implies that a kinetic model would need 10^6 reactions and reaction rate parameters. Identifying all of the reaction pathways and potential hazardous reaction products presents a serious challenge. Recently, however, reaction rules for defining chemical pathways and group contribution concepts for estimating rate parameters (Liguras and Allen, 1989a, b) have made it possible to develop molecular-level models of petroleum processes. Figure 36 presents an example of the use of reaction rules to establish a set of chemical pathways. Quann and Jaffe (1992) used a set of 7 rules to establish the hydrogenation pathways of the tetramethyl-chrysene shown in the figure. The multitude of potential products and reactions for the reactions of this single petroleum component are dramatic evidence of the complexity of detailed chemical kinetic models of natural products. The reaction network of Fig. 36 is useful in identifying formation pathways for undesired by-products, but to be useful in detailed process models, each of the reaction rates in the network must be estimated. For this purpose, group contribution approaches for estimating rate parameters, such as those described by

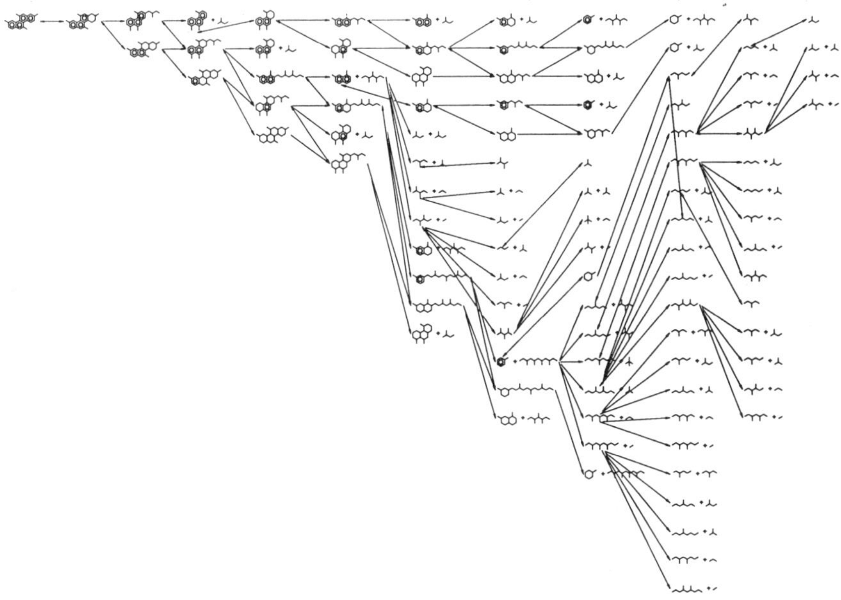

FIG. 36. Reaction pathway network generation for the hydrogenation of a methylated chrysene. The network was generated using seven rules (Quann and Jaffe, 1992).

Liguras and Allen (1989a, b), can be employed. Armed with molecular-level models of reaction pathways and reaction rates, it is now possible to perform studies identifying rates and routes to the formation of undesired by-products even in products as complex as petroleum.

V. Summary

The design of chemical processes and products that minimize waste and prevent the formation of pollutants is not new. Decades of work in chemical engineering have focused on this very topic. The results may have been called yield enhancement, energy efficiency, or by-product utilization, but the goal remained the same: to minimize raw material and energy utilization. Given that waste reduction and pollution prevention are not new concepts, their emergence as innovative compliance strategies may seem unusual. What has driven their increased importance are the dramatic increases in costs associated with waste treatment, disposal, and liability, and a better understanding of the role of individual chemical species in pollutant toxicity. The former has changed the economics of waste treatment versus prevention so that it is now more economical in many cases to prevent the formation of a pollutant rather than to treat it (for a quantitative case study, see Klee, 1992). The latter driving force for pollution prevention is requiring a much more detailed understanding of the chemistry of processes and products. When concentrations of 3,4,7,8-tetrachlorodibenzodioxin at the part-per-trillion level can significantly influence the economics of a process, it is necessary to understand processes occurring at rates and concentrations orders of magnitude smaller than considered in previous designs.

The challenges of pollution prevention—more mass-efficient designs, characterized at the molecular level—can be met with traditional and emerging chemical engineering tools. As pointed out in the National Research Council report on "Frontiers in Chemical Engineering" (1988), these tools can be applied at macro-, meso-, and microlevels. This review has attempted to summarize many of the approaches being used in pollution prevention at these three levels. At the macrolevel, the waste audits, life cycle analyses, and studies in industrial metabolism and industrial ecology are guiding waste-reduction efforts. At the mesolevel, the designs of traditional chemical process unit operations are being modified so that the units produce less waste; new flowsheeting techniques involving pinch technology are being used to assess the mass efficiency of processes.

Finally, at the microscale, wide-ranging studies are contributing to a molecular design of products and processes.

Because pollution prevention and waste reduction require all of the tools of chemical engineering, this review is not comprehensive. It should instead be viewed as a starting point for a set of challenges that will face chemical process and product design for the foreseeable future.

Acknowledgments

Preparation of this manuscript was made possible by support from the Ralph M. Parsons Foundation and the University of California Toxic Substances Research and Teaching Program. The author is also indebted to Professor Sheldon K. Friedlander of UCLA for sharing his considerable insight and vision.

References

Allen, D. T., The role of catalysis In industrial waste reduction. *In* "Industrial Environmental Chemistry: Waste Minimization in Industrial Processes and Remediation of Hazardous Wastes" (A. E. Martell and D. Sawyer, eds.), p. 89. Plenum, New York, 1992.

Allen, D. T., and Behmanesh, N., Wastes as raw materials. *In* Industrial Ecology (B. Allenby, ed.). National Academy Press, Washington, DC, 1994 (in press).

Allen, D. T., and Jain, R. K., eds., "Hazardous Waste and Hazardous Materials," Vol. 9, No. 1. Hazard. Waste Hazard. Mater., New York, 1992.

Allen, D. T., Rosselot, K. R., and Bakshani, N., "Pollution Prevention: Homework and Design Problems for Engineering Curricular," p. 82. Am. Inst. Chem. Eng., New York, 1992.

American Petroleum Institute, Waste minimization in the petroleum industry. *API Publ.* **849-00020** (1991).

Ayers, R. V., Industrial metabolism. *In* "Technology and Environment" (J. H. Ausubel and H. E. Sladovich, eds.). National Academy Press, Washington, DC, 1989.

Baker, R. D., Warren, J. L., Behmanesh, N., and Allen, D. T., Management of hazardous waste in the United States. *Hazard. Waste Hazard. Mater.*, **9**, 37 (1992).

Berglund, R. L., and Hansen, J. L., Fugitive emissions: An untapped application for TQC. *ASQC Qual. Congr. Trans.*, San Francisco, (1990).

Cairncross, F., "Costing the Earth." Harvard Business School Press, Cambridge, MA, 1992.

Chang, W. D., and Senkan, S. M., Chemical structure of fuel-rich, premixed, laminar flames of trichloroethylene. *Symp. (Int.) Combust.* [*Proc.*], **22**, 1453 (1988).

Chang, W. D., and Senkan, S. M., Detailed chemical kinetic modeling of the fuel rich flames of trichloroethylene. *Environ. Sci. Technol.* **23**, 442 (1989).

Chapman, J. L., and Tsou, E., The UCLA styrene process. *Prepr. Am. Chem. Soc. Environ. Div.*, **33**(2), 308 (1993).

Chemical Manufacturers Association, "CMA Hazardous Waste Survey '88." CMA, Washington, DC, 1990.

Chemical Manufacturers Association, "Preventing Pollution in the Chemical Industry 1987–1990." CMA, Washington, DC, 1992.

ChemSystems, Inc., "Vinyl Product Lifecycle Assessment." Prepared for the Vinyl Institute, Washington, DC, 1991.

Ciric, A. R., and Jia, T., "Economic Sensitivity Analysis of Waste Treatment Costs in Source Reduction Projects: Continuous Optimization Problems." University of Cincinnati, Cincinnati, OH, 1992.

Cusumano, J. A., Chairman of the Board of Catalytica, Inc., Designer catalysts: Hastemakers for a clean environment. *In* "Proceedings of Pollution Prevention the Chemical Process Industries, April 6–7, 1992." McGraw-Hill, New York, 1992.

Dorfman, M. H., Muir, W. R., and Miller, C. G., "Environmental Dividends: Cutting More Chemical Wastes." INFORM, Inc., New York, 1992.

Douglas, J. M., "Conceptual Design of Chemical Processes." McGraw-Hill, New York, 1988.

Douglas, J. M., Process synthesis for waste minimization. *Ind. Eng. Chem. Res.* **31**, 238 (1992).

El-Halwagi, M. M., and Manousiouthakis, V., Synthesis of mass exchange networks. *AIChE J.* **35**, 1233 (1989).

El-Halwagi, M. M., and Manousiouthakis, V., Automatic synthesis of mass exchange networks with single component targets. *Chem. Eng. Sci.* **45**, 2813 (1990).

Farman, J. C., Gardiner, G. B., and Shanklin, J. D., Large losses of total ozone in Antarctica reveal seasonal ClOx/NOx interaction. *Nature (London)* **315**, 207 (1985).

Fathi-Afshar, S., and Yang, J. C., Design the optimal structure of the petrochemical industry for minimum cost and least gross toxicity of chemical production. *Chem. Eng. Sci.* **40**, 781 (1985).

Franklin Associates, Ltd., "Comparative Energy and Environmental Impacts for Soft-drink Delivery Systems." Franklin Assoc., Prairie Village, KS, 1989.

Franklin Associates, Ltd., "Resource and Environmental Profile Analysis of Foamed Polystyrene and Bleached Paperboard Container." Franklin Assoc., Prairie Village, KS, 1990a.

Franklin Associates, Ltd., "Resource and Environmental Profile Analysis of Children's Disposable and Cloth Diapers." Franklin Assoc., Prairie Village, KS, 1990b.

Franklin Associates, Ltd., "Resource and Environmental Profile Analysis of Polyethylene and Unbleached Paper Grocery Sacks (report prepared for the Council for Solid Waste Solutions)." Franklin Assoc., Prairie Village, KS, 1990c.

Freeman, H., Harten, T., Springer, J., Randall, P., Curran, M. A., and Stone, K., Industrial pollution prevention: A critical review. *J. Air Waste Manage. Assoc.* **42**, 618 (1992).

Friedlander, S. K., The two faces of technology: Changing perspectives in design for environment. *In* "Industrial Ecology" (B. Allenby, ed.). National Academy Press, Washington, DC, 1994 (in press).

Frosch, R. A., and Gallopoulos, N. E., Strategies for manufacturing. *Sci. Am.* **261** (3), 144–152 (1989).

Gladfelter, W. L., Homogeneous catalytic carbonylation of nitroaromatics: An alternative to phosgene use. *Prepr. Am. Chem. Soc. Environ. Div.* **33**(2), 323 (1993).

Glas, J. P., Protecting the ozone layer: A perspective from industry. *In* "Technology and Environment" (J. H. Ausubel and H. E. Sladovich, eds.), p. 137. National Academy Press, Washington, DC, 1989.

Govind, R., Controlling hazardous waste: Computer assisted prediction of reaction byproducts. *Hazard. Subst.*, November, p. 26 (1985).

Hagh, B., and Allen, D. T., Catalytic hydrodechlorination. *In* "Innovative Hazardous Waste Treatment Technology" (H. M. Freeman, ed.), Vol. 2, p. 45. Technomic, Lancaster, PA, 1990.

Hocking, M. B., Paper versus polystyrene. *Science* **251**, 504 (1991); see also letters commenting on this paper, *ibid.*, p. 1361 (1991).

Hopper, J. R., Yaws, C. L., Ho, T. C., Vichailak, M., and Muninnimit, A., Waste minimization by process modification. *In* "Industrial Environmental Chemistry: Waste Minimization in Industrial Processes and Remediation of Hazardous Waste" (D. T. Sawyer and A. E. Martell, eds.), p. 25. Plenum, New York, 1992.

Hughes Aircraft Company Solvent Database, available through the South Coast Air Quality Management District, Diamond Bar, CA, 1991.

Hunt, R. G., and Franklin, W. E., "Resource and Environmental Profile Analysis of Beer Containers." Chemtech, American Chemical Soc., Washington, DC, 1975.

Joback, K. G., Designing molecules possessing desired physical properties. Ph.D. Thesis, Massachusetts Institute of Technology, Cambridge, MA, 1989.

Joback, K. G., "Pollution Prevention by Solvent Substitution." Presentation at New Jersey Institute of Technology, Newark, September 1992.

Kalnes, T. N., and James, R. B., Hydrogeneration and recycle of organic waste streams. *Environ. Progr.* **7**(3), 185 (1988).

Klee, H., "Executive Summary of the AMOCO/EPA Pollution Prevention Project." Copies available through American Petroleum Institute, Washington, DC, 1992.

Koch, D. G., and Kuta, C. C., Assessing environmental trade-offs: Procter & Gamble's approach to life cycle analysis. *In* "Inside Environment." 1991.

Liguras, D. K., and Allen, D. T., Structural models for catalytic cracking. Part I. Model compound reactions. *Ind. Eng. Chem. Res.* **28**, 665 (1989a).

Liguras, D. K., and Allen, D. T., Structural models for catalytic cracking. Part II. Reactions of a simulated oil mixture. *Ind. Eng. Chem. Res.* **28**, 674 (1989b).

Little, Arthur D., "Disposable versus Reusable Diapers—Health, Environmental and Economical Comparisons." Arthur D. Little, Cambridge, MA, 1990.

Molina, M., and Roland, F. S., Stratospheric sink for chlorofluoromethanes: Chlorine atom catalyzed destruction of ozone. *Nature (London)* **230**, 379 (1974).

MRI, Resource and environmental profile analysis of plastics and competitive materials. Prepared for the Society of the Plastic Industries, Kansas City, MO, 1974.

National Research Council, "Separation and Purification: Critical Needs and Opportunities," National Academy Press, Washington, DC, 1987.

National Research Council, "Frontiers in Chemical Engineering." National Academy Press, Washington, DC, 1988.

Nelson, K. E., Use these ideas to cut wastes. *Hydrocarbon Process.*, March (1990).

Quann, R. J., and Jaffe, S. B., Structure-oriented lumping: Describing the chemistry of complex hydrocarbon mixtures. *Ind. Eng. Chem. Res.* **31**, 2483 (1992).

Rudd, D. F., Fathi-Afshar, S. Trevino, A. A., and Stadtherr, M. A., "Petrochemical Technology Assessment." Wiley, New York, 1981.

Science Applications International Corporation, "Summary of Data on Industrial Nonhazardous Waste Disposal Practices," Contract 68-01-7050. U.S. Environ. Prot. Agency, Washington, DC, 1985.

Senkan, S. M., Kinetic models to predict and control minor constituents in process reactions. *In* "Industrial Environmental Chemistry: Waste Minimization in Industrial Processes and Remediation of Hazardous Waste (D. T. Sawyer and A. E. Martell, eds.), p. 45. Plenum, New York, 1992.

Society of Environmental Toxicology and Chemistry (SETAC), "A Technical Framework for Life-Cycle Assessments." SETAC Foundation for Environmental Education, Inc., Pensacola, FL, 1991.

Society of Environmental Toxicology and Chemistry (SETAC), "A Conceptual Framework for Life Cycle Impact Assessment." SETAE Foundation for Environmental Education, Inc., Pensacola, FL, 1993.

Tellus Institute, The Tellus Institute packaging study. Prepared for the Council of State Governments, Tellus Institute, Boston, MA, 1991a.

Tellus Institute, Alternative approaches to the financial evaluation of industrial pollution prevention investments. Prepared for the New Jersey Department of Environmental Protection Project P32250 (1991b).

United Nations Environment Program (UNEP), "Montreal Protocol on Substances that Deplete the Ozone Layer." UNEP, New York, 1987.

U.S. Congress, Office of Technology Assessment, "Green Products by Design: Choices for a Cleaner Environment," OTA-E-541. U.S. Govt. Printing Office, Washington, DC, 1992.

U.S. Department of Commerce, Bureau of the Census, "Manufacturer's Pollution Abatement Expenditures and Operating Costs," MA200(88)-1. U.S. Dept. of Commerce, Washington, DC, 1990.

U.S. Department of Commerce, Bureau of the Census, "Manufacturer's Pollution Abatement Costs and Expenditures," MA200-90-1. U.S. Dept. of Commerce, Washington, DC, 1992.

U.S. Department of Energy, Office of Industrial Technologies, "Industrial Waste Reduction Program: Program Plan." USDOE, Washington, DC, 1991.

U.S. Environmental Protection Agency (USEPA), "Resource and Environmental Profile Analysis of Nine Beverage Container Alternatives," EPA/530/WP-91c, prepared by MRI. USEPA, Washington, DC, 1974.

U.S. Environmental Protection Agency (USEPA), "Resource and Environmental Profile Analysis of Five Milk Container Systems," prepared by MRI, Chemtech. USEPA, Washington, DC, 1978.

U.S. Environmental Protection Agency (USEPA), "Compilation of Air Pollutant Emission Factors," 4th ed. with Supplements A-D, Publ. AP-42. USEPA, Research Triangle Park, NC, 1985.

U.S. Environmental Protection Agency (USEPA), "Report to Congress: Solid Waste Disposal in the United States," Vol. 1, EPA 530-SW-88-011. USEPA, Washington, DC, 1988.

U.S. Environmental Protection Agency (USEPA), "Characterization of Products Containing Lead and Cadmium in Municipal Solid Waste in the United States, 1970 to 2000," EPA/530-SW-89-015A. USEPA Washington, DC, 1989.

U.S. Environmental Protection Agency, "Characterization of Municipal Solid Waste in the United States: 1990 Update," EPA 530-SW-90-042. USEPA, Washington, DC, 1990.

U.S. Environmental Protection Agency (USEPA), Office of Solid Waste and Emergency Response, "National Survey of Hazardous Waste Generators and Treatment, Storage, Disposal and Recycling Facilities in 1986: Hazardous Waste Management in RCRA TSDR Units," EPA/530-SW-91-060. USEPA, Washington, DC, 1991a.

U.S. Environmental Protection Agency (USEPA), "Product Life Cycle Assessments: Inventory Guidelines and Principles." USEPA, Battelle, Columbus, OH, 1991b.

U.S. Environmental Protection Agency (USEPA), "Toxics in the Community," EPA 560/4-91/014. USEPA, Washington, DC, 1991c.

U.S. Environmental Protection Agency (USEPA), "Life Cycle Design Guidance Manual: Environmental Requirements and the Product System," EPA/600/R-92/226. USEPA, Cincinnati, OH, 1993a.

U.S. Environmental Protection Agency (USEPA), "Life Cycle Assessment: Inventory Guidelines and Principles," EPA/600/R-92/245. USEPA, Cincinnati, OH, 1993b.

Waste Advantage, Inc., "Industrial Waste Prevention." Waste Advantage, Inc., Southfield, MI, 1988.

Weekman, V. W., Lumps, models and kinetics in practice. *AIChE Monog. Ser.* **75** (1979).

TROPOSPHERIC CHEMISTRY

John H. Seinfeld,* Jean M. Andino,* Frank M. Bowman,* Hali J. L. Forstner,* and Spyros Pandis†

***Department of Chemical Engineering**
California Institute of Technology
Pasadena, California 91125

†Departments of Chemical Engineering
and Engineering and Public Policy
Carnegie Mellon University
Pittsburgh, Pennsylvania 15213

I. Introduction

The atmosphere is a giant chemical reactor, to which a wide spectrum of inorganic and organic chemical compounds are emitted from both anthropogenic and natural sources. Many, if not most, of these chemical compounds can undergo chemical transformation in the atmosphere, leading to products many of which are not themselves emitted directly by any sources. The emitted compounds may be in gaseous or particulate form. The major classes of problems that result from the emissions of species to the atmosphere are summarized in Table I. Regulatory issues that arise in association with these problems include those such as:

What levels of hydrocarbon and oxides of nitrogen emissions reductions are required to reduce urban ozone levels to desired standards?

What is the contribution of individual emitted species to visibility reduction?

What are the contributions of individual emitted species to acidity deposited at the earth's surface?

What level of stratospheric ozone depletion will result from projected global chlorofluorocarbon (CFC) emissions?

TABLE I
THE MAJOR PROBLEMS IN AIR POLLUTION

	Scale	Species
Urban ozone and smog	Urban (~ 100 km)	HC, NO_x, particulate matter
Toxic air pollutants		PAHs, metals, HC
Acid deposition	Regional (~ 1000 km)	SO_2, NO_x, HC
Regional ozone		HC, NO_x, biogenic HC
Climate change	Global	CO_2, CH_4, CFC, RSR′, SO_2
Stratospheric ozone		CFC, N_2O

What is the anticipated effect of continued emissions of CO_2 and other gases on global climate?

To assess human health impacts and other effects of compounds emitted to the atmosphere, it is necessary to know not just the identities and amounts of emitted species, but also their conversion products, and the physical state of the products. The study of atmospheric chemistry comprises the rates and mechanisms of reactions that occur in both the natural and the perturbed (polluted) atmosphere.

II. The Earth's Atmosphere

The earth's atmosphere is composed of a number of layers. The troposphere, the layer closest to the earth, extends from the earth's surface to the tropopause, the boundary between the troposphere and the stratosphere. The altitude of the tropopause varies from about 10 km to 18 km, depending on latitude and season; it is highest in the tropics and lowest in the polar regions. The temperature in the troposphere decreases with increasing altitude from an average of 290 K at the earth's surface to about 210 to 220 K at the tropopause. The stratosphere extends from the tropopause to an altitude of about 50 km; temperature increases with altitude in the stratosphere from the 210 to 220 K at the tropopause to about 270 K at the top of the stratosphere. Vertical mixing in the troposphere is relatively vigorous, with a characteristic time for mixing up to the tropopause of the order of 10 to 30 days. Because of the increasing temperature profile, the stratosphere is a relatively stable layer, and characteristic times for vertical mixing in the stratosphere are on the order of years. In the present chapter we restrict our attention to the chemistry of the troposphere.

The bottom layer of air in the troposphere, that 1 to 2 km of air closest to the earth's surface, can be called the atmospheric boundary layer. From the point of view of atmospheric chemistry, four regions of the atmospheric boundary layer can be identified:

1. the *urban* atmosphere—the region most strongly influenced by anthropogenic emissions
2. the *regional* atmosphere—a region influenced by both anthropogenic and natural emissions
3. the *remote, tropical forest* atmosphere—a region essentially free of anthropogenic emissions but strongly influenced by natural biogenic emissions

TABLE II
TYPICAL OZONE AND NO_x MIXING RATIOS IN REGIONS OF THE TROPOSPHERE

Regime	Summertime, daily max O_3 (ppb)	NO_x (ppb)
Urban	100–400	10–1000
Regional	50–120	0.2–10
Remote tropical forest	10–40	0.02–0.08
Remote marine	10–40	0.02–0.04

4. the *remote*, *marine* atmosphere—a region free of both anthropogenic and land-based biogenic emissions, in some sense the purest air in the troposphere.

Ozone is, for all practical purposes, not emitted from any sources; its presence in the background troposphere is the result of downward mixing of air from the stratosphere, where it is produced chemically, and of *in situ* chemical production in the troposphere from the oxidation of methane (Logan, 1985, 1989). In the clean, unpolluted marine atmosphere, ozone mixing ratios are in the range of 10 to 40 parts per billion (ppb), and those of the oxides of nitrogen are 20 to 40 parts per trillion (ppt). The presence of oxides of nitrogen concentrations higher than these is indicative of the presence of natural or anthropogenic sources. In polluted urban regions ozone can reach mixing ratios as high as 400 ppb, and oxides of nitrogen can attain values close to 1000 ppb.

Table II gives typical ozone and oxides of nitrogen levels in these four regions. Urban- and regional-scale atmospheric chemistry is characterized by the definitive influence of anthropogenic emissions. The goals of a study of urban- and regional-scale atmospheric chemistry are to understand the atmospheric transformations of emitted species to be able to predict the formation of ozone and other pollutants, and to predict the pathways of removal of emitted species and their transformation products from the atmosphere.

III. Atmospheric Physical Removal Processes

Compounds emitted into the atmosphere are removed from it by a variety of physical and chemical processes. The rates of removal depend on the chemical nature of the compound, its susceptibility to chemical attack, its solubility in water, and its physical state (vapor or particulate form). The characteristic times for the chemical transformations and removal processes vary widely, with lifetimes varying from less than one minute for the most chemically reactive compounds to months or even years for the most inert species.

This chapter is devoted to chemical removal processes in the troposphere. In this section, however, we briefly discuss physical removal processes. Gases and particles are physically removed from the atmosphere by deposition at the earth's surface (so-called *dry deposition*) and by absorption into droplets followed by transfer of the drops to the surface in the form of precipitation (so-called *wet deposition*).

A. Dry Deposition

Because the processes by which a molecule, or particle, is transported to the surface of the earth and absorbed by the surface are quite complex, the dry deposition process is represented by an overall transfer coefficient. It is generally assumed that the dry deposition flux is proportional to the local pollutant concentration [at a known reference height (z_r), typically 10 m], resulting in the expression $F = -v_d C$, where F represents the dry deposition flux (the amount of pollutant depositing to a unit surface area per unit time) and C is the local pollutant concentration at the reference height. The proportionality constant, v_d, has units of length per unit time and is known as the deposition velocity.

It is customary to interpret the dry deposition process in terms of the electrical resistance analogy, where transport of material to the surface is assumed to be governed by three resistances in series: the aerodynamic resistance (r_a), the quasi-laminar layer resistance (r_b), and the surface or canopy resistance (r_s) (Wu *et al.*, 1992). The aerodynamic resistance characterizes the turbulent transport through the atmosphere from reference height z_r down to a thin layer of stagnant air very near the surface. The molecular-scale diffusive transport across the thin quasi-laminar sublayer near the surface is characterized by r_b. The chemical interaction between the surface and the pollutant of interest once the gas molecules have reached the surface is characterized by r_s. The total resistance (r_t) is the sum of the three individual resistances, and is, by definition, the inverse of the deposition velocity, $v_d^{-1} = r_t = r_a + r_b + r_s$. Note that the deposition velocity is small when any one of the resistances is large. Hence, either meteorological factors or the chemical interactions on the surface can govern the rate of dry deposition.

Dry deposition velocities for gases to a variety of surfaces are available in the literature (see, for example, Dolske and Gatz, 1985; Colbeck and

Harrison, 1985; Huebert and Robert, 1985; Shepson *et al.*, 1992). Gases that are removed readily by dry deposition have deposition velocities of order 1 cm s^{-1} or larger. Examples include nitric acid (HNO_3) and sulfur dioxide (SO_2). Ozone deposition velocities are about 0.5 cm s^{-1}. With a 1 km deep atmospheric boundary layer, a gas with a deposition velocity of 1 cm s^{-1} has a timescale for dry deposition of the order of 1 day. Dry deposition will be an important removal process for species whose timescale for dry deposition is comparable to or smaller than that for chemical transformation.

The rate of dry deposition of particles depends on the particle size. Particles are transported down to the quasi-laminar layer near the surface by the same mechanisms of turbulent transport as are gases. The rate of transfer across the laminar layer is determined by the particle diffusivity, which depends on particle size. Particles with sizes in the range of 0.1 to 1.0 μm diameter have atmospheric lifetimes with respect to dry deposition of about 10 days.

B. Wet Deposition

Wet deposition encompasses the removal of gases and particles from the atmosphere by precipitation events, through incorporation into rain, snow, cloud, and fog water, followed by precipitation (Hales, 1986). As in the case of dry deposition, wet deposition is a complex phenomenon which in this particular case involves transport to the surface of a droplet, absorption, and possible aqueous-phase chemical conversion. Wet removal of gases is frequently approximated by assuming that the species is in equilibrium between the gas and aqueous phases. The equilibrium partitioning is represented in terms of a washout ratio, $W_g = [C]_{drop}/[C]_{air}$, where $[C]_{drop}$ and $[C]_{air}$ are the concentrations of the chemical in the aqueous and gas phases (Mackay, 1991).

Wet deposition is an important removal route for highly water-soluble species with washout ratio values of $W_g \geq 10^4$. Examples of such species are HNO_3 and hydrogen peroxide (H_2O_2). Particles and particle-associated species are efficiently removed from the atmosphere by precipitation; washout ratios for particles, W_p, are typically in the range of 10^4 to 10^6 (Eisenreich, 1987; Bidleman, 1988). Note that the importance of wet deposition as a removal process may depend on whether the chemical is present in the gas phase or is associated with particles. For example, gas-phase alkanes have low values of W_g and are inefficiently removed by wet deposition, but if the same alkane is absorbed by a particle it can be efficiently removed through removal of the host particle.

IV. Agents of Chemical Attack in the Troposphere

Atmospheric (gas-phase) compounds undergo chemical transformation by three possible routes: (1) photolysis; (2) chemical attack by free radical and other species; and (3) dissolution in droplets followed by aqueous-phase chemical reaction. In this section we briefly discuss photolysis and then introduce the most important gas-phase species responsible for chemical attack in the troposphere. We will discuss aqueous-phase processes in Section X.

A. Photolysis

Atmospheric species may undergo transformation by photolysis. For this to occur the compound must absorb light in the so-called actinic portion of the spectrum, from 290 nm to 1000 nm, and, after absorption of a photon, undergo chemical change. For most compounds, breakage of chemical bonds requires energies in excess of about 40 kcal $mole^{-1}$ (Benson, 1976); photolytic wavelengths less than about 700 nm correspond to this limit.

The rate of photolysis for the process

$$A + h\nu \longrightarrow \text{products}$$

is expressed as first-order in the concentration of A with a first-order rate constant given by

$$k_{\text{photolysis}} = \int J_\lambda \sigma_\lambda \phi_\lambda \, d\lambda,$$

where J_λ is the radiation flux at wavelength λ, σ_λ is the absorption cross-section for the molecule A at wavelength λ, and ϕ_λ is the photolysis quantum yield for A at wavelength λ. The value of J_λ depends on latitude, time of year, time of day, and atmospheric conditions, such as cloud cover or existence of haze, while J_λ and ϕ_λ are molecule-specific and independent of atmospheric conditions or location. Tabulated values of J_λ and ϕ_λ as a function of wavelength exist for most of the important absorbing species in atmospheric chemistry (Demerjian *et al.*, 1980). Also, values of J_λ are tabulated as a function of latitude, day of the year, and time of day. When lists of atmospheric chemical reactions are compiled, together with their rate constants, a single value of a first-order photolysis rate constant is frequently given, reflecting that at, say, noon on a particular day, say June 21, at a particular latitude of interest. Computer codes for solving the rate equations arising from atmospheric chemical mechanisms often include data files of J_λ, σ_λ, and ϕ_λ that allow the direct calculation of the photolysis rate constant for given molecules for the conditions of interest.

B. Gas-Phase Oxidizing Species

Chemical attack on atmospheric compounds is frequently an oxidation step. Principal oxidizing species in the troposphere include the hydroxyl radical (OH), ozone (O_3), and the nitrate radical (NO_3).

1. The Hydroxyl Radical

Hydroxyl radicals are formed in the troposphere via the following processes (Ehhalt *et al.*, 1991):

a. Photolysis of O_3. At wavelengths less than 319 nm, O_3 photodissociates to yield, in part, electronically excited oxygen atoms, $O(^1D)$:

$$O_3 + h\nu\ (\lambda < 319\ \text{nm}) \longrightarrow O(^1D) + O_2(^1\Delta_g). \tag{1}$$

Most of the excited $O(^1D)$ atoms are physically quenched by N_2 and O_2 back to the ground state $O(^3P)$,

$$O(^1D) + M[M = \text{air}(N_2 + O_2)] \longrightarrow O(^3P) + M, \tag{2}$$

but a small fraction of $O(^1D)$ reacts chemically with other species. Notably, the reaction of $O(^1D)$ with water vapor,

$$O(^1D) + H_2O \longrightarrow 2\,OH, \tag{3}$$

is an important source of tropospheric OH because of the large concentration of water vapor. For a relative humidity of 50% at 298 K, about 0.2 OH radicals are formed for each $O(^1D)$ atom formed.

b. Photolysis of Nitrous Acid. Nitrous acid, HONO, which is present during nighttime hours in urban atmospheres, is rapidly photolyzed during daytime hours to yield OH radicals (Calvert *et al.*, 1994):

$$\text{HONO} + h\nu\ (\lambda \lesssim 400\ \text{nm}) \longrightarrow \text{OH} + \text{NO}. \tag{4}$$

Nitrous acid is formed from the reaction of OH radicals with NO:

$$\text{OH} + \text{NO} \xrightarrow{M} \text{HONO}. \tag{5}$$

The principal removal process of HONO is photodecomposition. Nitrous acid achieves its maximum concentrations during nighttime in the urban atmosphere. Calvert *et al.* (1994) summarize observations of HONO. Typical nighttime urban mixing ratios range from about 1 ppb to maximum values approaching 10 ppb. Values reported for remote areas are usually much lower than those for urban areas. The photodissociation lifetime of HONO ranges from about 10 min at high sun to about 1 h for early morning sun. If HONO accumulates overnight, its photodissociation can be a significant early-morning source of OH radicals before other sources become dominant.

c. Reaction of HO_2 Radicals with NO. Hydroperoxyl (HO_2) radicals, formed, for example, from the photodissociation of aldehydes, as well as from the reactions of various hydrocarbons with OH, O_3, or NO_3, react with NO to produce the OH radical:

$$HO_2 + NO \longrightarrow OH + NO_2. \tag{6}$$

The magnitude of tropospheric NO concentrations is highly important in the conversion of HO_2 to the more highly reactive OH radical.

Measurement of atmospheric OH radical levels has proven to be a difficult task. Long-path absorption of laser light in the UV portion of the spectrum has been used to reliably measure OH concentrations near Julich, Germany (Hofzumahaus *et al.*, 1992) on the order of 10^6 molecules cm^{-3}. Mount and Eisele (1992) report intercomparison measurements of OH at Fritz Peak Observatory, Colorado in summer 1991 using two independent instruments. Hydroxyl levels were found to vary diurnally, ranging between $1–4 \times 10^6$ molecules cm^{-3} on the days studied. Computer modeling studies (Crutzen, 1982) suggest that average tropospheric 24-h OH radical levels are $\sim 5 \times 10^5$ molecules cm^{-3} in the northern hemisphere and $\sim 6 \times 10^5$ molecules cm^{-3} in the southern hemisphere.

Under noontime conditions at 298 K, OH generation rates for these pathways (1)–(3) are approximately

$$\begin{aligned}
&(1)\ O_3 + h\nu \longrightarrow && 0.22 \text{ ppb min}^{-1}\\
&(2)\ HONO + h\nu \longrightarrow && 0.097 \text{ ppb min}^{-1}\\
&(3)\ HO_2 + NO \longrightarrow && 0.59 \text{ ppb min}^{-1}
\end{aligned}$$

$[O_3] = 50$ ppb (1.2×10^{12} molecule cm^{-3}); $[HO_2] = 10^{-3}$ ppb (2.5×10^7 molecule cm^{-3}); $[NO] = 40$ ppb (9.8×10^{11} molecule cm^{-3}); $[HONO] =$ 1 ppb (2.5×10^{10} molecule cm^{-3}).

2. Ozone

Ozone (O_3), which for all practical purposes is not emitted from any ground-level source, is formed in the troposphere from photolysis of NO_2:

$$NO_2 + h\nu\ (\lambda \lesssim 430\ \text{nm}) \longrightarrow NO + O(^3P), \tag{7}$$

followed by

$$O(^3P) + O_2 + M \longrightarrow O_3 + M, \tag{8}$$

and from downward transport from the stratosphere. As seen in Table II, in the clean troposphere, O_3 mixing ratios are typically $\sim 30 \pm 10$ ppb [$\sim 7 \times 10^{11}$ molecules cm^{-3}] at ground level, increasing with altitude (Logan, 1985).

3. The Nitrate Radical

The gaseous NO_3 radical is formed via the reactions [see Atkinson (1991) and Wayne *et al.*, (1991) for a comprehensive review of the nitrate radical]

$$NO_2 + O_3 \longrightarrow NO_3 + O_2, \tag{9}$$

$$NO_2 + NO_3 \underset{}{\overset{M}{\rightleftarrows}} N_2O_5, \tag{10, 11}$$

with N_2O_5 being in a relatively rapid (characteristic time ~ 1 min at 298 K) equilibrium with NO_2 and the NO_3 radical (Tuazon *et al.*, 1984).

NO_3 radicals photolyze rapidly via two paths:

$$NO_3 + h\nu\ (\lambda < 700\ \text{nm}) \longrightarrow NO + O_2, \tag{12a}$$

$$NO_3 + h\nu\ (\lambda < 580\ \text{nm}) \longrightarrow NO_2 + O(^3P), \tag{12b}$$

with a noontime lifetime of ~ 5 s (Magnotta and Johnston, 1980), and react with NO,

$$NO_3 + NO \longrightarrow 2\,NO_2, \tag{13}$$

sufficiently rapidly that NO and NO_3 cannot coexist at mixing ratios of a few parts-per-trillion (ppt) or higher. For typical daytime conditions of $[NO_2] = 40$ ppb, $[O_3] = 50$ ppb, $[NO] = 40$ ppb, the maximum NO_3 mixing ratio will be 0.6 ppt. At nighttime, however, when NO concentrations drop near zero because of reaction with O_3, the NO_3 mixing ratio will reach 100 ppt.

Nitric acid is formed, probably in the absorbed phase, from the heterogeneous hydrolysis of N_2O_5 (Tuazon *et al.*, 1983):

$$N_2O_5 + H_2O \xrightarrow{\text{heterogeneous}} 2\,HNO_3. \tag{14}$$

V. Nitrogen Oxides Chemistry

Nitrogen-containing compounds, particularly oxidized nitrogen compounds, play a central role in the chemistry of the troposphere. So-called active nitrogen, denoted NO_x, the sum of NO and NO_2, exerts a controlling influence on the abundance of the OH radical and is essential for the photochemical production of tropospheric ozone.

Logan (1983) has estimated the global inventory of NO_x emissions (emission rates expressed in units of 10^{12} g N yr^{-1}, with mean value given and range of estimates in parentheses):

Fossil fuel combustion	21 (14–28)
Biomass burning	12 (4–24)
Lightning	8 (2–20)
Microbial activity in soils	8 (4–16)
Oxidation of ammonia	1–10
Photolytic or biological processes in the ocean	< 1
Input from the stratosphere	0.5

The chief sources of reactive nitrogen in the troposphere are fossil-fuel combustion, biomass burning for land-clearing purposes, lightning, soil-microbial activity, and transport from the stratosphere. Although transport from the stratosphere is by far the smallest of these, it has been estimated to supply most of the reactive nitrogen concentrations in remote marine locations. Support for this estimate has been based in part on the vertical profiles of NO_x found over remote areas, which indicate a strong downward gradient suggestive of transport from the stratosphere. It is argued that the lifetime of NO_x from the much larger continental sources is too short (i.e., only a few days) to contribute significantly to abundances over remote oceanic regions.

In recent years, however, an alternative view has begun to develop. Measurements in the remote Pacific appear consistent with the long-range transport of reactive nitrogen (in this case nitrate) from North America (Galasyn *et al.*, 1987; Savoie *et al.*, 1988). Additionally, the approximate factor-of-two increase of nitrate deposition in ice cores from Greenland over the last several decades suggests that the increased fossil-fuel sources of nitrogen oxides over this period are responsible for the nitrate deposition in this remote region as well (Neftel *et al.*, 1985).

The emissions of NO_x from fossil fuel combustion and biomass burning are increasing. Recent simulations show that these anthropogenic sources of NO_x may have contributed to increases in NO_x concentration over vast portions of the marine atmosphere (Penner *et al.*, 1991), which would be expected to lead to an increase in ozone concentration in these areas.

Dignon and Penner (1991) have developed a gridded global inventory of the emissions of NO_x from biomass burning using estimates of the amount of biomass burned in each region, together with estimates of the dominant type of vegetation and its nitrogen content. Heavy burning for deforestation is responsible for most of the emissions in Brazil, and heavy burning to clear land for shifting agriculture is responsible for most of the emissions in Africa. These results indicate that the total emission rate is nearly 12 Tg N yr^{-1}, highlighting the importance of this source in perturbing the natural cycle of nitrogen oxides.

Total odd nitrogen, denoted NO_y, is the sum of NO_x, HNO_3, HO_2NO_2, HONO, NO_3, $2N_2O_5$, organic nitrates, and possibly other inorganic nitrates and particulate nitrate, NO_3^-. Ambient measurements of oxidized nitrogen compounds have been surveyed by Fehsenfeld *et al.* (1988) and Ridley (1991).

The oxides of nitrogen emitted into the atmosphere comprise NO, NO_2, N_2O, HONO, and, possibly, HNO_3. N_2O is chemically inert in the troposphere, being transported into the stratosphere where it photodissociates (Liu *et al.*, 1977).

Nitric oxide (NO) reacts rapidly with ozone (O_3) to yield NO_2:

$$NO + O_3 \longrightarrow NO_2 + O_2. \tag{15}$$

NO_2 photolyzes rapidly (with a lifetime of $\sim$ 2 min at solar noon) to yield NO and an oxygen atom,

$$NO_2 + h\nu\ (\lambda \lesssim 430\ \text{nm}) \longrightarrow NO + O(^3P), \tag{16}$$

with the oxygen atom reacting with O_2 to yield O_3:

$$O(^3P) + O_2 + M \longrightarrow O_3 + M. \tag{17}$$

Because of the rapidity of the NO–O_3 and $O(^3P)$–O_2 reactions, NO, NO_2, and O_3 are in a photostationary state (a steady state sustained by the influx of photons) at which the concentration of ozone is given by

$$[O_3] = \frac{j[NO_2]}{k_{15}[NO]}, \tag{18}$$

where $j[NO_2]$ is the photolysis rate of NO_2.

Further reactions of NO and NO_2 under atmospheric conditions involve the formation of NO_3 radicals, and of N_2O_5, which is formed from the reaction of NO_2 with O_3 (see Section IV, B, 3).

NO and NO_2 also react with HO_2 radicals:

$$NO + HO_2 \longrightarrow NO_2 + OH, \qquad (19)\ (\text{also } 6)$$

$$NO_2 + HO_2 \overset{M}{\rightleftharpoons} HO_2NO_2, \qquad (20, 21)$$

with the latter process being reversible due to the rapid (~ 10 s lifetime at 298 K and 760 torr total pressure) back-decomposition of pernitric acid, HO_2NO_2 (Atkinson and Lloyd, 1984), and with OH radicals,

$$OH + NO \xrightarrow{M} HONO, \qquad (22)$$

$$OH + NO_2 \xrightarrow{M} HNO_3. \qquad (23)$$

The formation of HONO is balanced during daytime hours (when OH radicals are present at appreciable concentrations) by its rapid (~ 10–15 min lifetime at solar noon) photolysis:

$$HONO + h\nu\ (\lambda < 400\ \text{nm}) \longrightarrow OH + NO. \qquad (24)\ (\text{also } 4)$$

The major tropospheric loss process of NO_x involves the formation of nitric acid via reaction of OH radicals with NO_2 or by heterogeneous/homogeneous hydrolysis of N_2O_5, with nitric acid being removed from the troposphere mainly by dry and wet deposition.

VI. Chemistry of the Background Troposphere: The Methane Oxidation Cycle

The simplest alkane is methane (CH_4). Methane oxidation is the essential chemistry of the background troposphere (Logan *et al.*, 1981; Thompson and Cicerone, 1986). Ice-core records show that methane concentrations in the atmosphere have more than doubled since pre-industrial times (Khalil and Rasmussen, 1987), reaching a rate of increase of 1% yr^{-1} in the last decade (Khalil *et al.*, 1989). Methane is emitted to the atmosphere by ruminants, wetlands, tundra, open waters, termites, rice paddies, biomass burning, natural gas production, and coal mining [see Jacob (1991) for a review of the literature on methane sources]; the principal sink of CH_4 is reaction with OH.

The principal removal path for CH_4 is reaction with the OH radical. At prevailing estimated OH levels, the lifetime of CH_4 is about 10 yrs. Hydroxyl radical attack proceeds by H-atom abstraction to form the methyl radical,

$$CH_4 + OH \longrightarrow CH_3\cdot + H_2O. \tag{25}$$

Under atmospheric conditions the methyl radical reacts exclusively with O_2 to yield the methylperoxy ($CH_3O_2\cdot$) radical,

$$CH_3\cdot + O_2 \xrightarrow{M} CH_3O_2\cdot. \tag{26}$$

The methylperoxy radical can react with NO, NO_2, HO_2 radicals, and itself (also other organic peroxy radicals $RO_2\cdot$). The reaction with NO, analogous to reaction (6) (and 19),

$$CH_3O_2\cdot + NO \longrightarrow CH_3O\cdot + NO_2, \tag{27}$$

leads to formation of the methoxy ($CH_3O\cdot$) radical. Reaction with the HO_2 radical leads to the formation of methyl hydroperoxide (CH_3OOH),

$$CH_3O_2\cdot + HO_2\cdot \longrightarrow CH_3OOH + O_2. \tag{28}$$

Methyl hydroperoxide can photolyze,

$$CH_3OOH + h\nu \longrightarrow CH_3O\cdot + OH, \tag{29}$$

or react with the OH radical,

$$CH_3OOH + OH \longrightarrow CH_3O_2\cdot + H_2O \tag{30a}$$

$$\longrightarrow \cdot CH_2OOH + H_2O, \tag{30b}$$

where $\cdot CH_2OOH$ decomposes rapidly to formaldehyde (HCHO) and OH,

$$\cdot CH_2OOH \longrightarrow HCHO + OH. \tag{31}$$

The methoxy radical reacts virtually exclusively with O_2 to form formaldehyde and the HO_2 radical,

$$CH_3O\cdot + O_2 \longrightarrow HCHO + HO_2\cdot. \tag{32}$$

Formaldehyde can photolyze to yield non-radical and radical products,

$$HCHO + h\nu \longrightarrow H_2 + CO, \tag{33a}$$

$$\longrightarrow H\dot{C}O + H, \tag{33b}$$

where, at noontime conditions, reaction (33a) constitutes about 55% of the total photolysis reaction. Formaldehyde also reacts with OH,

$$HCHO + OH \longrightarrow H\dot{C}O + H_2O. \tag{34}$$

The hydrogen atom and formyl radical ($H\dot{C}O$) react exclusively with O_2 to produce the HO_2 radical,

$$H + O_2 \xrightarrow{M} HO_2\cdot, \tag{35}$$

$$H\dot{C}O + O_2 \longrightarrow HO_2\cdot + CO. \tag{36}$$

The lifetime of HCHO from photolysis is about 4 h; that from OH reaction is about 1.6 days.

Carbon monoxide reacts exclusively with the OH radical,

$$CO + OH \longrightarrow CO_2 + H, \tag{37}$$

where the H atom is immediately converted to $HO_2\cdot$ by reaction (35).

The tropospheric lifetime of CO is about 3 months. CO_2 is chemically stable under tropospheric conditions, and its loss processes involve transport to the stratosphere and absorption into the oceans.

The methane oxidation cycle is depicted in Fig. 1. A fundamental feature of the behavior of the methane oxidation chain is the competition

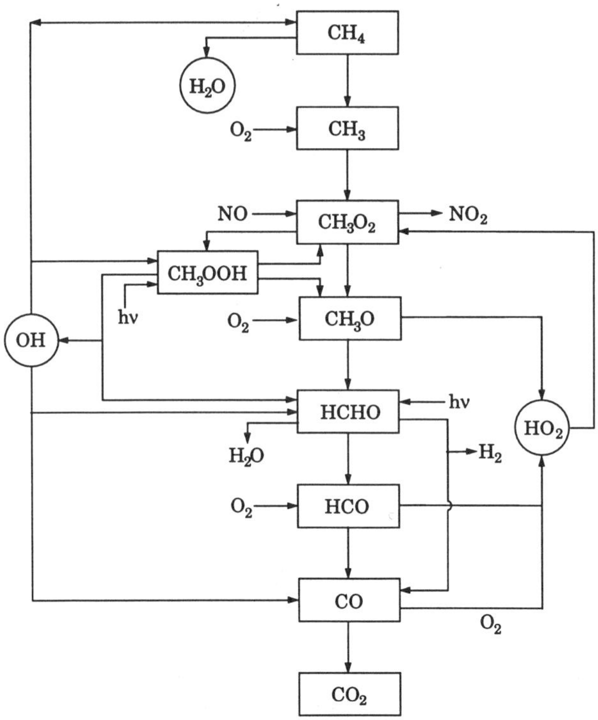

FIG. 1. Atmospheric methane oxidation cycle.

between NO and the HO_2 radical for reaction with the CH_3O_2 radical. Since the rate constants for reactions (27) and (28) are comparable, which of the two reactions predominates in a particular situation depends on the relative concentrations of NO and HO_2. Based on estimated HO_2 radical concentrations in the troposphere, reaction (27) is predominant for NO mixing ratios greater than about 30 ppt; otherwise, reaction (28) predominates. The HO_2 radical, in addition to reaction (6), can react with O_3 and with itself, the latter reaction constituting the principal source of gaseous hydrogen peroxide (H_2O_2),

$$HO_2 + O_3 \longrightarrow OH + 2O_2, \tag{38}$$

$$HO_2 + HO_2 \longrightarrow H_2O_2 + O_2. \tag{39}$$

Hydrogen peroxide is the dominant oxidant in clouds, fogs, or rain in the atmosphere. Photochemical activity largely determines the diurnal, seasonal, and latitudinal variations of the H_2O_2 concentration. H_2O_2 levels have been found to be higher in the afternoon, during the summer and in the southern latitudes (Sakugawa *et al.*, 1990). The major gas-phase destruction pathways for H_2O_2 are its reaction with OH and its photolysis:

$$H_2O_2 + OH \longrightarrow H_2O + HO_2, \tag{40}$$

$$H_2O_2 + h\nu \longrightarrow 2OH. \tag{41}$$

The destruction of H_2O_2 in the aqueous phase, mainly by reacting with dissolved SO_2, is discussed subsequently. Measured gas-phase mixing ratios of H_2O_2 range from 0.2 to 4.1 ppb during the fall in the eastern U.S. (Heikes *et al.*, 1987), from 0.1 to 1.0 ppb during the winter over the southern U.S. (Van Valin *et al.*, 1987), 0.2 to 2.4 ppb during winter in the eastern U.S. (Barth *et al.*, 1989), and from 0 to 2 ppb in Southern California (Sakugawa and Kaplan, 1989). Modeling studies have indicated that high concentrations of NO_x tend to inhibit H_2O_2 formation by scavenging free radical species from the air. High concentrations of VOC favor the H_2O_2 generation, because of the higher production of free radical species (Calvert and Stockwell, 1983). For a review of the current understanding of the atmospheric role of H_2O_2, the reader is referred to Sakugawa *et al.* (1990).

Whether the methane oxidation cycle leads to a net production or consumption of ozone depends on the NO level. For a net production of O_3 to exist, reaction (6), which propagates the chain, must compete effectively with reaction (15), which simply consumes an O_3 molecule to regenerate NO_2. Reaction (6) competes with reaction (15); at tropospheric O_3 levels, reaction (6) dominates over reaction (15) for NO mixing ratios exceeding about 10 ppt. At this level of NO, reaction (6) also dominates the HO_2 self-reaction (39).

When HO_2 radicals react with NO preferentially, OH radicals are regenerated and the chain leads to net ozone formation. Under sufficiently low NO conditions, where reactions (38) and (39) predominate, a net loss of O_3 occurs. In the remote marine boundary layer NO levels are sufficiently low (Table II) that methane oxidation leads to a net consumption of O_3. In the upper troposphere and in urban and regional areas, NO levels are sufficiently high to lead to a net production of O_3.

The methane oxidation cycle can be summarized as follows. In the high-NO_x regime, the net result of the cycle is

$$CH_4 + 4O_2 \longrightarrow HCHO + H_2O + 2O_3.$$

Thus, the oxidation of CH_4 under high-NO_x conditions leads to a net formation of two molecules of O_3 for each CH_4 that reacts with OH. Under low-NO_x conditions, the CH_3O_2 radical, produced by OH attack on CH_4, will react with HO_2 rather than NO to give the net reaction,

$$CH_4 + OH + HO_2 \longrightarrow CH_3OOH + H_2O.$$

The net reaction of the formaldehyde formed under high NO_x conditions can be written as

$$HCHO + 0.2OH + 0.92NO \xrightarrow{O_2} 0.92NO_2 + 0.92OH + CO + 0.44H_2 + 0.2H_2O.$$

Atmospheric formaldehyde oxidation thus represents a net source of OH radicals.

Globally, the methane oxidation chain results in an estimated net annual loss of about 0.22 molecules of OH for every CH_4 molecule destroyed (Tie *et al.*, 1992). The average annual yield of CO from methane oxidation is about 0.82 molecules of CO per molecule of CH_4 destroyed. The methane oxidation chain also produces about 1.15 molecules of ozone for each molecule of CH_4 destroyed. The increase of atmospheric CH_4 could be attributable, in part, to a decrease of global OH concentrations, resulting from increasing emissions of anthropogenic compounds, principally CO, that compete with CH_4 for the available OH.

VII. Chemistry of the Urban and Regional Atmosphere

The urban and regional atmosphere is characterized by anthropogenic emissions of NO_x and non-methane organic compounds. Also, biogenic organic compounds are emitted from vegetation. The chemistry of the urban and regional atmosphere, while far more complex than that of the methane oxidation cycle, has the same essential features—that is, oxidation initiated by the OH radical, and O_3 formation from a chain process involving HO_2 and RO_2 radicals. Hydrocarbon classes that are important in the urban and regional atmosphere are alkanes, alkenes, and aromatics; oxygen-containing organics include aldehydes, ketones, ethers, acids, and alcohols (Seila *et al.*, 1989). For example, the top 30 non-methane organic compounds measured during the 1987 Southern California Air Quality Study, ordered with respect to percentage of the total non-methane organic compounds on a carbon-atom concentration basis were (Lurmann and Main, 1992):

Propane	7.88 %
Toluene	7.876
Isopentane	7.841
n-Butane	6.166
Ethane	4.538
Ethene	4.202
n-Pentane	3.709
Acetylene	3.007
Isobutane	2.820
Benzene	2.776
2-Methylpentane	2.545
p-Xylene	2.442
m-Xylene	2.442
Acetone	2.359
o-Xylene	1.805
3-Methylpentane	1.789
n-Hexane	1.750
Methylcyclopentane	1.721
Propene	1.680
1,2,4-Trimethylbenzene	1.656
2,2,4-Trimethylpentane	1.414
Ethylbenzene	1.292
Acetaldehyde	1.226
3-Methylhexane	1.167
Methylcyclohexane	1.100
Pentanal	1.088
Formaldehyde	1.042
Methyl ethyl ketone	1.035
C6 carbonyl	1.034
m-Ethyltoluene	1.008

Warneck (1988) has estimated the annual global emission rates of non-methane organic compounds, expressed in units of 10^{12} g yr^{-1}:

Anthropogenic sources		
Combustion and chemical industry	36	(alkanes, alkenes, aromatics)
Natural gas	5	(light alkanes)
Organic solvents	15	(higher alkanes, aromatics)
Biomass burning	40	(light alkanes, alkenes)
Biogenic sources		
Foliage	830	(isoprene, monoterpenes)
Grasslands	47	(light alkanes and higher)
Soils	< 3	(ethene)
Ocean waters	6–10	(light alkanes/alkenes)

We now discuss briefly the essential features of the atmospheric chemistry of the different organic compound classes.

A. Alkanes

Under tropospheric conditions, the alkanes react with OH radicals during daylight hours and with the NO_3 radical during nighttime hours, with the latter process being of minor ($\lesssim 10\%$) importance as an atmospheric loss process.

Both reactions proceed via H-atom abstraction from C — H bonds,

$$RH + OH \longrightarrow R\cdot + H_2O, \tag{42}$$

$$RH + NO_3 \longrightarrow R\cdot + HNO_3, \tag{43}$$

where R is an alkyl group.

The total alkane–OH rate constant for a particular alkane can be determined from a structure–activity relationship that accounts for the numbers of primary, secondary, and tertiary hydrogen atoms (Atkinson, 1987). Atkinson (1989) notes that primary hydrogen atoms in alkanes typically react with OH with a rate constant of 1.75×10^{-13} cm^3 molecule^{-1} s^{-1} per carbon atom, while secondary hydrogen atoms typically react with OH with a rate constant of about 10.7×10^{-13} cm^3 molecule^{-1} s^{-1} per carbon atom. As with the methyl radical, the resulting alkyl (R) radical reacts rapidly, and exclusively, with O_2 under atmospheric conditions to yield an alkyl peroxy radical [see the comprehensive reviews of the chemistry of RO_2 radicals by Lightfoot *et al.* (1992) and Wallington *et al.* (1992)]:

$$R\cdot + O_2 \xrightarrow{M} RO_2\cdot. \tag{44}$$

These alkyl peroxy radicals can be classed as primary, secondary, or tertiary depending on the availability of H-atoms: $RCH_2OO\cdot$ (primary); $RR'CHOO\cdot$ (secondary): $RR'R''COO\cdot$ (tertiary).

Under tropospheric conditions, these alkyl peroxy (RO_2) radicals react with NO, via two pathways:

$$RO_2\cdot + NO \longrightarrow RO\cdot + NO_2, \tag{45a}$$

$$\xrightarrow{M} RONO_2; \tag{45b}$$

with HO_2 radicals:

$$RO_2\cdot + HO_2\cdot \longrightarrow ROOH + O_2; \tag{46}$$

or with other RO_2 radicals (including the same RO_2 species):

$$RO_2\cdot + RO_2\cdot \longrightarrow 2RO\cdot + O_2, \tag{47a}$$

$$\longrightarrow R'CHO + ROH + O_2, \tag{47b}$$

$$\longrightarrow ROOR + O_2. \tag{47c}$$

Similarly, for $RO_2\cdot + HO_2\cdot$,

$$RO_2\cdot + HO_2\cdot \longrightarrow ROOH\cdot + O_2\cdot, \tag{48a}$$

$$\longrightarrow R'CHO + H_2O + O_2, \tag{48b}$$

where pathway (48b) is generally negligible.

Under polluted urban atmospheric conditions, and indeed possibly for much of the lower troposphere in populated continental regions, reaction with NO is probably the dominant reaction pathway for RO_2 radicals.

For the alkyl peroxy radicals, reaction (45a) can form the corresponding alkoxy (RO) radical together with NO_2, or the corresponding alkyl nitrate, reaction (45b), with the yield of the alkyl nitrate increasing with increasing pressure and with decreasing temperature. For secondary alkyl peroxy radicals at 298 K and 760 torr total pressure, the alkyl nitrate yields increase monotonically from < 0.014 for a C_2 alkane up to ~ 0.33 for a C_8 alkane (Atkinson, 1990).

The resulting alkoxy radicals react under tropospheric conditions via a variety of processes: unimolecular decomposition, unimolecular isomerization, or reaction with O_2. Alkoxy radicals with fewer than five carbon atoms do not undergo isomerization; for these, the competitive processes are unimolecular decomposition versus reaction with O_2. The general alkoxy radical—O_2 reaction is

$$RO\cdot + O_2 \longrightarrow R'CHO + HO_2\cdot. \tag{49}$$

Unimolecular decomposition, on the other hand, proceeds as follows:

$$RCH_2O\cdot \longrightarrow R\cdot + HCHO, \tag{50}$$

$$RR_1CHO\cdot \longrightarrow R\cdot + R_1CHO, \tag{51}$$

$$RR_1R_2CHO\cdot \longrightarrow R\cdot + R_1C(O)R_2. \tag{52}$$

Rate constants for the alkoxy–O_2 reaction are as follows:

primary RO: 7.9×10^{-15} cm^3 molecule^{-1} s^{-1}
secondary RO: 7.5×10^{-15} cm^3 molecule^{-1} s^{-1}.

Tertiary alkoxy radicals are not expected to react with O_2 because of the absence of a readily available hydrogen atom. Assuming a ground-level O_2 concentration of 4.9×10^{18} molecules cm^{-3}, the two rate constants shown lead to the following pseudo first-order reaction rate constants: 3.87×10^4 s^{-1} (primary RO); 3.68×10^4 s^{-1} (secondary RO). These pseudo first-order rate constants can be compared with those for unimolecular decomposition (Atkinson, 1990). Generally, reaction with O_2 is the preferred path for the smaller alkoxy radicals.

B. Alkenes

Alkenes are removed from the troposphere via reaction with $O(^3P)$ atoms, OH radicals, NO_3 radicals, and O_3. Of these, reaction with $O(^3P)$ atoms is essentially negligible under atmospheric conditions.

1. Alkene–OH Reaction

Alkene–OH reactions generally proceed via OH radical addition to the double bond (Atkinson, 1989):

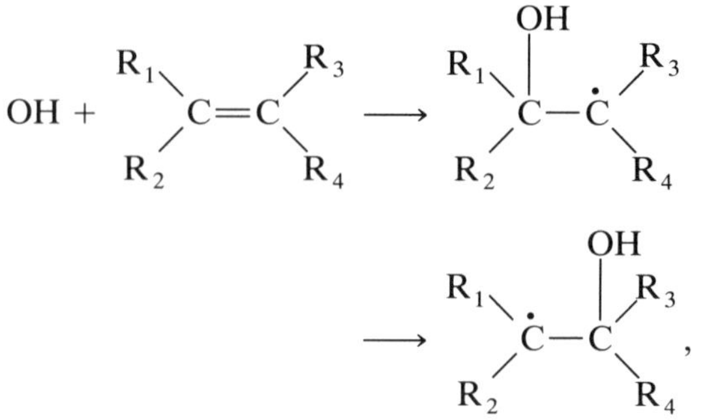

followed by rapid addition of O_2 to yield the corresponding hydroxyalkyl–peroxy radicals,

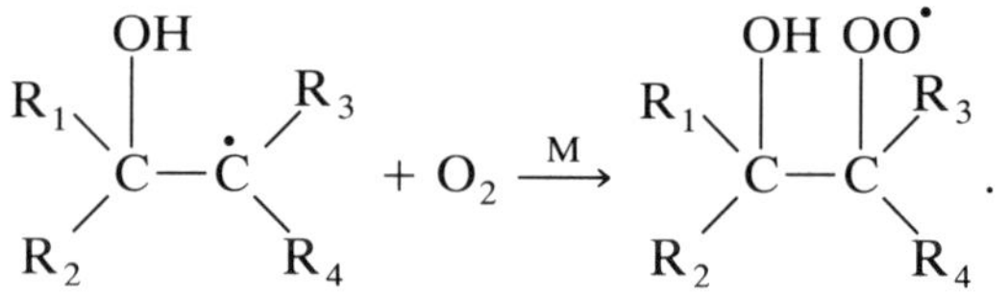

H-atom abstraction is a minor path. Reaction with NO yields the β-hydroxylalkoxy radical or the hydroxynitrate:

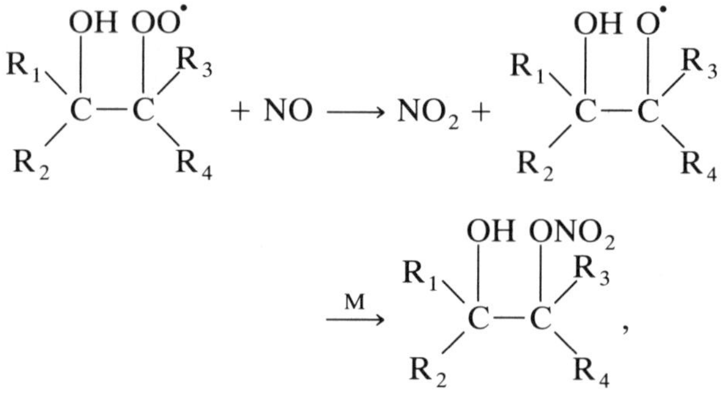

with the hydroxynitrate formation pathway accounting for ~ 1–1.5% of the overall NO reaction pathway at ~ 298 K for the propene system (Shepson *et al.*, 1985).

The dominant removal processes of the β-hydroxylalkoxy radicals are reactions with O_2, unimolecular decomposition, and unimolecular isomerization:

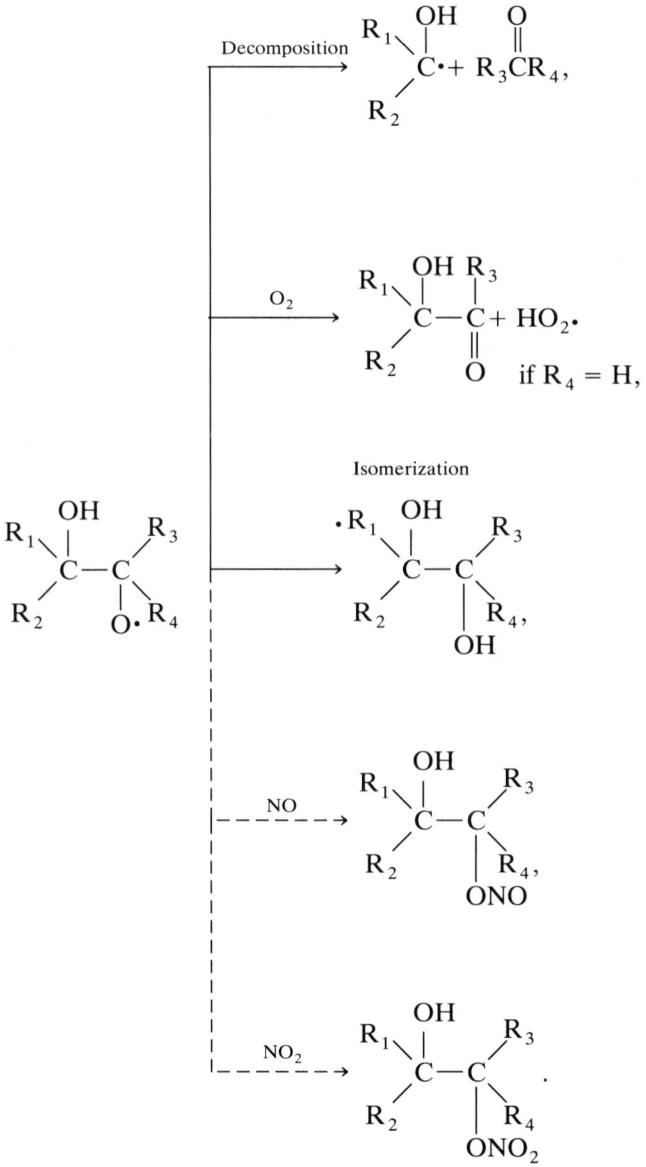

The ethene–OH reaction mechanism is

$$C_2H_4 + OH\cdot \longrightarrow HOCH_2CH_2\cdot, \tag{53}$$

$$HOCH_2CH_2\cdot + O_2 \longrightarrow HOCH_2CH_2O_2\cdot, \tag{54}$$

$$HOCH_2CH_2O_2\cdot + NO \longrightarrow HOCH_2CH_2O\cdot + NO_2, \tag{55}$$

$$HOCH_2CH_2O\cdot + O_2 \longrightarrow HOCH_2CHO + HO_2\cdot, \tag{56}$$

$$HOCH_2CH_2O\cdot \longrightarrow HCHO + \cdot CH_2OH \tag{57}$$

$$\cdot CH_2OH + O_2 \longrightarrow HCHO + HO_2\cdot. \tag{58}$$

Decomposition of the $HOCH_2CH_2O\cdot$ radical and reaction with O_2 are competitive processes with about 72% of the reaction proceeding by the decomposition path. For alkenes with carbon numbers greater than 3, reaction of the β-hydroxyalkoxy radical with O_2 is negligible compared with decomposition.

The net reaction of ethene with OH can be written as follows:

$$C_2H_4 + OH\cdot + NO \xrightarrow{2O_2} NO_2 + 0.28\, HOCH_2CHO + 1.44\, HCHO + HO_2\cdot. \tag{59}$$

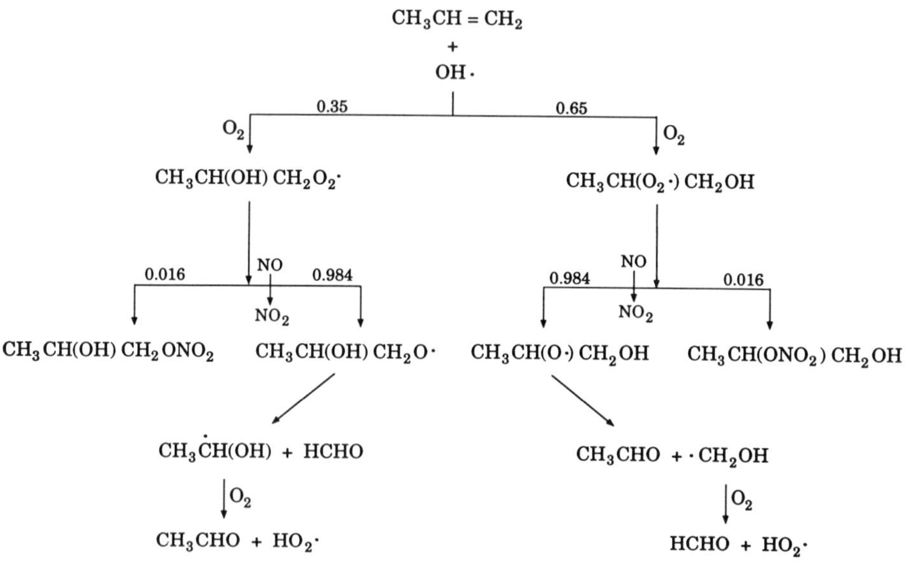

FIG. 2. Propene–OH reaction mechanism.

The propene–OH reaction mechanism is shown in Fig. 2. The net reaction of propene with OH is

$$C_3H_6 + OH\cdot + NO \xrightarrow{2O_2}$$
$$NO_2 + 0.984\,[CH_3CHO + HCHO + HO_2\cdot\,]$$
$$+ (0.016)(0.65)CH_3CH(ONO_2)CH_2OH$$
$$+ (0.016)(0.35)CH_3CH(OH)CH_2ONO_2. \quad (60)$$

2. Alkene-NO_3 Reaction (Hjorth et al., 1990; Atkinson, 1991)

As in OH–alkene reactions, NO_3 adds to the double bond and H-atom abstraction is relatively insignificant,

$$\underset{R_2}{\overset{R_1}{>}}C=C\underset{R_4}{\overset{R_3}{<}} + NO_3 \longrightarrow \underset{R_2}{\overset{R_1}{>}}\overset{ONO_2}{\underset{}{C}}-\overset{\cdot}{C}\underset{R_4}{\overset{R_3}{<}}.$$

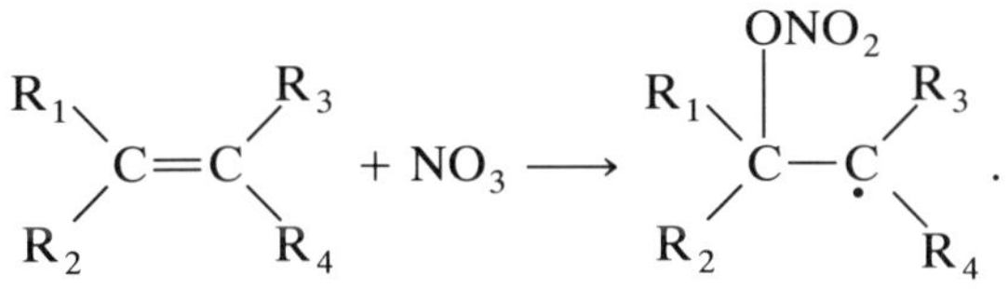

This is followed by rapid O_2 addition:

$$\underset{R_2}{\overset{R_1}{>}}\overset{ONO_2}{\underset{}{C}}-\overset{\cdot}{C}\underset{R_4}{\overset{R_3}{<}} + O_2 \longrightarrow \underset{R_2}{\overset{R_1}{>}}\overset{ONO_2}{\underset{}{C}}-C\underset{\underset{OO\cdot}{R_4}}{\overset{R_3}{<}},$$

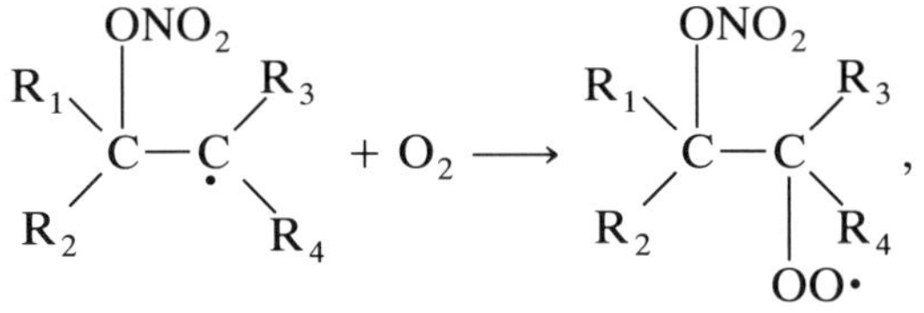

to produce the β-nitratoalkyl peroxy radical, subsequent reactions of which are

$$\underset{R_2}{\overset{R_1}{>}}\overset{ONO_2}{\underset{}{C}}-C\underset{\underset{OO\cdot}{R_4}}{\overset{R_3}{<}} + NO \longrightarrow \underset{R_2}{\overset{R_1}{>}}\overset{ONO_2}{\underset{}{C}}-C\underset{\underset{O\cdot}{R_4}}{\overset{R_3}{<}} + NO_2,$$

$$\longrightarrow \underset{R_2}{\overset{R_1}{>}}\overset{ONO_2}{\underset{}{C}}-C\underset{\underset{ONO_2}{R_4}}{\overset{R_3}{<}}.$$

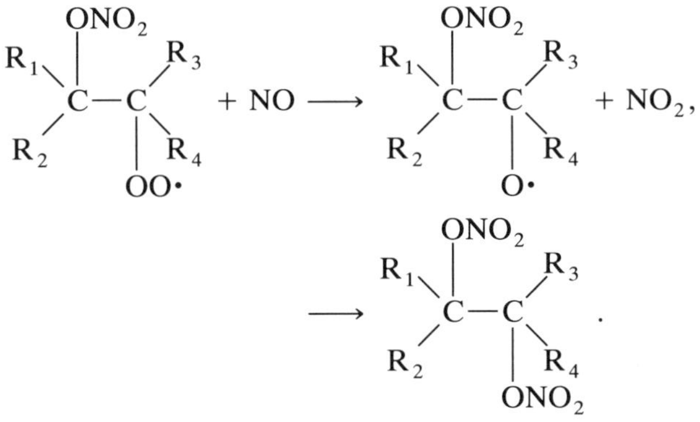

dinitrate

Further reactions of β-nitratoalkoxy radicals include

$$\underset{R_2}{\overset{R_1}{>}}\underset{|}{\overset{ONO_2}{C}}-\underset{\underset{O\cdot}{|}}{\overset{R_3}{C}}\underset{R_4}{\overset{}{<}} + O_2 \longrightarrow \underset{R_2}{\overset{R_1}{>}}\underset{|}{\overset{ONO_2}{C}}-\underset{\overset{\|}{O}}{\overset{R_4}{C}} + HO_2\cdot,$$

if $R_3 = H$

$$\underset{R_2}{\overset{R_1}{>}}\underset{|}{\overset{ONO_2}{C}}-\underset{\underset{O\cdot}{|}}{\overset{R_3}{C}}\underset{R_4}{\overset{}{<}} \overset{\Delta}{\longrightarrow} R_1\overset{O}{\underset{\|}{C}}R_2 + R_3\overset{}{\underset{\|}{C}}R_4 + NO_2,$$

$$\underset{R_2}{\overset{R_1}{>}}\underset{|}{\overset{ONO_2}{C}}-\underset{\underset{O\cdot}{|}}{\overset{R_3}{C}}\underset{R_4}{\overset{}{<}} + NO_2 \longrightarrow \underset{R_2}{\overset{R_1}{>}}\underset{|}{\overset{ONO_2}{C}}-\underset{\underset{ONO_2}{|}}{\overset{R_3}{C}}\underset{R_4}{\overset{}{<}}.$$

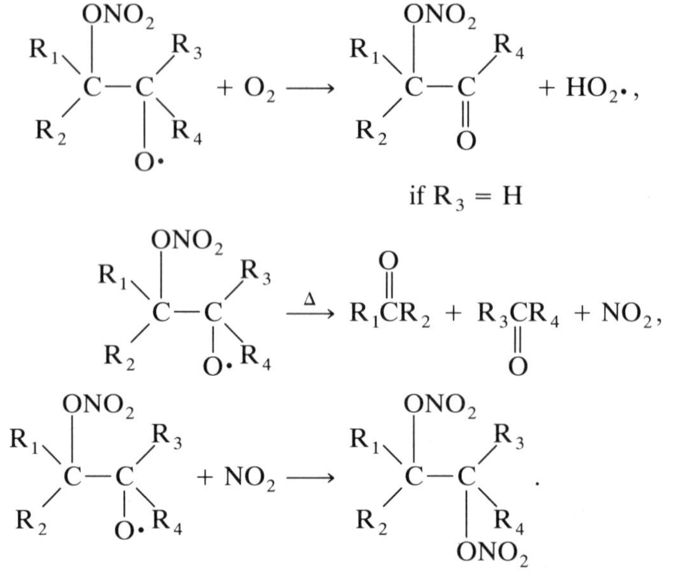

3. Alkene–O_3 Reaction

Reactions with ozone are competitive with the daytime OH radical reactions and the nighttime NO_3 radial reactions as a tropospheric loss process for the alkenes. These reactions have been shown to proceed via initial O_3 addition to the olefinic double bond, followed by rapid decomposition of the resulting "molozonide" (Atkinson, 1990):

$$\underset{R_2}{\overset{R_1}{>}}C=C\underset{R_4}{\overset{R_3}{<}} + O_3 \longrightarrow \left(\underset{R_2}{\overset{R_1}{>}}\overset{O-O-O}{\underset{C-C}{|\quad\quad|}}\underset{R_4}{\overset{R_3}{<}} \right)^{\neq}$$

$$\overset{a}{\swarrow} \quad\quad\quad \overset{b}{\searrow}$$

$$R_1-\overset{O}{\underset{\|}{C}}-R_2 \quad\quad\quad R_3-\overset{O}{\underset{\|}{C}}-R_4$$
$$+ \quad\quad\quad\quad\quad\quad\quad +$$
$$[R_3R_4\overset{\cdot}{C}OO\cdot]^{\neq}, \quad\quad [R_1R_2\overset{\cdot}{C}OO\cdot]^{\neq},$$

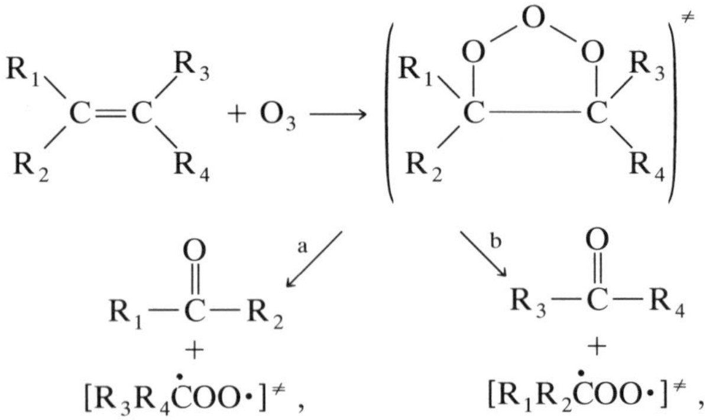

with the relative importance of the reaction pathways (a) and (b) being generally assumed to be approximately equal (Atkinson and Carter, 1984).

The major uncertainty concerns the fate under atmospheric conditions of the initially energy-rich Criegee biradical, which can be collisionally deactivated or can undergo unimolecular decomposition:

$$[R_3R_4\dot{C}OO\cdot]^{\ddagger} \xrightarrow{M} R_3R_4\dot{C}OO\cdot$$

$$\longrightarrow \text{products.}$$

The fraction of biradicals that are stabilized is pressure-dependent. At 1 atm., the fractional yields of stabilized biradicals are (Atkinson, 1990)

Ethene	0.39
2,-3-Dimethyl-2-butene	0.25–0.30
Propene	0.254
trans-2-Butene	0.185
2-Methylpropene	0.174

The decomposition pathways of Criegee biradicals are generally well established for the first three compounds in the series (Horie and Moortgat, 1992):

$$[\dot{C}H_2OO\cdot]^{\ddagger} \xrightarrow{M} \dot{C}H_2OO\cdot \qquad 37\%, \quad (61a)$$

$$\longrightarrow CO_2 + H_2 \qquad \sim 13\%, \quad (61b)$$

$$\longrightarrow CO + H_2O \qquad \sim 44\%, \quad (61c)$$

$$\xrightarrow[O_2]{} 2HO_2\cdot + CO_2 \qquad \sim 6\%, \quad (61d)$$

$$[CH_3\dot{C}HOO\cdot]^{\ddagger} \longrightarrow CH_3\dot{C}HOO\cdot \qquad 18\%, \quad (62a)$$

$$\xrightarrow{O_2} CH_3O_2\cdot + CO + OH\cdot \qquad \sim 30\%, \quad (62b)$$

$$\xrightarrow{O_2} CH_3O_2\cdot + CO_2 + HO_2\cdot \qquad \sim 32\%, \quad (62c)$$

$$\longrightarrow H\dot{C}O + CH_3O\cdot \qquad 6\%, \quad (62d)$$

$$\longrightarrow CH_4 + CO_2 \qquad 14\%. \quad (62e)$$

The stabilized biradicals react with a number of species:

$$\dot{R}CHO\dot{O} + H_2O \longrightarrow RCOOH + H_2O,$$

$$+ NO \longrightarrow RCHO + NO_2,$$

$$+ NO_2 \longrightarrow RCHO + NO_3,$$

$$+ SO_2 \xrightarrow{H_2O} RCHO + H_2SO_4,$$

$$+ CO \longrightarrow \text{products},$$

$$+ R'CHO \longrightarrow$$

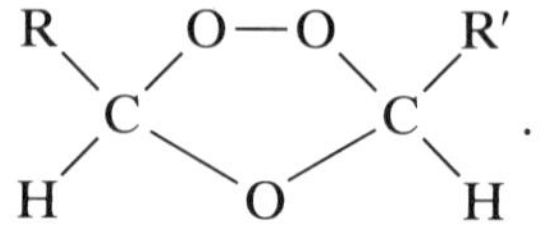

In addition, biradicals such as $(CH_3)_2\dot{C}OO\cdot$ may undergo unimolecular isomerization:

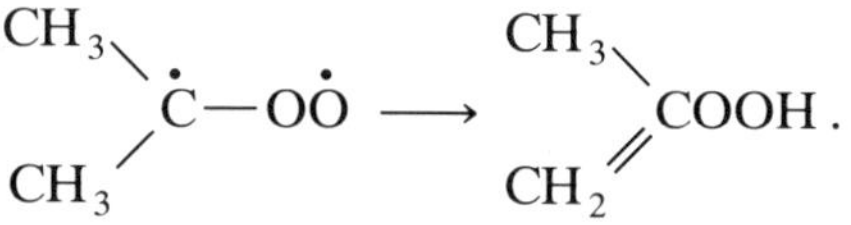

C. Aromatics

Of the classes of atmospheric hydrocarbons, aromatics have the greatest uncertainty concerning atmospheric oxidation mechanisms. Because of the importance of aromatics to ambient ozone and aerosol formation and as constituents of gasoline, this uncertainty has a significant effect on our ability to accurately simulate atmospheric chemistry. While rate constants (OH and NO_3) for most of the common aromatics are now available, as much as half of the carbon-containing products of their photooxidation remain unidentified. The aromatic compounds of concern in polluted urban atmospheres are the aromatic hydrocarbons (benzene, alkyl-substituted benzenes, and styrene) and their aromatic ring-retaining products (aromatic aldehydes and phenolic compounds). Additionally, there is interest in the atmospheric chemistry of the two- through four-ring polycyclic aromatic hydrocarbons (PAHs) and their derivatives.

The monocyclic aromatic hydrocarbons react in the atmosphere virtually solely with the OH radical (Atkinson, 1989). For example, rate constants for aromatic reactions with OH, O_3, and NO_3 are in the ranges: $k_{OH} \approx 10^{-12} - 10^{-11}$ cm^3 molecule^{-1} s^{-1}; $k_{O_3} < 10^{-20}$ cm^3 molecule^{-1} s^{-1}; $k_{NO_3} \approx 10^{-17} - 10^{-16}$ cm^3 molecule^{-1} s^{-1}. The aromatic–OH radical reaction proceeds via two reaction pathways: (a), a minor one involving H-atom abstraction from C–H bonds of, for benzene, the aromatic ring, or for alkyl-substituted aromatic hydrocarbons, the alkyl-substituent groups, and (b) a major reaction pathway involving OH radical addition to the aromatic ring. For example, for toluene these reaction pathways are

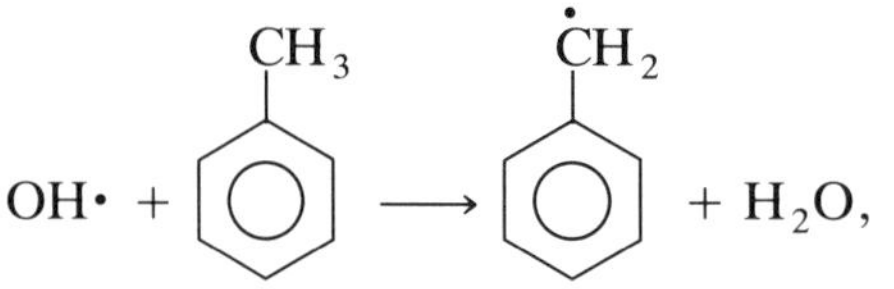

(63a)

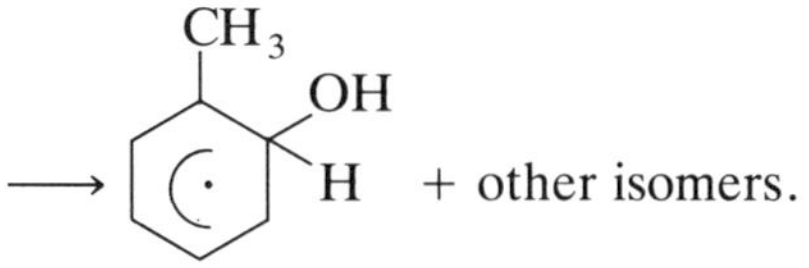

(63b)

The H-atom abstraction pathway leads mainly to the formation of aromatic aldehydes:

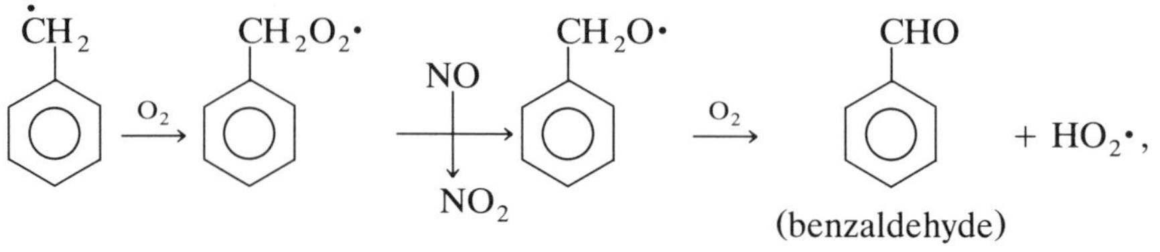

(64)

with subsequent reactions of these aromatic aldehydes with OH radicals leading to the formation of peroxyacyl nitrates and nitrophenols. This H-atom abstraction pathway is minor, accounting for $< 10\%$ of the overall OH radical reaction for benzene and the alkyl-substituted aromatic hydrocarbons.

The major OH radical reaction pathway is OH radical addition to the aromatic ring to yield hydroxycyclohexadienyl or alkyl-hydroxycyclohexadienyl radicals [reaction (63b)]. The reported rate constants for the reactions of the hydroxycyclohexadienyl-type radicals are in reasonable agreement, and the most recent data (Knispel *et al.*, 1990; Zetzsch *et al.*, 1990; Goumri *et al.*, 1990, 1992) show that the hydroxycyclohexadienyl and methylhydroxycyclohexadienyl radicals both react rapidly with NO_2 with similar room-temperature rate constants of $\sim 3 \times 10^{-11}$ cm^3 molecule^{-1} s^{-1}. The corresponding reactions with O_2 have much lower reported room temperature rate constants, of $\sim 1.8 \times 10^{-16}$ cm^3 molecule^{-1} s^{-1} for the hydroxycyclohexadienyl radical and $\sim 5 \times 10^{-16}$ cm^3 molecule^{-1} s^{-1} for the methylhydroxycyclohexadienyl radical (Knispel *et al.*, 1990). The absolute rate constant data indicate that at room temperature and atmospheric pressure of air, the potentially important reactions of the hydroxycyclohexadienyl-type radicals are with O_2 and NO_2, with the NO_2 reactions being of significance for NO_2 concentrations $> 3 \times 10^{12}$ molecules cm^{-3} for the OH–benzene adduct and $> 9 \times 10^{12}$ molecules cm^{-3} for the OH–toluene adduct.

The products arising from the OH radical addition pathways are still not totally understood. The initially formed OH-aromatic adduct is expected to react under atmospheric conditions mainly with O_2, again via two reaction pathways. For example, for the toluene–OH adduct,

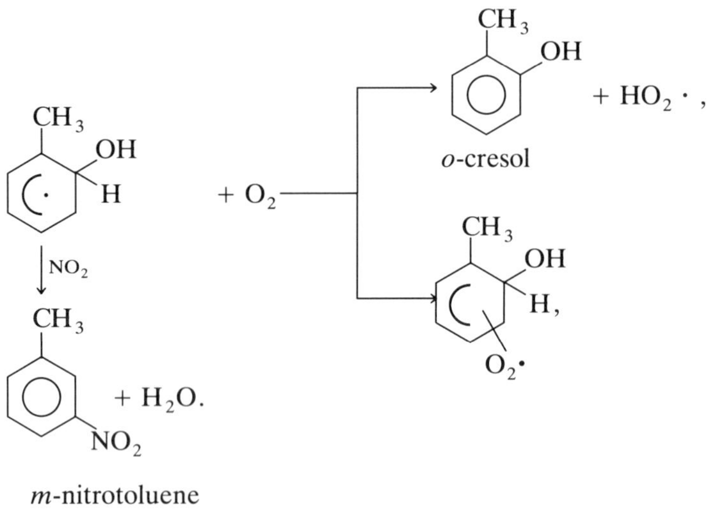

The H-atom abstraction reaction of the OH–aromatic adduct to yield phenolic compounds, such as *o*-cresol, has been shown to be relatively minor, accounting for ~ 16% of the overall OH radical reaction mechanism for toluene (Atkinson, 1990). The major reaction pathway is then that involving other reactions of the OH–aromatic–O_2 adducts, and these have been shown to involve ring cleavage. The α-dicarbonyls glyoxal, methylglyoxal, and biacetyl have been identified as products from benzene and the methyl-substituted benzenes (Bandow *et al.*, 1985; Bandow and Washida, 1985a, b; Tuazon *et al.*, 1986). The yields of these α-dicarbonyls, together with those of the theoretical, but so far unobserved, co-products, the 1,4-unsaturated dicarbonyls (such as CHOCH$=$CHCHO), and the initial H-atom abstraction process and that giving rise to phenol products do not fully account for 30–50% of the overall reaction products.

Phenol, the cresols, and the dimethylphenols are formed from the atmospheric degradation of benzene, toluene, and the xylenes, respectively, and data are available concerning the atmospheric reactions of these compounds. The potential atmospheric loss processes of phenolic compounds are reaction with NO_3, OH radicals, and O_3, together with wet and dry deposition (these compounds are readily incorporated into rain- and cloud-water and fog). The OH radical reactions proceed by OH radical addition to the aromatic ring and by H-atom abstraction from the substituent –OH and $-CH_3$ groups (Atkinson, 1989):

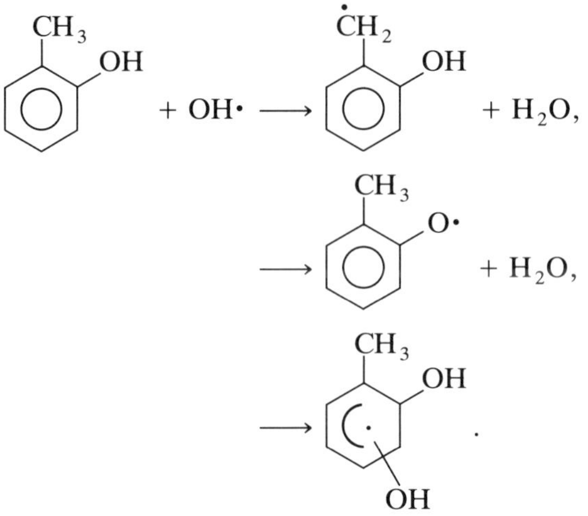

(65a)

(65b)

(65c)

At 298 K, kinetic studies indicate that the H-atom abstraction processes account for ~ 9% of the overall OH radical reaction for phenol [via pathway (65b)] and ~ 7% of the overall OH radical reaction for *o*-cresol [via pathways (65a) and (65b)] (Atkinson, 1989).

D. Aldehydes

Aldehydes are emitted by combustion processes and also are formed in the atmosphere from the photochemical degradation of other organic compounds. Aldehydes undergo photolysis, reaction with OH radicals, and reaction with NO_3 radicals in the troposphere. Reaction with NO_3 radicals is of relatively minor importance as a loss process for these compounds, but can be a minor contributor to the HO_2 (from formaldehyde) and peroxyacetyl nitrate (PAN) formation during nighttime hours (Stockwell and Calvert, 1983; Cantrell *et al.*, 1985). Thus, the major loss processes involve photolysis and reaction with OH radicals.

For formaldehyde, the OH reaction yields the formyl (HCO) radical, which subsequently reacts rapidly with O_2 to form HO_2 and CO [reactions (34) and (36)]. For the higher aldehydes, the acyl ($R\dot{C}O$) radical initially formed,

$$OH + RCHO \longrightarrow H_2O + R\dot{C}O, \tag{66}$$

rapidly adds O_2 to yield an acylperoxy radical,

$$R\dot{C}O + O_2 \longrightarrow RC(O)OO\cdot . \tag{67}$$

Under polluted atmospheric conditions these acylperoxy radicals then react with NO or NO_2:

$$RC(O)OO\cdot + NO \longrightarrow RC(O)O\cdot + NO_2, \tag{68}$$

$$RC(O)O\cdot \longrightarrow R\cdot + CO_2, \tag{69}$$

$$RC(O)OO\cdot + NO_2 \rightleftharpoons \underset{\text{peroxyacyl nitrates}}{RC(O)OONO_2}. \tag{70, 71}$$

The first member of the peroxyacyl nitrate series is $CH_3C(O)OONO_2$, peroxyacetyl nitrate (PAN). The lifetime of PAN is strongly temperature-dependent and ranges from ~ 30 min at 303 K to ~ 8 h at 273 K. Under urban conditions at fairly warm temperatures, the concentration of PAN is governed by the steady-state concentration of the peroxyacetyl radical, $CH_3C(O)OO$. With PAN formation proportional to NO_2 and competitive with peroxyacetyl radical reaction with NO, the steady-state concentration of PAN is proportional to the NO_2/NO ratio. From the $NO/NO_2/O_3$ photostationary state relation (18), since the steady-state concentration of O_3 is also proportional to the NO_2/NO ratio, the steady-state PAN concentration is proportional to the O_3 concentration.

E. Ketones

This class of organic emissions is exemplified by acetone and its higher homologues. As for the aldehydes, photolysis and reaction with the OH radical are the major atmospheric loss processes (Atkinson, 1989). The limited experimental data available indicate that, with the exception of acetone, photolysis is probably of minor importance. Reaction with the OH radical is then the major tropospheric loss process. For example, for methyl ethyl ketone:

$$\mathrm{OH\cdot + CH_3CH_2C(O)CH_3 \xrightarrow{O_2} H_2O + CH_3\overset{\overset{\displaystyle OO\cdot}{|}}{C}HC(O)CH_3}, \quad (72a)$$

$$\xrightarrow{O_2} \mathrm{H_2O + CH_3CH_2C(O)CH_2OO\cdot}, \quad (72b)$$

$$\xrightarrow{O_2} \mathrm{H_2O + \cdot OOCH_2CH_2C(O)CH_3}, \quad (72c)$$

with (72a) being the major reaction pathway (Atkinson, 1989). Subsequent reaction of this particular radical leads to

$$\mathrm{CH_3\overset{\overset{\displaystyle OO\cdot}{|}}{C}HC(O)CH_3 + NO \longrightarrow NO_2 + CH_3\overset{\overset{\displaystyle O\cdot}{|}}{C}HC(O)CH_3} \quad (73)$$

$$\downarrow$$

$$\mathrm{CH_3CHO + CH_3\dot{C}O}. \quad (74)$$

The major reaction products from the atmospheric reactions of the ketones are aldehydes and PAN precursors, although bifunctional oxygen-containing compounds will probably be formed in small yield.

F. α,β-Unsaturated Carbonyls

These compounds, exemplified by acrolein, crotonaldehyde, and methyl vinyl ketone, are known to react with ozone and with OH radicals. Photolysis and NO_3 radical reaction are of minor importance. Under atmospheric conditions the O_3 reactions are also of minor significance (Atkinson and Carter, 1984), leaving the OH radical reaction as the major loss process. For the aldehydes, OH radical reaction can proceed via two reaction pathways: OH radical addition to the double bond and H-atom abstraction from the –CHO group (Atkinson, 1989). For crotonaldehyde, for example, the OH reaction mechanism is given in Fig. 3. As can be noted from Fig. 3, these α,β-unsaturated aldehydes are expected to ultimately give rise to α-dicarbonyls such as glyoxal and methylglyoxal. For the α,β-unsaturated ketones such as methyl vinyl ketone, the major

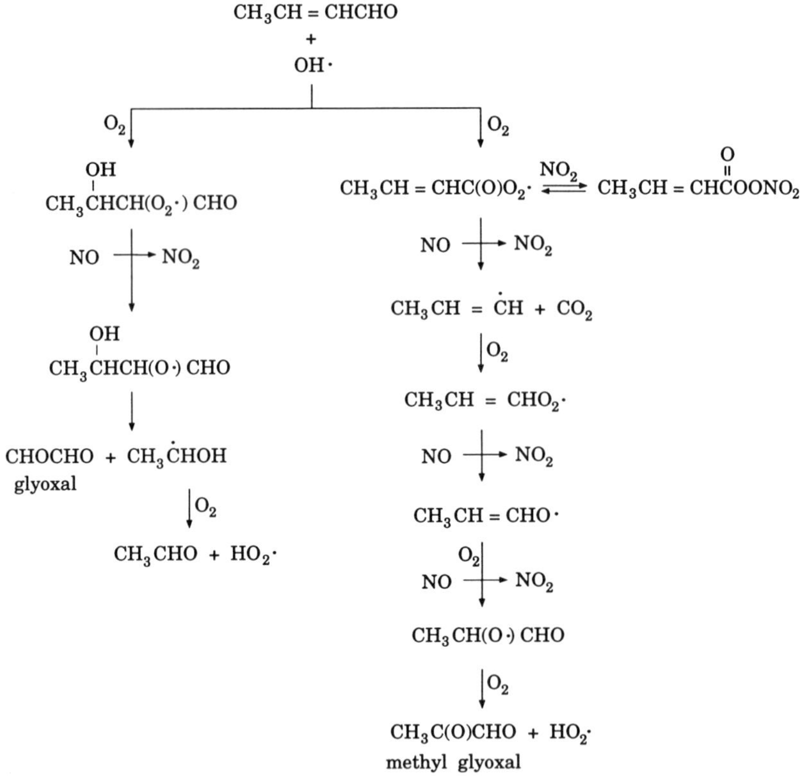

FIG. 3. Crotonaldehyde–OH reaction mechanism.

atmospheric reaction with the OH radical occurs only by OH radical addition to the double bond (Fig. 4). Again, α-dicarbonyls, together with aldehydes and hydroxyaldehydes, are formed as products.

G. ETHERS

The aliphatic ethers such as dimethyl ether and diethyl ether react under atmospheric conditions essentially solely with the OH radical, via H-atom abstraction from C–H bonds (Atkinson, 1989; Japar *et al.*, 1990, 1991). The dimethyl ether–OH mechanism is shown in Fig. 5. The net reaction is

$$CH_3OCH_3 + OH\cdot + NO \xrightarrow{2O_2} NO_2 + HC(O)OCH_3 + HO_2\cdot + H_2O, \quad (75)$$

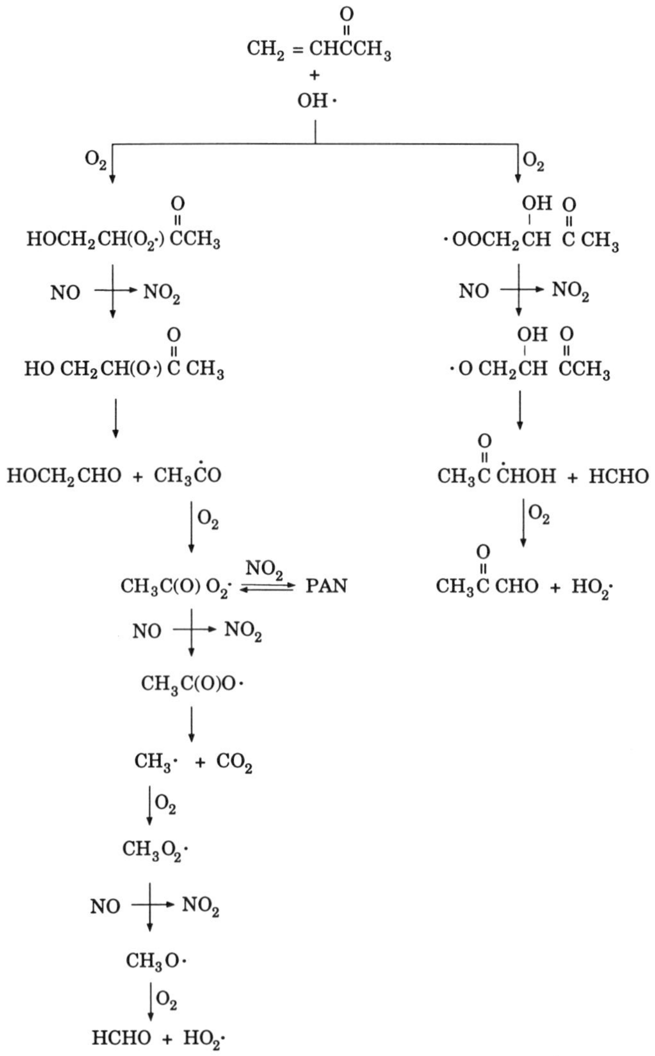

FIG. 4. Methyl vinyl ketone–OH reaction mechanism.

where the carbon-containing product is methyl formate. The diethyl ether–OH mechanism is also given in Fig. 5, and the net reaction is

$$C_2H_5OC_2H_5 + OH\cdot + 2NO \xrightarrow{2O_2} 2NO_2 + HC(O)OC_2H_5 + HCHO + HO_2\cdot + H_2O, \tag{76}$$

where the carbon-containing products are ethyl formate and formaldehyde.

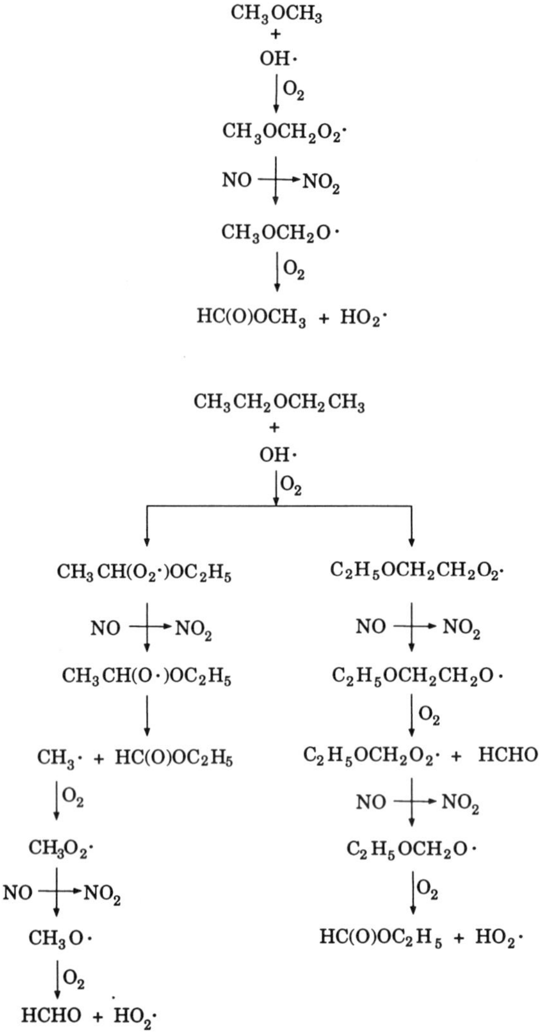

FIG. 5. Dimethyl ether–OH and diethyl ether–OH reaction mechanisms.

H. ALCOHOLS

The reaction sequences for the simpler aliphatic alcohols under atmospheric conditions are known (Atkinson, 1989); these involve H-atom abstraction, mainly from the αC–H bonds. For example, the methanol–OH reaction is

$$CH_3OH + OH\cdot \longrightarrow H_2O + \dot{C}H_2OH, \quad (77a)$$

$$\longrightarrow H_2O + CH_3O\cdot, \quad (77b)$$

with the first reaction pathway accounting for $\sim 85\%$ of the overall reaction at 298 K. Since, as shown earlier, both the $\dot{C}H_2OH$ and $CH_3O\cdot$ radicals react with O_2 to yield formaldehyde and HO_2, the overall reaction can be written as

$$CH_3OH + OH\cdot \xrightarrow{O_2} H_2O + HO_2\cdot + HCHO. \quad (78)$$

The ethanol–OH reaction proceeds as follows:

$$OH\cdot + CH_3CH_2OH \longrightarrow H_2O + \dot{C}H_2CH_2OH \quad (\sim 5\%), \quad (79a)$$

$$\longrightarrow H_2O + CH_3\dot{C}HOH \quad (\sim 90\%), \quad (79b)$$

$$\longrightarrow H_2O + CH_3CH_2O\cdot \quad (\sim 5\%), \quad (79c)$$

where the branching ratios are those at 298 K. The second two channels result in identical products under atmospheric conditions, HO_2 + CH_3CHO. The first channel forms the intermediate $\dot{C}H_2CH_2OH$, which, under atmospheric conditions, leads to the same products as the OH + ethene reaction. Using the ethene–OH mechanism given earlier, the overall ethanol–OH reaction mechanism can be written as

$$C_2H_5OH + OH\cdot + 0.05\ NO \longrightarrow 0.05\ NO_2$$
$$+ 0.014\ HOCH_2CHO + 0.072\ HCHO$$
$$+ 0.95\ CH_3CHO + HO_2\cdot + H_2O, \quad (80)$$

with the principal products being acetaldehyde and the HO_2 radical.

I. Gasoline Components

Oxygenated hydrocarbons can be added to gasoline to replace traditional gasoline hydrocarbon components in an effort to lower the atmospheric reactivity of automotive tailpipe and evaporative emissions. Oxygenates that are currently being added to gasolines or are being

TABLE III
OH Rate Constants for Oxygenated Hydrocarbons That Are Possible Gasoline Components

Compound	k_{OH} (298 K) 10^{12} cm^3 molecule^{-1} s^{-1}	Reference
Methanol	0.9	Wallington and Kurylo (1987)
Ethanol	3.4	Atkinson (1989)
t-Butyl alcohol	1.1	Wallington *et al.* (1988c)
Dimethyl ether	2.5	Wallington *et al.* (1988a)
Diethyl ether	14	Wallington *et al.* (1988a) Wallington and Japar (1991)
Methyl *t*-butyl ether	3.2	Wallington *et al.* (1988c, 1989)
Ethyl *t*-butyl ether	8.5	Wallington *et al.* (1989) Wallington and Japar (1991)
t-Amyl methyl ether	6.4	Wallington *et al.* (1988b)

considered include the following alcohols and ethers:

Methanol	CH_3OH
Ethanol	C_2H_5OH
t-Butyl alcohol (TBA)	$(CH_3)_3COH$
Dimethyl ether (DME)	CH_3OCH_3
Diethyl ether (DEE)	$C_2H_5OC_2H_5$
Methyl *t*-butyl ether (MTBE)	$CH_3OC(CH_3)_3$
Ethyl *t*-butyl ether (ETBE)	$C_2H_5OC(CH_3)_3$
t-Amyl methyl ether (TAME)	$CH_3OC(CH_3)_2CH_2CH_3$

Table III summarizes OH rate constants for these oxygenated hydrocarbons, and products of the OH radical reaction are listed in Table IV.

J. Carboxylic Acids and Esters

The formic acid–OH reaction proceeds via a complex that decomposes to CO_2 and H:

$$OH + H\overset{\overset{\displaystyle O}{\|}}{C}OH \longrightarrow H_2O + \underset{\displaystyle \downarrow \atop \displaystyle CO_2 + H.}{[COOH]} \qquad (81)$$

TABLE IV
PRODUCTS OF OH RADICAL REACTION WITH OXYGENATED HYDROCARBONS THAT ARE POSSIBLE GASOLINE COMPONENTS

Compound		Principal products: Stable species	Principal products: Free radicals
Methanol	CH_3OH	HCHO	HO_2
Ethanol	C_2H_5OH	CH_3CHO	HO_2
t-Butyl alcohol	$(CH_3)_3COH$	$(CH_3)_2CO$ HCHO	HO_2
Dimethyl ether	CH_3OCH_3	$HC(O)OCH_3$	HO_2
Diethyl ether	$C_2H_5OC_2H_5$	$HC(O)OC_2H_5$ HCHO	HO_2
Methyl *t*-butyl ether	$CH_3OC(CH_3)_3$	$HC(O)OC(CH_3)_3$ $(CH_3)_2CO$ HCHO	HO_2
Ethyl *t*-butyl ether	$C_2H_5OC(CH_3)_3$	$HC(O)OC(CH_3)_3$ $C_2H_5OC(O)CH_3$ HCHO	HO_2
t-Amyl methyl ether	$CH_3OC(CH_3)_2CH_2CH_3$	$HC(O)OC(CH_3)_2CH_2CH_3$ $CH_3C(O)OC_2H_5$ $CH_3C(O)OCH_3$ CH_3CHO	HO_2

The reaction dynamics and products formed from the reactions of OH radicals with the higher carboxylic acids are presently not known.

The esters RC(O)OR′ again react essentially totally with the OH radical under atmospheric conditions (Atkinson, 1989). Figure 6 gives the methyl acetate–OH mechanism.

K. BIOGENIC HYDROCARBONS

Biogenic hydrocarbons are principally emitted by trees. Isoprene and α- and β-pinene are the most abundant biogenic hydrocarbons which are emitted (Dimitriades, 1981) (see Fig. 7). The rate constants of the reactions of the biogenics with OH, ozone, and nitrate radicals have been well investigated (Atkinson, 1991; Atkinson *et al.*, 1990). However, limited data are available concerning the products of biogenic reactions in the atmosphere.

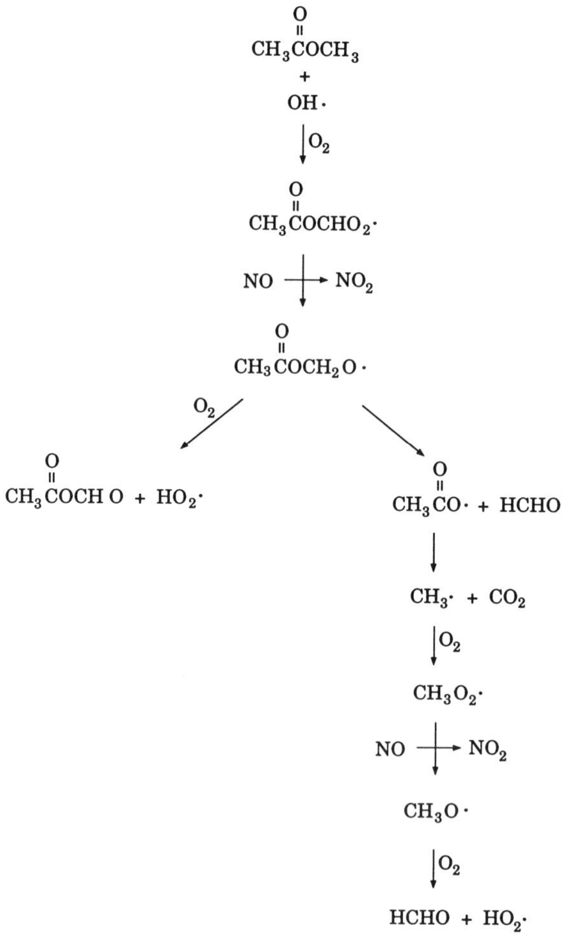

FIG. 6. Methyl acetate–OH reaction mechanism.

1. Hydroxyl Radical Reaction

The most important daytime loss process for the biogenics is reaction with OH radicals. Rate constants for the OH reaction with isoprene, α- and β-pinene are 1.01×10^{-10} cm^3 molecule^{-1} s^{-1}, 5.37×10^{-11} cm^3 molecule^{-1} s^{-1}, and 7.89×10^{-11} cm^3 molecule^{-1} s^{-1}, respectively. Hydroxyl radical reactions with dialkenes and monoterpenes proceed primarily via OH addition across the double bond. Subsequent addition of oxygen to the radical produces a peroxy radical. The reactions of the resulting peroxy radical proceed in a manner similar to those of alkyl peroxy radicals.

Isoprene

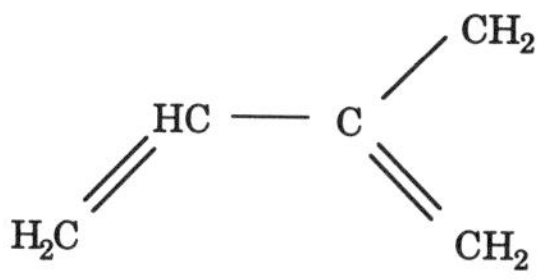

α-pinene

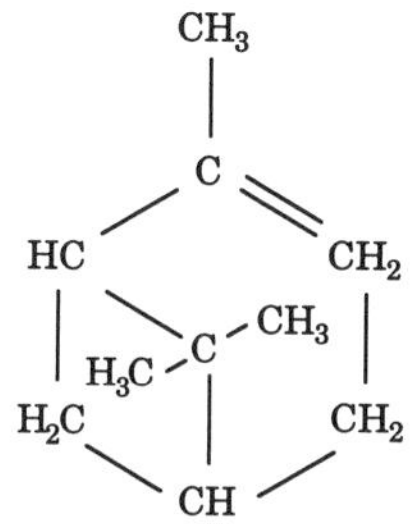

β-pinene

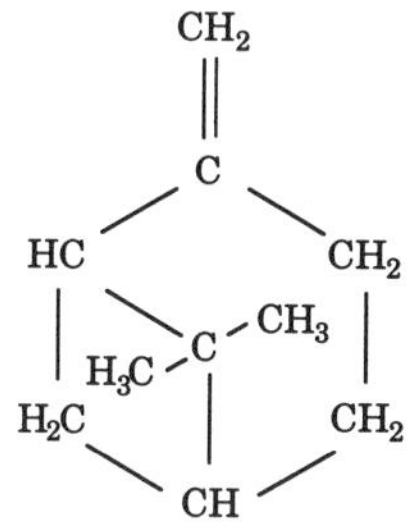

FIG. 7. Biogenic hydrocarbons.

In the presence of NO_x, the OH radical photooxidation of isoprene leads to methacrolein {$O=CHC(CH_3)=CH_2$}, methyl vinyl ketone {$CH_2=CHC(O)CH_3$}, and 3-methylfuran, in yields of 35.5%, 25%, and 5.1%, respectively (Paulson *et al.*, 1991a). Similar yields were obtained by Gu *et al.* (1985) and Tuazon and Atkinson (1990). A variety of other species, including organic nitrates and multisubstituted hydrocarbons, are also possible products. The yields of these remaining products have not been reported in the literature. Clearly, further work is needed to account for the remaining carbon.

The photooxidation products of the α- and β-pinene reaction with OH radicals have been studied by Arey *et al.* (1990) and Hatakeyama *et al.* (1991). In the presence of NO, the major gas-phase product of the

α-pinene reaction is pinonaldehyde, with a yield of 29% (Arey *et al.*, 1990). Similarly, the major gas-phase product of the β-pinene reaction is 6.6-dimethylbicyclo[3.1.1]heptan-2-one, with a yield of 30%. In both cases, the products have sufficiently low vapor pressures that they can condense into the aerosol phase.

2. *Ozone Reaction*

In addition to the reaction with OH, ozone reactions play a significant role in daytime loss processes for isoprene and α- and β-pinene. Room-temperature rate constants for the ozone reactions with these olefins are 1.43×10^{-17} cm^3 molecule^{-1} s^{-1}, 8.5×10^{-18} cm^3 molecule^{-1} s^{-1}, and 1.6×10^{-17} cm^3 molecule^{-1} s^{-1}, respectively.

These reactions proceed by initial ozone attack on the $C=C$ bond of the olefin. An intermediate ozonide is formed, which rapidly decomposes to a carbonyl and a biradical. The biradical can be stabilized, or it can decompose. Paulson *et al.* (1991b) found the products methacrolein, methyl vinyl ketone, and propene, in yields of 68%, 25%, and 7%, respectively. Based on the presence of epoxides in the ozone/isoprene system, Paulson *et al.* concluded that $O(^3P)$ was being formed. Calculations indicated that 0.45 $O(^3P)$ radicals were formed for every ozone/isoprene reaction. However, Atkinson *et al.* (1993) recently showed that the epoxides were formed directly from the reaction with ozone rather than the reaction with $O(^3P)$. The epoxides formed were 1,2-epoxy-2-methyl-3-butene and 1,2-epoxy-3-methyl-3-butene, in yields of 0.028 and 0.011, respectively. There was also definite evidence for the formation of OH radicals in the ozone system, thus causing difficulties in product analyses. Each ozone/isoprene reaction yielded 0.68 OH radicals (Paulson *et al.*, 1991b).

The product distribution of the monoterpene reactions with ozone has not been fully elucidated. However, studies by Hatakeyama *et al.* (1989) indicate the formation of pinonaldehyde, nor-pinonaldehyde, formaldehyde, CO, and CO_2 from the reaction of α-pinene with ozone. The β-pinene/ozone reaction led to the formation of 6,6-dimethylbicyclo-[3.1.1]heptane-2-one, formaldehyde, and CO_2. Aerosol accounted for approximately 14–18% of the overall reaction in each case.

3. *Nitrate Radical Reaction*

Nitrate radical reactions are the dominant nighttime loss process for biogenics in the troposphere. The room-temperature (298 K) rate constants of the nitrate radical reaction with isoprene and α- and β-pinene are 6.78×10^{-13} cm^3 molecule^{-1} s^{-1}, 6.16×10^{-12} cm^3 molecule^{-1} s^{-1}, and 2.51×10^{-12} cm^3 molecule^{-1} s^{-1}, respectively. In general, reactions with rate constants $> 1 \times 10^{-13}$ cm^3 molecule^{-1} s^{-1} are too fast to proceed via H-atom abstraction. Instead, they proceed by an addition mechanism. Thus, the NO_3 radical adds to the double bond in isoprene and the monoterpenes, forming a nitroxyperoxy radical in the presence of O_2):

$$NO_3 + >C{=}C< \longrightarrow >C-C-ONO_2,$$

$$>C-C-ONO_2 + O_2 \longrightarrow OO{=}C-C-ONO_2.$$

This nitroxyperoxy radical can react with NO_2 to form a thermally unstable nitroxyperoxynitrate compound; react with itself to form a nitroxyalkoxy radical, hydroxy nitrate, and nitroxy-aldehyde/ketone; or react with NO to form a nitroxyalkoxy radical or dinitrate. The nitroxyalkoxy radical can decompose to form an aldehyde/ketone and NO_2, or can react with O_2 to form a nitroxy aldehyde/ketone.

Limited product data are available for the nitrate radical reaction with isoprene and α- and β-pinene. For the isoprene reaction, Barnes *et al.* (1990) determined molar yields of total nitrates of 80%, CO of 4%, and formaldehyde of 11%. Methacrolein was also detected, but an accurate product yield could not be determined. Additional work with α- and β-pinene was not conclusive. Although nitrate features were observed as initial reaction products, these compounds quickly transferred into aerosols, thus preventing identification via the methods employed in the study (FTIR spectroscopy).

L. Atmospheric Lifetimes of Organics

Organic compounds react in the troposphere with the OH radical, the NO_3 radical, and O_3. In addition, the carbonyls may also photolyze. Given an estimate of ambient concentrations of OH, NO_3, and O_3, and of light intensity, it is possible to estimate the chemical lifetimes of organic compounds (since the reaction rate constants with OH, NO_3, and O_3 are available for virtually all compounds of interest). Table V summarizes estimates of the tropospheric lifetimes of organic compounds. For the compounds listed, in most cases, OH reaction is the controlling factor determining the lifetime of the species. Exceptions include the NO_3 reactions of the biogenic hydrocarbons, isoprene and α-pinene, and photolysis of formaldehyde.

TABLE V
ESTIMATED TROPOSPHERIC LIFETIMES OF ORGANIC COMPOUNDS RESULTING FROM PHOTOLYSIS AND REACTION WITH OH, NO_3, AND O_3

	Lifetime due to reaction with[a]			
Organic	OH	NO_3	O_3	$h\nu$
Methane	9.6 yr	> 120 yr		
Ethane	60 d	> 12 yr		
Propane	13 d	> 2.5 yr		
n-Butane	6.1 d	~ 2.5 yr		
Ethene	1.8 d	225 d	9.7 d	
Propene	7.0 h	4.9 d	1.5 d	
Isoprene	1.8 h	50 min	1.2 d	
α-Pinene	3.4 h	5 min	1.0 d	
Formaldehyde	1.6 d	77 d	> 4.5 yr	4 h
Acetaldehyde	1.0 d	17 d	> 4.5 yr	5 d
Methanol	17 d	> 77 d		
Ethanol	4.7 d	> 51 d		
Methyl-*t*-butyl ether	5.5 d			
Benzene	12.5 d	> 6 yr	> 4.5 yr	
Toluene	2.6 d	1.9 yr	> 4.5 yr	
m-Xylene	7.8 h	200 d	> 4.5 yr	

[a] $[OH] = 1.5 \times 10^6$ molecules/cm^3 (avg. 12-h concentration); $[NO_3] = 5 \times 10^8$ molecules/cm^3 (avg. 12-h concentration); $[O_3] = 7 \times 10^{11}$ molecules/cm^3 (avg. 24-h concentration).

M. POLYCYCLIC AROMATIC HYDROCARBONS (PAHs)

Polycyclic aromatic hydrocarbons (PAHs) are formed during combustion of carbonaceous materials (Fig. 8). Carcinogenicity and mutagenicity exhibited by many PAHs in laboratory studies have led to widespread concern that they are also human carcinogens [International Association for Research on Cancer (IARC), 1987]. Menichini (1992) presents a comprehensive review of ambient data on urban PAH levels. The PAHs and their analogues and derivatives have relatively low vapor pressures and are distributed between the gas and particulate phase. [For reviews of partitioning of semi-volatile organic compounds between the gas and particulate phases, see Pankow (1987, 1993).] The 2–4-ring PAHs are, in temperate climates, primarily associated with the gas phase; this distribution will change markedly towards the particulate phase with the reduced temperatures typical of mid-continental wintertime conditions. As presently understood, the atmospheric transformations of these PAHs and their derivatives depend upon the phase with which they are associated. The available data obtained to date show that for the PAHs present in the gas phase, reaction with the OH radical and, to a lesser extent, N_2O_5, will

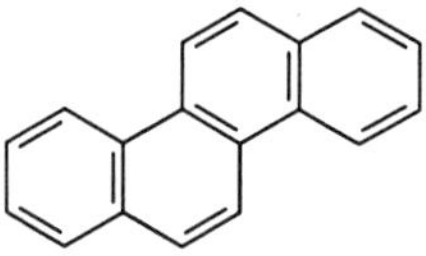

chrysene

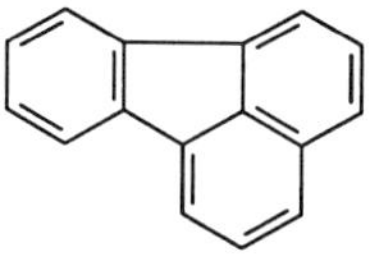

fluoranthene

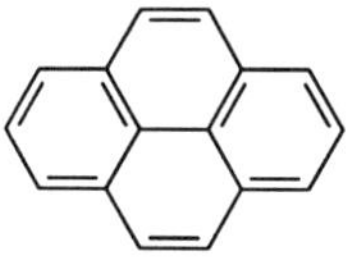

pyrene

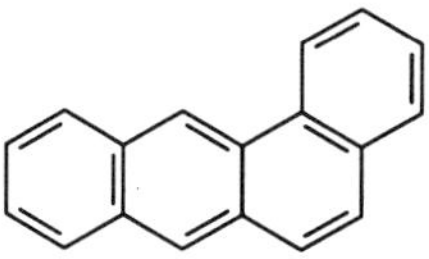

benz[*a*]anthracene

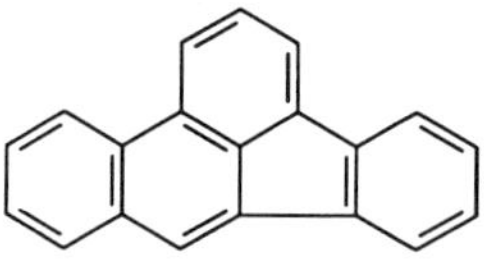

benzo[*b*]fluoranthene

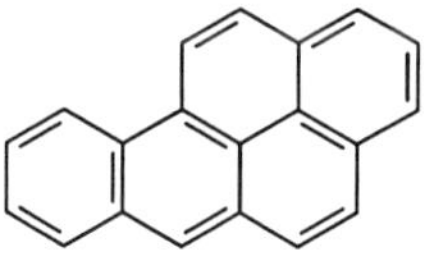

benzo[*a*]pyrene

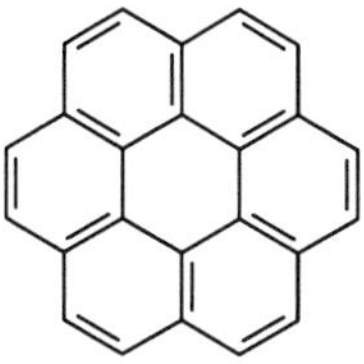

coronene

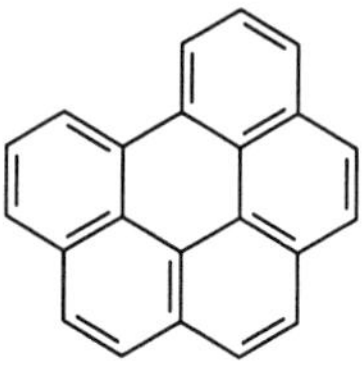

benzo[*ghi*]perylene

FIG. 8. Polycyclic aromatic hydrocarbons.

predominate, leading to PAH lifetimes in the atmosphere of a few hours or less.

VIII. Atmospheric Reactions of Selected Nitrogen and Sulfur Compounds

A. Reduced Nitrogen Compounds

Reduced nitrogen compounds emitted into the atmosphere include ammonia (NH_3) and hydrogen cyanide (HCN), and possibly their higher homologues such as the aliphatic and aromatic amines RNH_2, RR′NH, and RR′R″N and the nitriles RCN, where R, R′, R″ ≡ alkyl or aryl group.

1. Amines

The major atmospheric reactions of the amines identified to date involve the gas-phase reaction with the OH radical:

$$NH_3 + OH \longrightarrow H_2O + \dot{N}H_2, \tag{82}$$

$$CH_3NH_2 + OH \longrightarrow H_2O + CH_3\dot{N}H, \tag{83}$$

$$(CH_3)_2NH + OH \longrightarrow H_2O + (CH_3)_2N\cdot, \tag{84a}$$

$$\longrightarrow H_2O + \dot{C}H_2NHCH_3, \tag{84b}$$

$$(CH_3)_3N + OH \longrightarrow H_2O + \dot{C}H_2N(CH_3)_2, \tag{85}$$

and with gaseous nitric acid to form the corresponding nitrate salts. The reaction of ammonia and nitric acid vapor to give ammonium nitrate is a major route to form particulate nitrate (Stelson *et al.*, 1979),

$$NH_3 + HNO_3 \rightleftharpoons NH_4NO_3. \tag{86, 87}$$

The reactions of amines with the OH radial are rapid, with lifetimes during daylight hours being on the order of hours. Ammonia, however, being highly soluble and reactive with atmospheric acids, will be removed preferentially by those routes rather than through reaction with the OH radical. Particulate–nitrate salts will undergo dry and/or wet deposition to surfaces.

2. *Nitriles*

The available experimental data suggest that this class of reduced nitrogen compounds will react mainly with OH radicals under tropospheric conditions. Hydrogen cyanide (HCN) reacts only slowly with OH radicals, with a room-temperature rate constant at atmospheric pressure of 3×10^{-14} cm^3 molecule^{-1} s^{-1} (Atkinson, 1989). For the organic nitriles, the available evidence shows that the OH reaction occurs via H-atom abstraction from the alkyl groups, for example,

$$CH_3CN + OH \longrightarrow H_2O + \dot{C}H_2CN, \tag{88}$$

probably leading ultimately to the formation of CN radicals.

3. *Nitrites*

Methyl nitrite is the first member of this class of organic compounds, and photolysis is its only important loss process:

$$CH_3ONO + h\nu \longrightarrow CH_3O\cdot + NO, \tag{89}$$

with a photolysis lifetime of ~ 10–15 min at solar noon (Taylor *et al.*, 1980).

B. Sulfur Oxides

Sulfur dioxide (SO_2) reacts under tropospheric conditions via both gas- and aqueous-phase processes (see Section X) and is also removed physically via dry and wet deposition. With respect to chemical removal, reaction with the OH radical is dominant:

$$SO_2 + OH \xrightarrow{M} HSO_3, \tag{90}$$

followed by the regeneration of the chain-carrying HO_2 radical:

$$HSO_3 + O_2 \longrightarrow HO_2 + SO_3. \tag{91}$$

Sulfur trioxide, even if emitted directly from a source, in the presence of water vapor, is converted rapidly to sulfuric acid:

$$SO_3 + H_2O \longrightarrow H_2SO_4. \tag{92}$$

SO_2 is the principal sulfur-containing compound emitted into the atmosphere from anthropogenic sources. Once emitted, SO_2 can be removed from the atmosphere by gas-phase reaction with the OH radical [reaction (90)], dry deposition, and absorption into cloud droplets. The lifetime of SO_2 based on reaction with the OH radical, at typical atmospheric levels of OH, is about 15 days. As was noted earlier, SO_2 is one of the gases that is reasonably efficiently removed from the atmosphere by dry deposition. At its dry deposition velocity of about 1 cm s^{-1}, the lifetime of SO_2 by dry deposition in a 1 km deep boundary layer is about 1 day. When clouds are present, the removal of SO_2 can be enhanced even beyond that attributable to dry deposition. Such processes will be discussed in Section X.

Sulfuric acid exists essentially totally in the particulate phase under atmospheric conditions, and it is generally neutralized by reaction with metal cations or ammonia, to form salts such as Na_2SO_4, $CaSO_4$, $(NH_3)_2SO_4$, and NH_3HSO_4. Wet and dry deposition lead to sulfate removal from the troposphere.

C. Reduced Sulfur Compounds

Reduced sulfur-containing species RSH react with OH radicals during daytime hours and with NO_3 radicals during nighttime hours. For H_2S, the NO_3 radical reaction is probably relatively slow, and hence the dominant tropospheric removal process involves OH radical reaction (NASA, 1985):

$$H_2S + OH \longrightarrow H_2O + SH. \qquad (93)$$

While it appears that the SH radical undergoes a series of reactions resulting in the ultimate formation of SO_2, the details of the reaction sequence are still not totally understood (Friedl *et al.* 1985).

For the aliphatic thiols, OH radical and NO_3 radical reactions are both important. For example, for CH_3SH, both OH and NO_3 reactions lead to the group $CH_3S(OH)H$, which is thought to proceed, through CH_3S, to HCHO, SO_2, and CH_3SO_3H.

Cloud condensation nuclei (CCN) concentrations in remote marine regions may be controlled by dimethylsulfide, CH_3SCH_3 (DMS), emissions from marine phytoplankton (Charlson *et al.*, 1987). After DMS is emitted from the ocean, it undergoes photochemical oxidation via a series of gas-phase reactions (OH radical and NO_3 radical) to produce, as major sulfur-containing products, methanesulfonic acid, CH_3SO_3H (MSA), and SO_2 (Yin *et al.*, 1990a, b; Jensen *et al.*, 1991, 1992; Tyndal and Ravishankara, 1991).

Sulfur dioxide undergoes further oxidation to form sulfuric acid (H_2SO_4). Oxidation of SO_2 to sulfate may occur either via gas-phase reactions (initiated by the reaction of OH with SO_2) or by heterogeneous processes in fogs and clouds. In the latter process, SO_2 is absorbed into the drop and reacts primarily with H_2O_2 or O_3 to form sulfate (see Section X). If the droplet then evaporates (rather than forming precipitation), a sulfate-rich aerosol remains. This conversion process creates SO_4^{2-} and aerosol mass, but does not form new particles, because cloud droplets form on pre-existing particles (CCN). After evaporation, larger, more sulfate-rich aerosol particles remain, but no new ones.

The formation of new particles from the gas-phase oxidation of DMS to form MSA and H_2SO_4 depends on the chemical pathway for degradation of DMS. Because MSA and H_2SO_4 are the only known condensable species formed in the reaction sequence that oxidizes DMS, these are the species that may form new aerosols and CCN. If the emissions are anthropogenic SO_2, gas-phase oxidation will also produce H_2SO_4. Whether new particles form depends on the vapor concentrations of MSA and H_2SO_4, as well as on the concentrations of pre-existing particles, since condensation onto existing particles competes with new particle formation for available condensable vapors.

IX. Tropospheric Aerosols and Gas-to-Particle Conversion

Compounds are emitted into the atmosphere in both gaseous and particulate forms. In addition, gas-phase oxidation of a number of compounds can lead to products that condense into the particulate phase. The subject of tropospheric aerosols—their sources, chemistry, and removal—is a significant one and beyond the scope of the present chapter.

Table VI summarizes aerosol mass concentrations and composition in different regions of the troposphere. It is interesting to note that average total fine particle mass (that associated with particles of diameter less than about 2 μm) in non-urban continental, i.e., regional, aerosols is only a factor of two lower than urban values. This reflects the relatively long residence time of particles (recall the estimate of a lifetime of fine particles by dry deposition of 10 days). Correspondingly, the average composition of non-urban continental and urban aerosols is roughly the same. The average mass concentration of remote aerosols is a factor of three lower than that of non-urban continental aerosols. The elemental carbon component, a direct indicator of anthropogenic combustion sources, drops to 0.3% in the remote aerosols, but sulfate is still a major compo-

TABLE VI
MASS CONCENTRATIONS AND COMPOSITION OF TROPOSPHERIC AEROSOLS

Region	Mass ($\mu g/m^3$)	Percentage composition				
		C (elem)	C (org)	NH_4	NO_3	SO_4
Remote (11 areas)[a]	4.8	0.3	11	7	3	22
Non-urban continental (14 areas)[a]	15	5	24	11	4	37
Urban (19 areas)[a]	32	9	31	8	6	28
Rubidoux, California[b] (1986 annual average)	87.4	3	18	6	20	6

[a] Heintzenberg (1989).
[b] Solomon *et al.* (1989).

nent. This is attributable to a global average concentration of non-sea salt sulfate of about 0.5 $\mu g\ m^{-3}$. Rubidoux, California, located about 100 km east of downtown Los Angeles, routinely experiences some of the highest particulate matter concentrations in the U.S.

Figure 9 depicts the chemical paths of conversion of gaseous to particulate species. Gas-phase oxidation of certain organics, such as aromatics and the terpenes, can lead to products that condense. To accumulate in

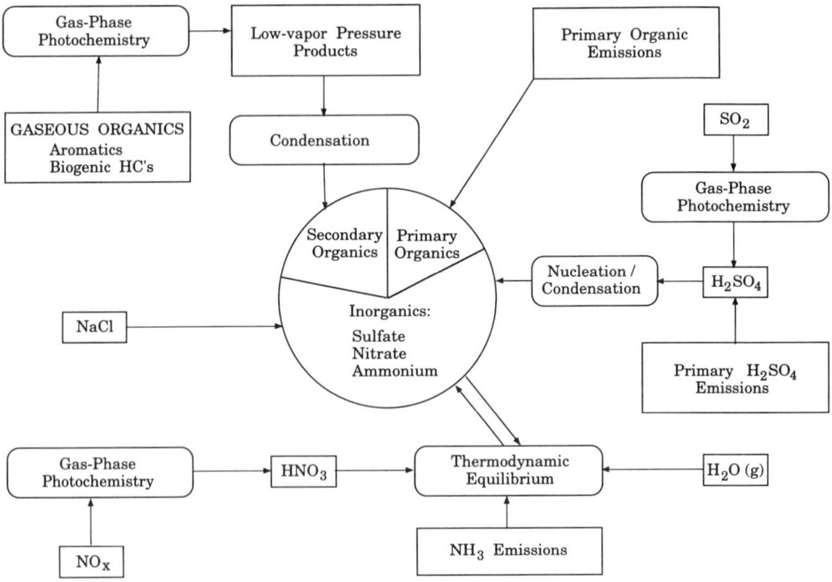

FIG. 9. Chemical paths of conversion of gaseous to particulate species.

the condensed phase, a reaction product must first be formed in the gas phase at a concentration equal to its saturation level. Generally, compounds whose pure component vapor pressures are less than 10^{-6} torr are candidates for gas-to-particle conversion (Grosjean and Seinfeld, 1989; Pandis *et al.*, 1991, 1992; Wang *et al.*, 1992a, b).

The chemical composition of atmospheric aerosols is complex. The following major aerosol components can generally be expected to be present, in varying amounts, depending on the source and history of the air mass involved: carbonaceous material (elemental and organic); nitrate; sulfate; ammonium; soil-related material; sea-salt material (for regions near the sea); and water. In addition, aerosol chemical composition is known to vary significantly with particle size. For example, most of the sulfate, ammonium, organic, and elemental carbon are in particles of diameters less than 2 μm, while most of the crustal material resides in larger particles. Nitrate may occur in both small and large particles. Chemical constituents of aerosols can be classified as nonvolatile or volatile. The inert nonvolatile species primarily consist of particulate organic and elemental carbon from combustion sources, tire wear, and crustal material such as road dust. These materials form a core upon which other chemical species may condense. For example, sodium and sulfate have such low vapor pressures that they can be considered nonvolatile. Sodium originates in sodium chloride (NaCl) salt in sea spray that has been advected inland in regions near oceans. Some sulfate originates from sea salt, but a major source of sulfate is atmospheric oxidation of SO_2. Sulfate is formed either by gas-phase oxidation of SO_2 or by aqueous-phase oxidation in aerosol particles or fog droplets, where it reduces the vapor pressure of NH_3. Sulfate formed in the gas phase rapidly condenses because of its low vapor pressure. NaCl in the aerosol phase reduces the equilibrium vapor pressures of nitric acid, while increasing the vapor pressure of HCl. Both NaCl and H_2SO_4 shift the equilibrium concentrations of the active and volatile species, which affects aerosol mass. Ammonium, sulfate, nitrate, sodium, and chloride typically account for 25% to 50% of the nonwater atmospheric aerosol mass. The mass of these inorganics in an aerosol particle, the ambient temperature, and the relative humidity determine the mass of water in the aerosol. Under conditions of low relative humidity, little or no water may exist in atmospheric aerosol, but under conditions of high relative humidity, water may make up over half of the total aerosol mass (Pilinis *et al*, 1989). Ammonia, chloride, nitrate, and water are the primary active volatile chemical species in atmospheric aerosols. The inorganics (ammonia, chloride, and nitrate) react with each other and with the two nonvolatile active species (sodium and sulfate) to form ammonium and sodium salts. If the relative humidity is sufficiently high, the aerosol inorganics will form a pure aqueous solution. If the relative humidity is sufficiently low, the aerosol inorganics will form solid salts, and water may only be present in salt hydrates. For intermediate relative humidities, the aerosol may form an aqueous solution in equilibrium with one or more salts. The volatile organic species consist of primary and secondary volatile organic compounds and organic nitrates. These species condense if their saturation vapor pressure is exceeded in the gas phase, but they are not expected to undergo significant chemical reaction in the aerosol phase.

X. Aqueous-Phase Atmospheric Chemistry

Relative to the levels of the species we have been considering, water vapor is at a high concentration in the atmosphere. Liquid water, in the form of clouds and fog, is frequently present. Small water droplets can themselves be viewed as microscopic chemical reactors where gaseous species are absorbed, reactions take place, and species evaporate back to the gas phase. Droplets themselves do not always leave the atmosphere as precipitation; more often than not, in fact, cloud droplets evaporate before coalescing to a point where precipitation can occur. In terms of atmospheric chemistry, droplets can both alter the course of gas-phase chemistry through the uptake of vapor species and act as a medium for production of species that otherwise would not be produced in the gas phase or would be produced by different paths at a lower rate in the gas phase (Fig. 10). Concentrations of dissolved species in cloud, fog, and rain droplets are in the micromolar range, and therefore one usually assumes that the atmospheric aqueous phase behaves as an ideal solution.

Cloud processes have been predicted to have a significant effect on the chemistry of the clean troposphere (Lelieveld and Crutzen, 1990, 1991; Warneck, 1991, 1992). For example, the uptake of HCHO, HO_2 radicals, and N_2O_5 into cloud droplets can lead to a decrease in the production of ozone. Removal of HCHO reduces the rate of gas-phase production of HO_2 radicals, and N_2O_5 into cloud droplets can lead to a decrease in the production of ozone. Removal of HCHO reduces the rate of gas-phase production of HO_2 radicals [reactions (33)–(36)], and consequent conversion of NO to NO_2. Also, aqueous-phase reactions of $H_2C(OH)_2$, the hydrated form of HCHO, lead to the formation of O_2^-, which can react with dissolved O_3 to enhance the rate of transfer of O_3 to the liquid phase over that based solely on physical solubility. Absorption of N_2O_5 into

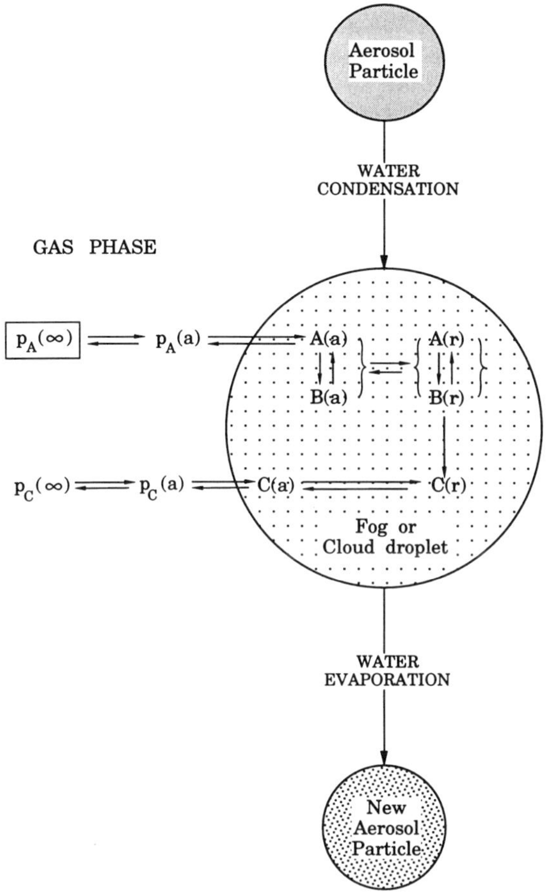

FIG. 10. Role of water droplets in atmospheric chemistry.

droplets is followed by rapid hydrolysis to nitric acid [reaction (14)], preventing the reformation of NO_2 by reaction (11).

The chemistry that occurs in cloud and fog droplets in the atmosphere has been shown, in the last decade or so, to be highly complex. Most atmospheric species are soluble to some extent, and the liquid-phase reactions that are possible lead to a diverse spectrum of products. The aspect of atmospheric aqueous-phase chemistry that has received the most attention is that involving dissolved SO_2. Sulfur dioxide is not particularly soluble in pure water, but the presence of other dissolved species such as H_2O_2 or O_3 displaces the dissolution equilibrium for SO_2, effectively enhancing the solubility of SO_2. Once dissolved, SO_2 can be oxidized to sulfate, a principal contributor to acidic deposition.

A. Aqueous-Phase Equilibria

The liquid water content of the atmosphere, w_L, is usually expressed either in grams of water per cubic meter of air, or as a dimensionless volume fraction L (e.g., cubic meters of liquid water per cubic meter of air). Typical liquid water content values are 0.1 to 1 g m^{-3} ($L = 10^{-7}$–10^{-6}) for clouds, 0.05 to 0.5 g m^{-3} ($L = 5 \times 10^{-7}$–5×10^{-6}) for fogs, and only 10^{-5} to 10^{-4} g m^{-3} ($L = 10^{-11}$–10^{-10}) for aerosols.

TABLE VII
Henry's Law Coefficients of Some Atmospheric Gases Dissolving in Liquid Water

Species	H (M/atm) (298 K)	Reference
O_2	1.3×10^{-3}	Wagman *et al.* (1982)
NO	1.9×10^{-3}	Schwartz and White (1981)
C_2H_4	4.8×10^{-3}	Wagman *et al.* (1982)
NO_2	1.0×10^{-2}	Schwartz (1984)
O_3	1.13×10^{-2}	Kozac-Channing and Helz (1983)
N_2O	2.5×10^{-2}	Loomis (1928)
CO_2	3.4×10^{-2}	Smith and Martell (1976)
H_2S	0.12	Wagman *et al.* (1982)
SO_2	1.23	Smith and Martell (1976)
CH_3ONO_2	2.6	Lee *et al.* (1983)
$CH_3C(O)O_2NO_2$	2.9	Lee (1984b)
CH_3O_2	6.0	Jacob (1986)
OH	25.0	Jacob (1986)
HNO_2	49.0	Schwartz and White (1981)
NH_3	75.0	Hales and Drewes (1979)
CH_3OH	220.0	Snider and Dawson (1985)
CH_3OOH	227.0	Lind and Kok (1986)
$CH_3C(O)OOH$	473.0	Lind and Kok (1986)
HCl	727.0	Marsh and McElroy (1985)
HO_2	2.0×10^3	Jacob (1986)
HCOOH	3.5×10^3	Latimer (1952)
HCHO	6.3×10^3	Ledbury and Blair (1925)
CH_3COOH	8.7×10^3	Wagman *et al.* (1982)
H_2O_2	7.45×10^4	Lind and Kok (1986)
HNO_3	2.1×10^5	Schwartz (1984)
NO_3	2.1×10^5	Jacob (1986)

For dilute solutions, the equilibrium distribution of a reagent gas A between the gas and aqueous phases is given by Henry's law,

$$[A] = H_A p_A, \tag{94}$$

where p_A is the partial pressure of A in the gas-phase, [A] is the equilibrium aqueous-phase concentration of A, and H_A is the Henry's law coefficient for species A. The customary units of H_A are mole L^{-1} atm^{-1}. H_A can be viewed as the equilibrium constant of the reaction

$$A(g) \rightleftarrows A(aq). \tag{95}$$

Table VII gives the Henry's law coefficients of some atmospheric gases in liquid water at 298 K. The values given reflect only the physical solubility of the gas regardless of the subsequent fate of the dissolved species A. Some of the species included in Table VII dissociate after dissolution or react with water. The Henry's law constants of Table VII do not account for these processes, and the modifications necessary will be discussed in the next paragraph. Henry's law coefficients generally decrease for increasing temperatures, resulting in lower solubilities at higher temperatures (Seinfeld, 1986).

Several gases, after dissolving in the aqueous-phase, ionize and establish an aqueous-phase chemical equilibrium system. For example, for SO_2,

$$SO_2(g) \rightleftarrows SO_2 \cdot H_2O, \tag{96}$$

$$SO_2 \cdot H_2O \rightleftarrows HSO_3^- + H^+, \tag{97}$$

$$HSO_3^- \rightleftarrows SO_3^{2-} + H^+, \tag{98}$$

with

$$H_{SO_2} = \frac{[SO_2 \cdot H_2O]}{p_{SO_2}}, \qquad K_{s1} = \frac{[HSO_3^-][H^+]}{[SO_2 \cdot H_2O]},$$

$$K_{s2} = \frac{[SO_3^{2-}][H^+]}{[HSO_3^-]}. \tag{99}$$

K_{s1} and K_{s2} are the first and second dissociation constants for SO_2. It is convenient to consider the total dissolved sulfur in oxidation state IV as a single entity and refer to it as S(IV),

$$[S(IV)] = [SO_2 \cdot H_2O] + [HSO_3^-] + [SO_3^{2-}]. \tag{100}$$

The three sulfur species are in rapid equilibrium, and therefore [S(IV)] changes only when SO_2 is transferred between the gas and aqueous phases. The total dissolved sulfur, S(IV), can be expressed as a function of only the pH and the partial pressure of SO_2 over the solution by

$$[S(IV)] = H_{SO_2} p_{SO_2} \left[1 + \frac{K_{s1}}{[H^+]} + \frac{K_{s1} K_{s2}}{[H^+]^2} \right]. \tag{101}$$

The preceding equation can be expressed in a form similar to Henry's law as

$$[S(IV)] = H^*_{S(IV)} p_{SO_2}, \tag{102}$$

where $H^*_{S(IV)}$ is the effective (or modified) Henry's law coefficient given for S(IV) by

$$H^*_{S(IV)} = H_{SO_2} \left[1 + \frac{K_{s1}}{[H^+]} + \frac{K_{s1} K_{s2}}{[H^+]^2} \right]. \tag{103}$$

The modified Henry's law coefficient relates the total dissolved S(IV) (and not only $SO_2 \cdot H_2O$) with the SO_2 vapor pressure over the solution. The effective Henry's law coefficient always exceeds the Henry's law coefficient, indicating that the dissociation of a species enhances its solubility in the aqueous phase.

The major reactions taking place in the atmospheric aqueous phase are presented in Table VIII. Several of these species that are in rapid equilibrium can be also considered as single entities:

$$\begin{aligned}
[S(VI)] &= [H_2SO_4(aq)] + [HSO_4^-] + [SO_4^{2-}], \\
[N(V)] &= [HNO_3(aq)] + [NO_3^-], \\
[HO_2^T] &= [HO_2(aq)] + [O_2^-], \\
[HCHO^T] &= [HCHO] + [H_2C(OH)_2].
\end{aligned}$$

Equations relating the total concentrations of these aqueous-phase species with the corresponding equilibrium concentrations of the gas-phase species can be derived similarly to those for S(IV).

B. S(IV) to S(VI) Transformation and Sulfur Chemistry

The aqueous-phase conversion of dissolved SO_2 to sulfate is probably the most important chemical transformation in cloudwater. Dissolution of SO_2 in water results in the formation of three chemical species: hydrated $SO_2(SO_2 \cdot H_2O)$, the bisulfite ion (HSO_3^-), and the sulfite ion (SO_3^{2-}). At

TABLE VIII
AQUEOUS-PHASE ATMOSPHERIC CHEMISTRY

	Reaction	Rate expression $M^n\ (s)^{-1}$	$-E/R$	Reference
1.	$H_2O_2 \xrightarrow{h\nu} 2OH$			Graedel and Weschler (1981)
2.	$OH + HO_2 \rightarrow H_2O + O_2$	7.0×10^9	−1500	Sehested *et al.* (1968)
3.	$OH + O_2^- \rightarrow OH^- + O_2$	1.0×10^{10}	−1500	Sehested *et al.* (1968)
4.	$OH + H_2O_2 \rightarrow H_2O + HO_2$	2.7×10^7	−1700	Christensen *et al.* (1982)
5.	$HO_2 + HO_2 \rightarrow H_2O_2 + O_2$	8.6×10^5	−2365	Bielski (1978)
6.	$HO_2 + O_2^- \xrightarrow{H_2O} H_2O_2 + O_2 + OH^-$	1.0×10^8	−1500	Bielski (1978)
7.	$O_2^- + O_3 \xrightarrow{H_2O} OH + 2O_2 + OH^-$	1.5×10^9	−1500	Sehested *et al.* (1983)
8.	$H_2O_2 + O_3 \rightarrow H_2O + 2O_2$	$7.8 \times 10^{-3}[O_3]^{-0.5}$	0	Martin (1984)
9.	$HCO_3^- + OH \rightarrow H_2O + CO_3^-$	1.5×10^7	−1910	Weeks and Rabani (1966)
10.	$HCO_3^- + O_2^- \rightarrow HO_2^- + CO_3^-$	1.5×10^6	0	Schmidt (1972)
11.	$CO_3^- + O_2^- \xrightarrow{H_2O} HCO_3^- + O_2 + OH^-$	4.0×10^8	−1500	Behar *et al.* (1970)
12.	$CO_3^- + H_2O_2 \rightarrow HO_2 + HCO_3^-$	8.0×10^5	−2820	Behar *et al.* (1970)
13.	$Cl^- + OH \rightarrow ClOH^-$	4.3×10^9	−1500	Jayson *et al.* (1973)
14.	$ClOH^- \rightarrow Cl^- + OH$	6.1×10^9	0	Jayson *et al.* (1973)
15.	$ClOH^- \xrightarrow{H^+} Cl + H_2O$	$2.1 \times 10^{10}[H^+]$	0	Jayson *et al.* (1973)
16.	$Cl \xrightarrow{H_2O} ClOH^- + H^+$	1.3×10^3	0	Jayson *et al.* (1973)
17.	$O_2^- + Cl_2^- \rightarrow 2Cl^- + O_2$	1.0×10^9	−1500	Ross and Neta (1979)
18.	$H_2O_2 + Cl_2^- \rightarrow 2Cl^- + HO_2 + H^+$	1.4×10^5	−3370	Hagesawa and Neta (1978)
19.	$H_2O_2 + Cl \rightarrow Cl^- + HO_2 + H^+$	4.5×10^7	0	Graedel and Goldberg (1983)
20.	$OH^- + Cl_2^- \rightarrow 2Cl^- + OH$	7.3×10^6	−2160	Hagesawa and Neta (1978)
21.	$NO_2^- + OH \rightarrow NO_2 + OH^-$	1.0×10^{10}	−1500	Treinin and Hayon (1970)
22.	$NO_2^- + O_3 \rightarrow NO_3^- + O_2$	5.0×10^5	−6950	Damschen and Martin (1983)
23.	$NO_3^- \xrightarrow{h\nu,\ H_2O} NO_2 + OH + OH^-$			Graedel and Weschler (1981)
24.	$NO_3 + O_2^- \rightarrow NO_3^- + O_2$	1.0×10^9	−1500	Jacob (1986)
25.	$NO_3 + Cl^- \rightarrow NO_3^- + Cl$	1.0×10^8	−1500	Ross and Neta (1979)

Continues

TABLE VIII—*Continued*

	Reaction	Rate expression M^n (s)$^{-1}$	$-E/R$	Reference
26.	$H_2C(OH)_2 + OH \xrightarrow{O_2} HCOOH + HO_2 + H_2O$	2.0×10^9	−1500	Bothe and Schulte-Frohlinde (1980)
27.	$HCOOH + OH \xrightarrow{O_2} CO_2 + HO_2 + H_2O$	1.6×10^8	−1500	Scoles and Willson (1967)
28.	$HCOO^- + OH \xrightarrow{O_2} CO_2 + HO_2 + OH^-$	2.5×10^9	−1500	Anbar and Neta (1967)
29.	$HCOO^- + CO_3^- \xrightarrow{O_2,\, H_2O} CO_2 + HCO_3^- + HO_2 + OH^-$	1.1×10^5	−3400	Chen *et al.* (1973)
30.	$HCOO^- + Cl_2^- \xrightarrow{O_2} CO_2 + HO_2 + 2Cl^-$	1.9×10^6	−2600	Hagesawa and Neta (1978)
31.	$CH_3C(O)O_2NO_2 \rightarrow NO_3^- +$ products	4.0×10^{-4}	0	Lee (1984b)
32.	$CH_3O_2 + HO_2 \rightarrow CH_3OOH + O_2$	4.3×10^5	−3000	Jacob (1986)
33.	$CH_3O_2 + O_2^- \xrightarrow{H_2O} CH_3OOH + O_2 + OH^-$	5.0×10^7	−1600	Jacob (1986)
34.	$CH_3OOH + OH \rightarrow CH_3O_2 + H_2O$	2.7×10^7	−1700	Jacob (1986)
35.	$CH_3OH + OH \rightarrow HCHO + HO_2 + H_2O$	4.5×10^8	−1500	Anbar and Neta (1967)
36.	$CH_3OOH + OH \rightarrow HCHO + OH + H_2O$	1.9×10^7	−1800	Jacob (1986)
37.[a]	$S(IV) + O_3 \rightarrow S(VI) + O_2$	2.4×10^4		
		3.7×10^5	−5530	Hoffmann and
		1.5×10^9	−5280	Calvert (1985)
38.[a]	$S(IV) + H_2O_2 \rightarrow S(VI) + H_2O$	1.3×10^6	−4430	McArdle and Hoffmann (1983)
39.[a]	$S(IV) + \frac{1}{2}O_2 \xrightarrow{Mn^{2+},\, Fe^{3+}} S(VI)$	4.7	−13,700	
		0.82	−11,000	
		5.0×10^3	−13,700	
		1.0×10^7	−11,000	Martin (1984)
40.	$SO_3^{2-} + OH \xrightarrow{O_2} SO_5^- + OH^-$	4.6×10^9	−1500	Huie and Neta (1987)
41.	$HSO_3^- + OH \xrightarrow{O_2} SO_5^- + H_2O$	4.2×10^9	−1500	Huie and Neta (1987)

42.	$SO_5^- + HSO_3^- \xrightarrow{O_2} HSO_5^- + SO_5^-$	3.0×10^5	-3100	Huie and Neta (1987)
	$SO_5^- + SO_3^{2-} \xrightarrow{O_2} HSO_5^- + SO_5^-$	1.3×10^7	-2000	Huie and Neta (1987)
43.	$SO_5^- + O_2^- \xrightarrow{H_2O} HSO_5^- + OH^- + O_2$	1.0×10^8	-1500	Jacob (1986)
44.	$SO_5^- + HCOO^- \xrightarrow{O_2} HSO_5^- + CO_2 + O_2^-$	1.4×10^4	-4000	Jacob (1986)
45.	$SO_5^- + SO_5^- \rightarrow 2SO_4^- + O_2$	2.0×10^8	-1500	Jacob (1986)
46.	$HSO_5^- + HSO_3^- \xrightarrow{H^+} 2SO_4^{2-} + 3H^+$	7.5×10^7	-4755	Jacob (1986)
47.	$HSO_5^- + OH \rightarrow SO_5^- + H_2O$	1.7×10^7	-1900	Jacob (1986)
48.	$SO_4^- + HSO_3^- \xrightarrow{O_2} SO_4^{2-} + H^+ + SO_5^-$	1.3×10^9	-1500	Jacob (1986)
49.	$SO_4^- + HO_2 \rightarrow SO_4^{2-} + H^+ + O_2$	5.0×10^9	-1500	Jacob (1986)
50.	$SO_4^- + O_2^- \rightarrow SO_4^{2-} + O_2$	5.0×10^9	-1500	Jacob (1986)
51.	$SO_4^- + H_2O_2 \rightarrow SO_4^{2-} + H^+ + HO_2$	1.2×10^7	-2000	Ross and Neta (1979)
52.	$SO_4^- + NO_2^- \rightarrow SO_4^{2-} + NO_2$	8.8×10^8	-1500	Jacob (1986)
53.	$SO_4^- + HCOO^- \xrightarrow{O_2} SO_4^{2-} + CO_2 + HO_2$	1.7×10^8	-1500	Jacob (1986)
54.	$SO_4^- + Cl^- \rightarrow SO_4^{2-} + Cl$	2.0×10^8	-1500	Ross and Neta (1979)
55.	$HSO_3^- + CH_3OOH \xrightarrow{H^+} SO_4^{2-} + 2H^+ + prd$	1.9×10^7	-3800	Hoffmann and Calvert (1985)
56.[a]	$HSO_3^- + CH_3C(O)OOH \rightarrow SO_4^{2-} + H^+ + prd$	5.0×10^7	-4000	
		6.0×10^2		Hoffmann and Calvert (1985)
57.	$S(IV) + HO_2 \rightarrow S(VI) + OH$	1.0×10^6	0	Hoffmann and Calvert (1985)
	$S(IV) + O_2^- \xrightarrow{H_2O} S(VI) + OH + OH^-$	1.0×10^5	0	Hoffmann and Calvert (1985)
58.	$2NO_2 + HSO_3^- \xrightarrow{H_2O} SO_4^{2-} + 3H^+ + 2NO_2^-$	2.0×10^6	0	Lee and Schwartz (1983)
59.	$HCHO + HSO_3^- \rightarrow HOCH_2SO_3^-$	2.9×10^2	-4900	Boyce and Hoffmann (1984)
	$HCHO + SO_3^{2-} \xrightarrow{H_2O} HOCH_2SO_3^- + OH^-$	2.5×10^7	-1800	Boyce and Hoffmann (1984)
60.	$HOCH_2SO_3^- + OH \xrightarrow{O_2} SO_5^- + HCHO + H_2O$	1.4×10^9	-1500	Jacob (1986)
61.	$HSO_3^- + Cl_2^- \xrightarrow{O_2} SO_5^- + 2Cl^- + H^+$	3.4×10^8	-1500	Huie and Neta (1987)
	$SO_3^{2-} + Cl_2^- \xrightarrow{O_2} SO_5^- + 2Cl^-$	1.6×10^8	-1500	Huie and Neta (1987)

[a] Reaction with "nonelementary" rate expression.

the pH range of atmospheric interest (pH 2–7), most of the S(IV) is in the form of HSO_3^-, whereas at low pH (pH < 2), all of the S(IV) occurs as $SO_2 \cdot H_2O$. At higher pH values (pH > 7), SO_3^{2-} is the preferred S(IV) state (Seinfeld, 1986). The individual dissociations (Table V) are fast, occurring on timescales of milliseconds or less (Martin, 1984; Schwartz and Freiberg, 1981; Seinfeld, 1986). Therefore, during a reaction consuming one of the three species, $SO_2 \cdot H_2O$, HSO_3^-, or SO_3^{2-}, the corresponding aqueous-phase equilibria are re-established instantaneously. The dissociation of dissolved SO_2 enhances its aqueous solubility, and the total amount of dissolved S(IV) always exceeds that predicted by Henry's law for SO_2 alone and is quite pH-dependent. The Henry's law coefficient for SO_2 alone, H_{SO_2}, is 1.23 M atm^{-1} at 298 K, while for the same temperature, the effective Henry's law coefficient for S(IV), $H^*_{S(IV)}$, is 16.4 M atm^{-1} for pH 3, 152 M atm^{-1} for pH 4, and 1,524 M atm^{-1} for pH 5. Equilibrium S(IV) concentrations for SO_2 gas-phase concentrations of 0.2–200 ppb, and over a pH range 1–6, vary approximately from 0.001 to 1000 μM.

Several pathways for S(IV) transformation to S(VI) have been identified involving reactions of S(IV) with O_3, H_2O_2, O_2 (catalyzed by Mn^{2+} and Fe^{3+}), OH, SO_5^-, HSO_5^-, SO_4^-, PAN, CH_3OOH, $CH_3C(O)OOH$, HO_2, NO_3, NO_2, N(III), HCHO, and Cl_2^- (Pandis and Seinfeld, 1989a).

1. *Oxidation of S(IV) by O_3*

Although ozone reacts very slowly with SO_2 in the gas phase, the aqueous-phase reaction is rapid. The possible importance of O_3 as an aqueous-phase oxidant for S(IV) was first suggested by Penkett (1972), and the kinetics of

$$S(IV) + O_3 \rightarrow S(VI) + O_2 \tag{104}$$

have been studied by several investigators (Erickson *et al.*, 1977; Penkett *et al.*, 1979; Maahs, 1983). Hoffmann and Calvert (1985), after a detailed investigation of existing experimental kinetic and mechanistic data, suggested the following expression for the rate of the reaction of S(IV) with dissolved ozone:

$$R_1 = -\frac{d[S(IV)]}{dt} = \left(k_0[SO_2 \cdot H_2O] + k_1[HSO_3^-] + k_2[SO_3^{2-}]\right)[O_3], \tag{105}$$

recommending the values $k_0 = 2.4 \times 10^4$ M^{-1} s^{-1}, $k_1 = 3.7 \times 10^5$ M^{-1} s^{-1}, and $k_2 = 1.5 \times 10^9$ M^{-1} s^{-1}. They also proposed that this reaction proceeds by nucleophilic attack on ozone by $SO_2 \cdot H_2O$, HSO_3^-, and SO_3^{2-}. An increase in the aqueous-phase pH results in an increase of all three, $[SO_2 \cdot H_2O]$, $[HSO_3^-]$, and $[SO_3^{2-}]$, equilibrium concentrations, and therefore in an increase of the overall reaction rate. For an ozone gas-phase concentration of 30 ppb, the reaction rate varies from less than 0.001 μM h^{-1} (ppb $SO_2)^{-1}$ at pH 2 [or less than 0.01% SO_2(g) h^{-1} (g water/m^3 air)$^{-1}$] to 3000 μM h^{-1} (ppb $SO_2)^{-1}$ at pH 6 [7000% SO_2(g) h^{-1} (g water/m^3 air)$^{-1}$]. The gas-phase SO_2 oxidation rate is of the order of 1% h^{-1}, and therefore the S(IV) heterogeneous oxidation by ozone is significant for pH values greater than 4. The strong positive dependence of the reaction rate on the pH renders this reaction self-limiting. The production of sulfate by this reaction lowers the pH and effectively decreases the rate of further reaction. The availability of atmospheric ozone guarantees that this reaction will play an important role both as a sink of gas-phase SO_2 and as a cause of cloudwater acidification as long as the pH of the atmospheric aqueous phase exceeds 4.

2. Oxidation by Hydrogen Peroxide and Organic Peroxides

Hydrogen peroxide, H_2O_2, is one of the most effective oxidants of S(IV) in clouds and fogs (Pandis and Seinfeld, 1989a). H_2O_2 is very soluble in water, and under typical ambient conditions its aqueous-phase concentration is approximately six orders of magnitude higher than that of ozone. This reaction has been studied in detail by several investigators (Hoffmann and Edwards, 1975; Penkett *et al.*, 1979; Martin and Damschen, 1981; Cocks *et al.*, 1982; Kunen *et al.*, 1983; McArdle and Hoffmann, 1983), and the reproducibility of the measurements suggests a lack of susceptibility of this reaction to influence of trace constituents. The proposed rate expression is (Hoffmann and Calvert, 1985)

$$R_2 = -\frac{d[\mathrm{S(IV)}]}{dt} = \frac{k[\mathrm{H^+}][\mathrm{H_2O_2}][\mathrm{HSO_3^-}]}{1 + K[\mathrm{H^+}]}, \tag{106}$$

with $k = 7.45 \times 10^7$ M^{-1} s^{-1} and $K = 13$ M^{-1} at 298 K. Noting that H_2O_2 is a very weak electrolyte, that $[H^+][HSO_3^-] = H_{SO_2} K_{s1} p_{SO_2}$, and that for pH > 2, $1 + K[H^+] \simeq 1$, one concludes that the rate of this reaction is practically pH-independent in the pH range of atmospheric interest. For a H_2O_2(g) concentration of 1 ppb, the rate is roughly 300 μM h^{-1} (ppb $SO_2)^{-1}$ [700% SO_2(g) h^{-1} (g water/m^3 air)$^{-1}$]. The near pH independence can also be viewed as the result of the cancellation of the pH dependence of the S(IV) solubility and the reaction rate constant. The reaction is very fast, and indeed both field measurements (Daum *et al.*,

1984) and theoretical studies (Pandis and Seinfeld, 1989b) have suggested that $H_2O_2(g)$ and $SO_2(g)$ rarely coexist in clouds and fogs. The species with the lowest concentration before the cloud or fog formation is the limiting reactant and is rapidly depleted inside the cloud or fog layer.

Organic peroxides have been also proposed as potential aqueous-phase oxidants (Graedel and Goldberg, 1983; Lind and Lazrus, 1983; Hoffmann and Calvert, 1985):

$$HSO_3^- + CH_3OOH \xrightarrow{H^+} SO_4^{2-} + 2H^+ + \text{product}, \qquad (107)$$

$$HSO_3^- + CH_3C(O)OOH \longrightarrow SO_4^{2-} + H^+ + \text{product}. \qquad (108)$$

Simulations for typical continental clouds suggested that these reactions are of minor importance for the S(IV) oxidation and represent small sinks for the gas-phase hydroperoxide (0.2% $CH_3OOH\ h^{-1}$) and peracetic acid [0.7% $CH_3C(O)OOH\ h^{-1}$].

3. O_2 Oxidation

The S(IV) oxidation by O_2 is known to be catalyzed by Fe^{3+} and Mn^{2+}:

$$S(IV) + \tfrac{1}{2}O_2 \xrightarrow{Mn^{2+},\ Fe^{3+}} S(IV). \qquad (109)$$

This reaction has been the subject of considerable interest (Hoffmann and Boyce, 1983; Martin, 1984; Hoffmann and Jacob, 1984; Hoffmann and Calvert, 1985; Clarke and Radojevic, 1987), and significantly different measured reaction rates, rate laws, and pH dependencies have been reported (Hoffmann and Jacob, 1984). Martin and Hill (1987a, b) have demonstrated that this reaction is inhibited as ionic strength increases, and is also self-inhibited. They explained most of the literature discrepancies by differences in experimental factors during the various laboratory studies.

In the presence of oxygen, iron in the ferric state, Fe(III), catalyzes the oxidation of S(IV) in aqueous solutions. Fe(II) appears not to directly catalyze the reaction and is first oxidized to Fe(III) before S(IV) oxidation can begin (Huss *et al.*, 1982a, b). The equilibria involving Fe(III) in aqueous solution are

$$Fe^{3+} + H_2O \rightleftarrows FeOH^{2+} + H^+, \qquad (110)$$

$$FeOH^{2+} + H_2O \rightleftarrows Fe(OH)_2^+ + H^+, \qquad (111)$$

$$Fe(OH)_2^+ + H_2O \rightleftarrows Fe(OH)_3(s) + H^+, \qquad (112)$$

$$2FeOH^{2+} \rightleftarrows Fe_2(OH)_2^{4+}, \qquad (113)$$

with Fe^{3+}, $FeOH^{2+}$, $Fe(OH)_2^+$, and $Fe_2(OH)_2^{4+}$ being soluble, and $Fe(OH)_3$ insoluble (Seinfeld, 1986). The concentration of Fe^{3+} can be calculated from the equilibrium with solid $Fe(OH)_3$ (Stumm and Morgan, 1981):

$$Fe(OH)_3(s) + 3H^+ \rightleftharpoons Fe^{3+} + 3H_2O \tag{114}$$

as

$$[Fe^{3+}] \simeq 10^3[H^+]^3 \text{ in M at 298 K,} \tag{115}$$

and for a pH of 4.5, $[Fe^{3+}] = 3 \times 10^{-11}$ M.

For pH values from 0 to 3.6, the iron-catalyzed S(IV) oxidation rate is first-order in iron, first-order in S(IV), and is inversely proportional to $[H^+]$ (Martin and Hill, 1987a),

$$r = -\frac{d[S(IV)]}{dt} = k_1 \frac{[Fe^{3+}][S(IV)]}{[H^+]}. \tag{116}$$

This reaction is inhibited by ionic strength and sulfate, and these effects are described by

$$k_1 = k_1^* 10^{-2\sqrt{I}/(1+\sqrt{I})} \tag{117}$$

and

$$k_1 = k_1^* \frac{1}{1 + 150[S(VI)]^{2/3}}, \tag{118}$$

where I is the ionic strength of the solution and [S(VI)] is in molar. A rate constant $k_1^* = 6\ s^{-1}$ has been recommended by Martin and Hill (1987a). Sulfite appears to be almost equally inhibiting as sulfate. This does not pose a problem for regular atmospheric conditions [S(IV) < 0.001 M], but the preceding rate expressions should not be applied to laboratory studies where the S(IV) concentrations exceed 0.001 M. This reaction is very slow under typical atmospheric conditions in this pH regime.

The rate expression for the same reaction changes completely above pH 3.6. This suggests that the mechanism of the reaction differs in the two pH regimes; it is probably a free radical chain at high pH, and a non-radical mechanism at low pH (Martin *et al.*, 1991). The low solubility of Fe(III) above pH 3.6 presents special experimental problems. At high pH the reaction rate depends on the amount of iron in solution, rather than on the total amount of iron present. At this range the reaction is second-order in dissolved iron (zero-order above the solution iron saturation point) and first-order in S(IV). The reaction is still not very well understood, and Martin *et al.* (1991) proposed the following phenomenological expressions (in M s^{-1}):

$$\text{pH 4.0:} \qquad -\frac{d[\mathrm{S(IV)}]}{dt} = 1 \times 10^{9}[\mathrm{S(IV)}][\mathrm{Fe}^{3+}]^2,$$

$$\text{pH 5.0–6.0:} \qquad -\frac{d[\mathrm{S(IV)}]}{dt} = 1 \times 10^{-3}[\mathrm{S(IV)}],$$

$$\text{pH 7.0:} \qquad -\frac{d[\mathrm{S(IV)}]}{dt} = 1 \times 10^{-4}[\mathrm{S(IV)}],$$

for the following conditions:

$$[\mathrm{S(IV)}] \simeq 10\ \mu\mathrm{M},\ [\mathrm{Fe}^{3+}] > 0.1\ \mu\mathrm{M},\ I < 0.01\ \mathrm{M},$$

$$[\mathrm{S(VI)}] < 100\ \mathrm{M},\ \text{and}\ T = 298\ \mathrm{K}.$$

Note that iron does not appear in the pH 5–7 rates because it is assumed that a trace of iron will be present under normal atmospheric conditions. This reaction is important in this high pH regime (Pandis and Seinfeld, 1989b; Pandis *et al.*, 1992).

Martin *et al.* (1991) also found that non-complexing organic molecules (e.g., acetate, trichloroacetate, ethylalcohol, isopropyl alcohol, formate, allyl alcohol, etc.) are highly inhibiting at pH values of 5 and above, and are not inhibiting at pH values of 3 and below. They calculated that for remote clouds, formate would be the main inhibiting organic, but by less than 10%. In contrast, near urban areas, formate could reduce the rate of the catalyzed oxidation by a factor of 10–20 in the high-pH regime.

The manganese-catalyzed S(IV) oxidation was initially thought to be inversely proportional to the H^+ concentration. Martin and Hill (1987b) suggested that ionic strength, not hydrogen ion, accounts for the pH dependence of the rate. These authors were also able to explain some unusual behavior described in the literature on this reaction and to partially reconcile some of the literature rates. The manganese-catalyzed reaction obeys zero-order kinetics in S(IV) in the concentration regime above 100 μM S(IV),

$$-\frac{d[\mathrm{S(IV)}]}{dt} = k_0[\mathrm{Mn}^{2+}]^2, \qquad k_0 = k_0^{*}10^{-4.07\sqrt{I}/(1+\sqrt{I})}, \tag{119}$$

with $k_0^* = 680\ \mathrm{M}^{-1}\ \mathrm{s}^{-1}$ (Martin and Hill, 1987b). For S(IV) concentrations below 1 μM, the reaction is first-order in S(IV),

$$-\frac{d[\mathrm{S(IV)}]}{dt} = k_0[\mathrm{Mn}^{2+}][\mathrm{S(IV)}], \qquad (120)$$

$$k_0 = k_0^* 10^{-4.07\sqrt{I}/(1+\sqrt{I})},$$

with $k_0^* = 1000\ \mathrm{M}^{-1}\ \mathrm{s}^{-1}$ (Martin and Hill, 1987b). It is still not clear which rate law is appropriate for use in atmospheric calculations, although Martin and Hill (1987b) suggested the provisional use of the first-order, low S(IV) rate.

When both Fe^{3+} and Mn^{2+} are present in atmospheric droplets, the overall rate of the S(IV) reaction is enhanced over the sum of the two individual rates. Martin (1984) reported that the rates measured were 3 to 10 times higher than expected from the sum of the independent rates. Martin and Good (1991) obtained at pH 3.0 and for [S(IV)] < 10 μM the following rate law:

$$-\frac{d[\mathrm{S(IV)}]}{dt} = 750[\mathrm{Mn(II)}][\mathrm{S(IV)}] + 2600[\mathrm{Fe(III)}][\mathrm{S(IV)}] + 1.0 \times 10^{10}[\mathrm{Mn(II)}][\mathrm{Fe(III)}][\mathrm{S(IV)}], \qquad (121)$$

and a similar expression for pH 5.0 in agreement with the work of Ibusuki and Takeuchi (1987).

4. *S(IV) Oxidation by Free Radicals*

Free radicals, such as OH and HO_2, either heterogeneously scavenged by the aqueous phase or produced in the aqueous phase, participate in a series of aqueous-phase reactions (Graedel and Weschler, 1981; Chameides and Davis, 1982; Graedel and Goldberg, 1983; Schwartz, 1984; Jacob, 1986; Pandis and Seinfeld, 1989a).

Huie and Neta (1987) suggested that the product of the OH attack on HSO_3^- and SO_3^{2-} is SO_3^-, which subsequently reacts rapidly with O_2 to produce SO_5^-,

$$\mathrm{HSO_3^-} + \mathrm{OH} \xrightarrow{\mathrm{O_2}} \mathrm{SO_5^-} + \mathrm{H_2O}, \qquad (122)$$

$$\mathrm{SO_3^{2-}} + \mathrm{OH} \xrightarrow{\mathrm{O_2}} \mathrm{SO_5^-} + \mathrm{H_2O}. \qquad (123)$$

The fate of SO_5^- is reaction via a series of pathways to produce HSO_5^-, SO_4^-, and S(VI), creating a relatively complicated reaction system. Pandis and Seinfeld (1989a), using the mechanism proposed by Jacob (1986), calculated that SO_5^- reacts mainly with O_2^- to produce HSO_5^-:

$$SO_5^- + O_2^- \xrightarrow{H_2O} HSO_5^- + OH^- + O_2, \tag{124}$$

but is also autoconverted to SO_4^-,

$$SO_5^- + SO_5^- \longrightarrow 2SO_4^- + O_2, \tag{125}$$

and acts as a catalyst transforming S(IV) to HSO_5^-,

$$SO_5^- + HSO_3^- \xrightarrow{O_2} HSO_5^- + SO_5^-, \tag{126}$$

$$SO_5^- + SO_3^{2-} \xrightarrow{O_2} HSO_5^- + SO_5^-. \tag{127}$$

The SO_4^- produced by reaction (125) is mainly converted to sulfate by reacting either with the chloride ion,

$$SO_4^- + Cl^- \longrightarrow SO_4^{2-} + Cl, \tag{128}$$

or with HSO_3^-,

$$SO_4^- + HSO_3^- \xrightarrow{O_2} HSO_4^{2-} + H^+ + SO_5^-. \tag{129}$$

In this last reaction one more molecule of S(IV) is oxidized, propagating the reaction chain. The SO_4^- can be converted to sulfate also by reacting with H_2O_2, HO_2 and O_2^-, and $HCOO^-$, but these reactions appear to be of minor significance (Pandis and Seinfeld, 1989a).

The HSO_5^- produced by reactions (124), (126), and (127) mainly reacts with HSO_3^- to produce sulfate,

$$HSO_5^- + HSO_3^- \xrightarrow{H^+} 2SO_4^{2-} + 2H^+. \tag{130}$$

Pandis and Seinfeld (1989a) proposed that under typical remote continental conditions there are two main radical pathways resulting in the conversion of S(IV) to S(VI):

$$S(IV)(+OH) \longrightarrow SO_5^-(+O_2^-) \longrightarrow HSO_5^-(+HSO_3^-) \longrightarrow S(VI), \tag{131}$$

$$S(IV)(+OH) \longrightarrow SO_5^- \longrightarrow SO_4^-(+Cl^-, HSO_3^-) \longrightarrow S(VI), \tag{132}$$

with the first of these two pathways typically being faster than the second.

5. *Oxidation of S(IV) by Oxides of Nitrogen*

Nitrogen dioxide has a low water solubility, and therefore its low resulting aqueous-phase concentrations suggests that its oxidation of S(IV),

$$2NO_2 + HSO_3^- \xrightarrow{H_2O} 3H^+ + 2NO_2^- + SO_4^{2-}, \tag{133}$$

should be of minor importance in most cases. This reaction has been studied by Lee and Schwartz (1983) at pH 5.0, 5.8, and 6.4 and was described as a reaction that is first-order in NO_2 and first-order in S(IV), with a pH-dependent rate constant. The evaluation of this rate expression was considered tentative by Lee and Schwartz, in view of evidence for the formation of a long-lived intermediate species. The apparent rate constant was found to increase with pH. This reaction is considered of secondary importance at the concentrations and pH values representative of clouds. However, Pandis and Seinfeld (1989b) reported that for fogs occurring in urban polluted areas with high NO_2 concentrations, this reaction could be a major pathway for the S(IV) oxidation, if the atmosphere has enough neutralizing capacity, e.g., high NH_3(g) concentrations.

6. S(IV) and HCHO Reaction

SO_3^{2-} reacts with formaldehyde to produce hydroxymethanesulfonate ion (HMSA) (Boyce and Hoffmann, 1984),

$$HCHO + SO_3^{2-} \rightleftarrows {}^{-}OCH_2SO_3^-, \qquad (134)$$

$$HCHO + HSO_3^- \rightleftarrows HOCH_2SO_3^-. \qquad (135)$$

The HMSA formed acts as a S(IV) reservoir protecting it from further oxidation, and its formation explains the high S(IV) concentrations that have been observed in clouds and fogs. The kinetics of the HCHO–S(IV) reaction in the pH range 0–3.5 has been shown to be slow, so that S(IV) and HCHO cannot reach the equilibrium state (Munger *et al.*, 1984). The effectiveness of HMSA as a S(IV) reservoir depends critically on its resistivity to OH attack,

$$HOCH_2SO_3^- + OH \xrightarrow{O_2} SO_5^- + HCHO + H_2O. \qquad (136)$$

Jacob (1986) suggested a reaction constant of $1.4 \times 10^9\ M^{-1}\ s^{-1}$ for this reaction.

C. Nitrite and Nitrate Chemistry

Nitrogen dioxide aqueous-phase oxidation by water (Lee, 1984a),

$$NO_2 + NO_2 \xrightarrow{H_2O} NO_2^- + NO_3^- + 2H^+, \qquad (137)$$

by NO (Lee, 1984a),

$$NO + NO_2 \xrightarrow{H_2O} 2NO_2^- + 2H^+, \tag{138}$$

by OH, etc., have all been found to proceed far too slowly under ambient conditions to contribute either to the removal of these nitrogen oxides or to cloudwater acidification.

The NO_3 radical (either directly or as N_2O_5) appears to be the most reactive nitrogen species in the aqueous phase,

$$N_2O_5 + H_2O \longrightarrow 2H^+ + 2NO_3^-, \tag{139}$$

$$NO_3 + Cl^- \longrightarrow NO_3^- + Cl. \tag{140}$$

The solubility of nitrogen(III) (that is, HONO + NO_2^-) is fairly high, and its aqueous chemistry is potentially interesting. Pandis and Seinfeld (1989a) suggested that its most important aqueous-phase reaction is with OH:

$$NO_2^- + OH \longrightarrow NO_2 + OH^-, \tag{141}$$

producing NO_2 that can return to the gas phase.

D. Organic Aqueous-Phase Chemistry

Several organic species (formaldehyde, formic acid, methanol, methylperoxide, etc.) are transferred from the gas to the aqueous-phase and contribute to the atmospheric aqueous-phase reaction system (Graedel and Weschler, 1981). The complex formation by S(IV) and aldehydes has already been discussed. Formaldehyde is very soluble in water because it hydrates to its diol form, methylene glycol:

$$HCHO \xrightarrow{H_2O} H_2C(OH)_2.$$

The equilibrium constant for this reaction is 1800, so that HCHO in cloud water is almost totally present as $H_2C(OH)_2$. Methylene glycol is rapidly oxidized by OH to produce HCOOH:

$$H_2C(OH)_2 + OH \xrightarrow{O_2} HCOOH + HO_2 + H_2O. \tag{142}$$

This reaction has been calculated to consume HCHO for typical continental clouds at a rate of 12% h^{-1}, and therefore clouds are expected to decrease the ambient HCHO(g) concentrations, and also to produce formic acid, enhancing its gas-phase concentration. Formaldehyde is also produced in the aqueous phase by reaction of OH with methanol:

$$CH_3OH + OH \longrightarrow HCHO + HO_2 + H_2O, \qquad (143)$$

but this source is almost a factor of 10 slower than reaction (142). Other minor aqueous-phase sources of HCHO are the reaction of CH_3OOH with OH, the photolysis of CH_3OOH, and the reaction of CH_3OH with SO_4^- (Pandis and Seinfeld, 1989a).

The main aqueous-phase sink of HCOOH is its reaction with OH:

$$HCOO^- + OH \xrightarrow{O_2} CO_2 + HO_2 + OH^-, \qquad (144)$$

$$HCOOH + OH \xrightarrow{O_2} CO_2 + HO_2 + H_2O. \qquad (145)$$

Note that reactions (144) and (145) can be considered as competitive with (142), as they both consume OH. The ratio of the HCOOH production to the HCOOH consumption can be expressed as a function of the pH and the gas-phase partial pressure ratio (p_{HCHO}/p_{HCOOH}) for a constant temperature. The ratio of the gas-phase partial pressures is under ordinary conditions over 10, and for all the pH of interest a net production of HCOOH is expected. Other minor sinks of formic acid are its reactions with SO_5^- and SO_4^- (Jacob, 1986).

The consumption rate of methanol in reaction (143) is typically around 0.1% $CH_3OH(g)$ per hour, and only a negligibly small decrease of the gas-phase methanol concentration is expected because of its cloud chemistry. Similarly, aqueous-phase reactions of CH_3OOH, CH_3O_2, and $CH_3C(O)OOH$ are too slow to influence either the corresponding gas-phase concentrations or the aqueous-phase reaction system.

E. Oxygen and Hydrogen Chemistry

While ozone is not produced in the aqueous phase, at least 12 different chemical pathways consuming ozone have been identified. As a result of the relatively small aqueous-phase solubility of ozone, none of these reactions is rapid enough to significantly influence gas-phase ozone concentrations (Pandis and Seinfeld, 1989a). The fastest of these reactions is that with O_2^-:

$$O_3 + O_2^- \xrightarrow{H_2O} OH + 2O_2 + OH^-. \qquad (146)$$

This reaction results in a lifetime of $O_3(aq)$ of the order of 1 s, but because of the small ozone solubility, this rate corresponds to a consumption of gas-phase ozone at only 0.1% h^{-1} (assuming Henry's law equilibrium for ozone).

The OH radical participates in a number of aqueous-phase reactions; at least 16 reactions producing OH and 19 consuming it have been proposed by various investigators. The principal sink for dissolved OH under conditions typical of remote continental clouds is reaction (142). Other sinks are the reactions with hydrogen peroxide, formic acid, and S(IV). The main aqueous-phase sources of OH are reaction (146) and the photolysis of dissolved hydrogen peroxide. Secondary sources are the photolysis of NO_3^- and the oxidation of S(IV) by HO_2.

The main aqueous-phase sources of the HO_2 radical are usually the principal sinks of OH, and vice versa. HO_2 is a major aqueous-phase source of hydrogen peroxide,

$$HO_2 + O_2^- \xrightarrow{H_2O} H_2O_2 + O_2 + OH^-, \tag{147}$$

and therefore it accelerates indirectly the oxidation of S(IV) to S(VI).

XI. Atmospheric Chemical Mechanisms

A chemical mechanism is the set of chemical reactions and associated rate constants that describes the conversion of emitted species into products. From the point of view of tropospheric chemistry, the starting compounds are generally the oxides of nitrogen and sulfur and organic compounds, and ozone is a product species of major interest. Chemical mechanisms are a component of atmospheric models that simulate emissions, transport, dispersion, chemical reactions, and removal processes (Seinfeld, 1986, 1988).

The mechanism development process begins with the assembly of reactions and rate parameters which are obtained from a consideration of chemical and thermodynamic theory, the chemical literature, recommendations and evaluations of kinetic data, and from consideration of the available literature data for the more complex portions of the overall mechanism (Carter, 1990). This step is subject to some limitations:

Not all rate data or mechanistic pathways of interest are available in the literature, and

laboratory kinetic measurements must often be performed at conditions significantly different from those in the atmosphere, thus frequently requiring extrapolation and introducing uncertainty.

Therefore, throughout the mechanism development process, some form of testing is used to determine the importance of inclusion or exclusion of a given reaction, and to assess the sensitivity of the mechanism's predictions to the choice of rate parameters, which have some uncertainty due either to the use of estimation techniques or to experimental measurement uncertainty.

Explicit chemical mechanisms in which every reaction is an elementary reaction are generally too detailed to be used in atmospheric models. Therefore, a process of generalization and deletion is applied to the explicit mechanism to produce a mechanism more practically sized for use in atmospheric models while not sacrificing accuracy of prediction.

Mechanisms developed to represent urban and regional-scale tropospheric chemistry are generally tested with data obtained in laboratory chambers. In the first testing phase, the so-called "core" mechanism or the inorganic and carbonyl reaction set, which includes the inorganic species, carbon monoxide (CO), formaldehyde (HCHO), acetaldehyde (CH_3CHO), and PAN, should be tested. Because the core mechanism is generally based on widely accepted recommendations, such as the NASA (1987) and IUPAC evaluations and review, the primary purpose of this phase is not to test the adequacy of the chemistry. Rather, the purpose of this phase of testing is to test and refine the representations of chamber-dependent phenomena such as solar radiation intensity and spectral distribution, and wall processes including ozone destruction, nitrous acid (HONO) production from NO_2, nitric acid (HNO_3) production from N_2O_5, and possible NO, NO_2, HCHO, HONO, and HO_2 production from chamber-related processes. A uniform treatment of photolytic processes should be used—that is, the photolytic rates should be derived from species cross-sections and quantum yields and from the spectral distribution of the radiation sources in the different chambers. To the extent that the processes are understood, a uniform treatment should also be used for chamber sources and sinks of reactants. Data from each chamber should be used to determine the parameters for the descriptions of these processes.

In the second phase, the mechanism's performance against more complex hydrocarbon HC–NO_x–air experiments is tested. The mechanism's reactions for other carbonyls, alkanes, alkenes, and aromatic species are first evaluated independently by testing against experiments with single organic compounds, and parameterization of uncertain reaction rate constants and product yields is generally carried out using these single HC–NO_x experiments. The mechanism's performance for complex mixtures of organics with NO_x is then evaluated using known mixtures. Additional evaluation using experiments with automobile exhaust and with urban air (i.e., captive air experiments) are recommended because these mixtures are most representative of ambient organic mixtures.

XII. Conclusion

A great deal has been learned over the past 20 years or so concerning atmospheric chemical processes of anthropogenically emitted compounds. For the majority of anthropogenic emissions, chemical reaction with the hydroxyl (OH) radical is the major atmospheric loss process, with photolysis and/or reaction with O_3 being of importance for some species. Reaction with the nitrate (NO_3) radical can be an important removal route, especially at night. Ozone is photochemically produced when nitrogen oxides react in the presence of CO, CH_4, non-methane hydrocarbons (NMHCs), and sunlight. There are several hydrocarbons that, together with CO, ultimately lead to ozone production. They may be divided into three categories. The first category consists of the most abundant and chemically simple hydrocarbon, CH_4, which has many natural and anthropogenic sources. The second category consists of biogenic hydrocarbons such as isoprene and terpenes, which are emitted by vegetation. These hydrocarbons are highly reactive and may be responsible for a significant portion of the ozone formed in non-urban regions. The third category of compounds contains many of the organics emitted by industrial and transportation processes, such as the alkanes, alkenes, aromatics, and aldehydes. Many of these are quite reactive and contribute to ozone formation on a local-to-regional scale. Some of the ozone produced regionally is also exported to remote continental and oceanic areas. In addition, many of the alkanes emitted from human activities, especially the lighter alkanes, have long chemical lifetimes, can be transported over long distances, and can contribute to *in situ* ozone production over remote areas. A knowledge of the atmospherically important loss processes and of the atmospheric lifetimes for anthropogenic emissions is of importance, since these lifetimes determine the geographical extent of the influence of the parent compound; a short lifetime leads to local exposure, while a long lifetime leads to regional or global exposure at correspondingly lower concentration levels.

In addition to the chemical loss processes in the troposphere, physical loss processes must also be taken into account. For particles, the atmospheric lifetime due to dry deposition for 0.1–1 μm particles is of the order of several days. The lifetimes with respect to dry deposition for many organic compounds are of the order of weeks or months. However, for certain species that have relatively slow gas-phase chemical loss rates, such as nitric acid and sulfur dioxide, dry deposition can be the major loss process under typical atmospheric conditions. For highly water-soluble gases such as SO_2, HNO_3, and H_2O_2, wet removal can be quite important, and in fog and cloud systems this process leads to removal of these compounds from the gas phase into the aqueous phase, where further reactions can occur, leading to the ultimate formation of acids and other oxygenated products. For species present in the particulate phase, dry and wet deposition constitute the physical loss processes, while photolysis and/or reaction with gas-phase and co-adsorbed reactive intermediates constitute the possible chemical loss processes.

The major uncertainties in understanding of gas-phase atmospheric chemistry concern reaction mechanisms and products of the oxidation of organic compounds. In general, aqueous-phase chemical processes occurring in droplets and submicron-sized particles are less well understood than those occurring in the gas phase. Virtually the full range of sulfur- and nitrogen-containing species reactions in the aqueous phase, along with those of dissolved organic species, require continued study.

Appendix: Supplementary References

There exist a number of recent comprehensive summaries of aspects of tropospheric chemistry. These include the following:

Hydroxyl radical-organic reactions	Atkinson (1989)
Mechanisms of gas-phase organic reactions	Atkinson (1990)
Nitrate radical chemistry	Atkinson (1991); Wayne *et al.* (1991)
Organic peroxy radical chemistry	Lightfoot *et al.* (1992); Wallington *et al.* (1992)
Rate constants	Atkinson *et al.* (1992)
Tropospheric chemistry literature 1987–1990	Jacob (1991)
Urban and regional ozone	National Research Council (1991)

In addition, the following books treat the general subject of atmospheric chemistry: Finlayson-Pitts and Pitts (1986); Seinfeld (1986); Warneck (1988); Wayne (1991).

References

Anbar, M., and Neta, P., A compilation of specific bimolecular rate constants for the reactions of hydrated electrons, hydrogen atoms and hydroxyl radicals with inorganic and organic compounds in aqueous solution. *Int. J. Appl. Radiat. Isot.* **18**, 493 (1967).

Arey, J., Atkinson, R., and Aschmann, S. M., Product study of the gas-phase reactions of the monoterpenes with the OH radical in the presence of NO_x. *J. Geophys. Res.* **95**, 18539 (1990).

Atkinson, R., A structure activity relationship for the estimation of rate constants for the gas-phase reactions of OH radicals with organic compounds. *Int. J. Chem. Kinet.* **19**, 799 (1987).

Atkinson, R., Kinetics and mechanisms of the gas-phase reactions of the hydroxyl radical with organic compounds. Monograph 1. *J. Phys. Chem. Ref. Data* (1989).

Atkinson, R., Gas-phase tropospheric chemistry of organic compounds: A review. *Atmos. Environ.* **24A**, 1 (1990).

Atkinson, R., Kinetics and mechanisms of the gas-phase reactions of the NO_3 radical with organic compounds. *J. Phys. Chem. Ref. Data* **20**, 459 (1991).

Atkinson, R., and Carter, W. P. L., Kinetics and mechanisms of the gas-phase reactions of ozone with organic compounds under atmospheric conditions. *Chem. Rev.* **84**, 437 (1984).

Atkinson, R., and Lloyd, A. C., Evaluation of the kinetics and mechanisms of kinetic and mechanistic data for modeling of photochemical smog. *J. Phys. Chem. Ref. Data* **13**, 315 (1984).

Atkinson, R., Hasegawa, D., and Aschmann, S. M., Rate constants for the gas-phase reactions of O_3 with a series of monoterpenes and related compounds at 296 ± 2K. *Int. J. Chem. Kinet.* **22**, 871 (1990).

Atkinson, R., Baulch, D. L., Cox, R. A., Hampson, R. F., Jr., Kerr, J. A., and Troe, J., Evaluated kinetic and photochemical data for atmospheric chemistry: Supplement IV. *Atmos. Environ.* **26A**, 1187 (1992).

Atkinson, R., Arey, J., Aschmann, S. M., and Tuazon, E. C., Formation of $O(^3P)$ atoms and epoxides from the gas-phase reaction of O_3 with isoprene. *Res. Chem. Intermed.* **20**, 385 (1994).

Bandow, H., and Washida, N., Ring-cleavage reactions of aromatic hydrocarbons studied by FT-IR spectroscopy. II. Photooxidation of o-, m-, and p-xylenes in the NO_x-air system. *Bull. Chem. Soc. Jpn.* **58**, 2541 (1985a).

Bandow, H., and Washida, N., Ring-cleavage reactions of aromatic hydrocarbons studied by FT-IR spectroscopy. III. Photooxidation of 1,2,3-, 1,2,4- and 1,3,5-trimethylbenzenes in the NO_x-air system. *Bull. Chem. Soc. Jpn.* **58**, 2549 (1985b).

Bandow, H., Washida, N., and Akimoto, H., Ring-cleavage reactions of aromatic hydrocarbons studied by FT-IR spectroscopy. I. Photooxidation of toluene and benzene in the NO_x-air system. *Bull. Chem. Soc. Jpn.* **58**, 2531 (1985).

Barnes, I., Bastian, V., Becker, K. H., and Tong, Z., Kinetics and products of reactions of NO_3 with monoalkenes, dialkenes, and monoterpenes. *J. Phys. Chem.* **94**, 2413 (1990).

Barth, M. C., Hegg, D. A., Hobbs, P. V., Walega, J. G., Kok, G. L., Heikes, B. G., and Lazrus, A. L., Measurements of atmospheric gas-phase and aqueous-phase hydrogen peroxide concentrations in winter on the east coast of the United States. *Tellus* **41B**, 61 (1989).

Behar, D., Czapski, G., and Duchovny, I., Carbonate radical in flash photolysis and pulse radiolysis of aqueous carbonate solutions. *J. Phys. Chem.* **74**, 2206 (1970).

Benson, S. W., "Thermochemical Kinetics," 2nd ed. Wiley, New York, 1976.

Bidleman, T. F., Atmospheric processes. *Environ. Sci. Technol.* **22**, 361 (1988).

Bielski, B. H. J., Reevaluation of the spectral and kinetic properties of HO_2 and O_2^- free radicals. *Photochem. Photobiol.* **28**, 645 (1978).

Bothe, E., and Schulte-Frohlinde, D., Reaction of dihydroxymethyl radical with molecular oxygen in aqueous solution. *Z. Naturforsch. B: Anorg. Chem., Org. Chem.* **35**, 1035 (1980).

Boyce, S. D., and Hoffmann, M. R., Kinetics and mechanism of the formation of hydroxymethanesulfonic acid at low pH. *J. Phys. Chem.* **88**, 4740 (1984).

Calvert, J. G., Yarwood, G., and Dunker, A., An evaluation of the mechanism of HONO formation in the urban atmosphere. Preprint (1994).

Calvert, J. R., and Stockwell, W. R., Acid generation in the troposphere by gas-phase chemistry. *Environ. Sci. Technol.* **17**, 2231 (1983).

Cantrell, C. A., Stockwell, W. R., Anderson, L. G., Busarow, K. L., Perner, D., Schmeltekopf, A., Calvert, J. G., and Johnston, H. S., Kinetic study of the NO_3-CH_2O reaction and its possible role in nighttime tropospheric chemistry. *J. Phys. Chem.* **89**, 139 (1985).

Carter, W. P. L., A detailed mechanism for the gas-phase atmospheric reactions of organic compounds. *Atmos. Environ.* **24**, 481 (1990).

Chameides, W. L., and Davis, D. D., The free radical chemistry of cloud droplets and its impact upon the composition of rain. *J. Geophys. Res.* **87**, 4863 (1982).

Charlson, R. J., Lovelock, J. E., Andreae, M. O., and Warren, S. G., Oceanic phytoplankton, atmospheric sulphur, cloud albedo and climate. *Nature (London)* **326**, 655 (1987).

Chen, S., Cope, V. W., and Hoffman, M. Z., Behavior of CO_3^- radicals generated in the flash photolysis of carbonatoamines complexes of cobalt (III) in aqueous solution. *J. Phys. Chem.* **77**, 1111 (1973).

Christensen, H., Sehested, K., and Corfitzen, H., Reactions of hydroxyl radicals with hydrogen peroxide at ambient and elevated temperatures. *J. Phys. Chem.* **86**, 1588 (1982).

Clarke, A. G., and Radojevic, M., Oxidation of SO_2 in rainwater and its role in acid rain chemistry. *Atmos. Environ.* **21**, 1115 (1987).

Cocks, A. T., McElroy, W. L., and Wallis, P. G., "The Oxidation of Sodium Sulphite Solutions by Hydrogen Peroxide," Rep. RD/L/2215N81. Central Electricity Research Laboratories, United Kingdom, 1982.

Colbeck, I., and Harrison, R. M., Dry deposition of ozone: Some measurements of deposition velocity and of vertical profiles to 100 metres. *Atmos. Environ.* **19**, 1807 (1985).

Crutzen, P. J., The global distribution of hydroxyl. *In* "Atmospheric Chemistry" (E. D. Goldberg, ed.), p. 313. Springer-Verlag, New York, 1982.

Damschen, D. E., and Martin, L. R., Aqueous aerosol oxidation of nitrous acid by O_2, O_3, and H_2O_2. *Atmos. Environ.* **17**, 2005 (1983).

Daum, P. H., Kelly, T. J., Schwartz, S. E., and Newman, L., Measurements of the chemical composition of stratiform clouds. *Atmos. Environ.* **18**, 2671 (1984).

Demerjian, K. L., Schere, K. L., and Peterson, J. T., Theoretical estimates of actinic (spherically integrated) flux and photolytic rate constants of atmospheric species in the lower troposphere. *Adv. Environ. Sci. Technol.* **10**, 369 (1980).

Dignon, J., and Penner, J. E., Biomass burning: A source of nitrogen oxides in the atmosphere. *In* "Global Biomass Burning" (J. Levine, ed.), p. 370. MIT Press, Cambridge, MA, 1991.

Dimitriades, B., The role of natural organics in photochemical air pollution: Issues and research needs. *J. Air Pollut. Control Assoc.* **3**, 229 (1981).

Dolske, D. A., and Gatz, D. F., A field intercomparison of methods for the measurement of particle and gas dry deposition. *J. Geophys. Res.* **90**, 2076 (1985).

Ehhalt, D. H., Dorn, H.-P., and Poppe, D., The chemistry of the hydroxyl radical in the troposphere. *Proc.—R. Soc. Edinburgh, Sect. B: Biol. Sci.* **97**, 17 (1991).

Eisenreich, S. J., Sources and fates of aquatic pollutants. *Adv. Chem. Ser.* **216**, 393 (1987).

Erickson, R. E., Yates, L. M., Clark, R. L., and McEwen, D., The reaction of sulfur dioxide with ozone in water and its possible atmospheric significance. *Atmos. Environ.* **11**, 813 (1977).

Fehsenfeld, F. C., Parrish, D. D., and Fahey, D. W., The measurement of NO_x in the nonurban troposphere. *In* "NATO Workshop on Tropospheric Ozone: Regional and Global Ozone and its Environmental Consequences" (I. Isaksen, ed.), p. 185. Reidel Publ., Hingham, MA, 1988.

Finlayson-Pitts, B. J., and Pitts, J. N., Jr., "Atmospheric Chemistry: Fundamentals and Experimental Techniques." Wiley, New York, 1986.

Friedl, R. R., Brune, W. H., and Anderson, J. G., Kinetics of SH with NO_2, O_3, O_2 and H_2O_2. *J. Phys. Chem.* **89**, 5505 (1985).

Galasyn, J. F., Tschudy, K. L., and Huebert, B. J., Seasonal and diurnal variability of nitric acid vapor and ionic aerosol species in the remote free troposphere at Mauna Loa, Hawaii. *J. Geophys. Res.* **92**, 3105 (1987).

Goumri, A., Sawerysyn, J.-P., Pauwels, J.-F., and Devolder, P., *In* "The Physico-Chemical Behavior of Atmospheric Pollutants," p. 315. Reidel Publ., Dordrecht, The Netherlands, 1990.

Goumri, A., Elmaimouni, L., Sawerysyn, J. P., and Devolder, P., Reaction rates at (297 ± 3)K of four benzyl-type radicals with O_2, NO, and NO_2 by discharge flow/laser induced fluorescence. *J. Phys. Chem.* **96**, 5395 (1992).

Graedel, T. E., and Goldberg, K. I., Kinetic studies of raindrop chemistry. 1. Inorganic and organic processes. *J. Geophys. Res.* **88**, 10865 (1983).

Graedel, T. E., and Weschler, C. J., Chemistry within aqueous atmospheric aerosols and raindrops. *Rev. Geophys.* **19**, 505 (1981).

Grosjean, D., and Seinfeld, J. H., Parameterization of the formation potential of secondary organic aerosols. *Atmos. Environ.* **23**, 1733 (1989).

Gu, C. L., Rynard, C. M., Hendry, D. G., and Mill, T., Hydroxyl radical oxidation of isoprene. *Environ. Sci. Technol.* **19**, 151 (1985).

Hagesawa, K., and Neta, P., Rate constants and mechanisms of reaction for Cl_2^- radicals. *J. Phys. Chem.* **82**, 854 (1978).

Hales, J. M., Air pollutants and their effects on the terrestrial ecosystem. *Adv. Environ. Sci. Technol.* 211–251 (1986).

Hales, J. M., and Drewes, D. R., Solubility of ammonia in water at low concentrations. *Atmos. Environ.*, **13**, 1133 (1979).

Hatakeyama, S., Izumi, K., Fukuyama, T., and Akimoto, H., Reactions of ozone with α-pinene and β-pinene in air: Yields of gaseous and particulate products. *J. Geophys. Res.* **94**, 13013 (1989).

Hatakeyama, S., Izumi, K., Fukuyama, T., Akimoto, H., and Washida, N., Reactions of OH with α-pinene and β-pinene in air: Estimate of global CO production from atmospheric oxidation of terpenes. *J. Geophys. Res.* **96**, 947 (1991).

Heikes, B. G., Kok, G. L., Walega, J. G., and Lazrus, A. L., H_2O_2, O_3 and SO_2 measurements in the lower troposphere over the eastern United States during fall. *J. Geophys. Res.* **92**, 915 (1987).

Heintzenberg, J., Fine particles in the global troposphere, a review. *Tellus* **41B** 149 (1989).

Hjorth, J., Lohse, C., Nielsen, C. J., Skov, H., and Restelli, G., Products and mechanisms of gas-phase reactions between NO_3 and a series of alkenes. *J. Phys. Chem.* **94**, 7494 (1990).

Hoffmann, M. R., and Boyce, S. D., Catalytic autooxidation of aqueous sulfur dioxide in relationship to atmospheric systems. *Adv. Environ. Sci. Technol.* **12**, 148 (1983).

Hoffmann, M. R., and Calvert, J. G., "Chemical Transformation Modules for Eulerian Acid Deposition Models. Vol. 2. The Aqueous-Phase Chemistry," EPA/600/3-85/017. U.S. Environ. Prot. Agency, Research Triangle Park, NC, 1985.

Hoffmann, M. R., and Edwards, J. O., Kinetics of oxidation of sulfite by hydrogen peroxide in acidic solution. *J. Phys. Chem.* **79**, 2096 (1975).

Hoffmann, M. R., and Jacob, D. J., Kinetics and mechanisms of the catalytic oxidation of dissolved sulfur dioxide in aqueous solution: An application to nighttime fog water chemistry. *In* "SO_2, NO, and NO_2 Oxidation Mechanisms: Atmospheric Considerations" (J. G. Calvert, ed.), p. 63. Butterworth, Stoneham, MA, 1984.

Hofzumahaus, A., Dorn, H.-P., Callies, J., Platt, U., and Ehhalt, D., Tropospheric OH concentration measurements by laser long-path absorption spectroscopy. *Atmos. Environ.* **25A**, 2017 (1992).

Horie, O., and Moortgat, G. K., Decomposition pathways of the excited Criegee intermediates in the ozonolysis of simple alkenes. *Atmos. Environ.* **25A**, 1881 (1992).

Huebert, B. J., and Robert, C. H., The dry deposition of nitric acid to grass. *J. Geophys. Res.* **90**, 2085 (1985).

Huie, R. E., and Neta, P., Rate constants for some oxidations of S(IV) by radicals in aqueous solutions. *Atmos. Environ.* **21**, 1743 (1987).

Huss, A., Jr., Lim, P. K., and Eckert, C. A., Oxidation of aqueous SO_2. 1. Homogeneous Manganese(II) and Iron(II) catalysis at low pH. *J. Phys. Chem.* **86**, 4224 (1982a).

Huss, A., Jr., Lim, P. K., and Eckert, C. A., Oxidation of aqueous SO_2. 2. High pressure studies and proposed reaction mechanisms. *J. Phys. Chem.* **86**, 4229 (1982b).

Ibusuki, T., and Takeuchi, K., Sulfur dioxide oxidation by oxygen catalyzed by mixtures of manganese(II) and iron(III) in aqueous solutions at environmental reaction conditions. *Atmos. Environ.* **21**, 1555 (1987).

International Agency for Research on Cancer (IARC), "Overall Evaluations of Carcinogenicity: An Updating of IARC Monographs. Vols. 1 to 42. Monographs on the Evaluation of the Carcinogenic Risk of Chemicals to Humans," Suppl. 7. Int. Agency Res. Cancer, Lyons, 1987.

Jacob, D. J., Chemistry of OH in remote clouds and its role in the production of formic acid and peroxymonosulfate. *J. Geophys. Res.* **91**, 9807 (1986).

Jacob, D. J., Tropospheric chemistry: 4 years of U.S. research, 1987–1990. *Rev. Geophys. Suppl.*, p. 2 (1991).

Japar, S. M., Wallington, T. J., Richert, J. F. O., and Ball, J. C., The atmospheric chemistry of oxygenated fuel additives: *t*-butyl alcohol, dimethyl ether, and methyl *t*-butyl ether. *Int. J. Chem. Kinet.* **22**, 1257 (1990).

Japar, S. M., Wallington, T. J., Rudy, S. J., and Chang, T. Y., Ozone-forming potential of a series of oxygenated organic compounds. *Environ. Sci. Technol.* **25**, 415 (1991).

Jayson, G. G., Parsons, B. J., and Swallow, A. J., Some simple, highly reactive, inorganic chlorine derivatives in aqueous-solution. *Trans. Faraday Soc.* **69**, 1597 (1973).

Jensen, N. R., Hjörth, J., Skov, H., and Restelli, G., Products and mechanism of the reaction between NO_3 and dimethylsulphide in air. *Atmos. Environ.* **25A**, 1897 (1991).

Jensen, N. R., Hjörth, J., Skov, H., and Restelli, G., Products and mechanism of the gas-phase reaction of NO_3 with CH_3SCH_3, CD_3SCD_3, CH_3SH and CH_3SSCH_3. *J. Atmos. Chem.* **14**, 95 (1992).

Khalil, M. A. K., and Rasmussen, R. A., Atmospheric methane: Trends over the last 10,000 years. *Atmos. Environ.* **21**, 2445 (1987).

Khalil, M. A., Rasmussen, R. A., and Shearer, M. J., Trends of atmospheric methane during the 1960's and 1970's. *J. Geophys. Res.* **94**, 18279 (1989).

Knispel, R., Koch, R., Siese, M., and Zetzsch, C., Adduct formation of OH radicals with benzene, toluene, and phenol and consecutive reactions of adducts with NO_x and O_2. *Ber. Bunsenges. Phys. Chem.* **94**, 1375 (1990).

Kozac-Channing, L. F., and Heltz, G. R., Solubility of ozone in aqueous solutions of 0-0.6 M ionic strength at 5-30°C. *Environ. Sci. Technol.* **17**, 145 (1983).

Kunen, S. M., Lazrus, A. L., Kok, G. L., and Heikes, B. G., Aqueous oxidation of SO_2 by hydrogen peroxide. *J. Geophys. Res.* **88**, 3671 (1983).

Latimer, W. M., "The Oxidation States of the Elements and Their Potentials in Aqueous Solutions," p. 70. Prentice-Hall, New York, 1952.

Ledbury, W., and Blair, E. W., The partial formaldehyde vapour pressure of aqueous solutions of formaldehyde. Part II. *J. Chem. Soc.* **127**, 2832 (1925).

Lee, Y. N., Atmospheric aqueous-phase reactions of nitrogen species. "Gas-Liquid Chemistry of Natural Waters," Vol. 1, BNL 51757, p. 20/1. Brookhaven Natl. Lab., Upton, NY, 1984a.

Lee, Y. N., Kinetics of some aqueous-phase reactions of peroxyacetyl nitrate. "Gas-Liquid Chemistry of Natural Waters," Vol. 1, BNL 51757, p. 21/1. Brookhaven Natl. Lab., Upton, NY, 1984b.

Lee, Y. N., and Schwartz, S. E., Kinetics of oxidation of aqueous sulfur(IV) by nitrogen dioxide. *In* "Precipitation Scavenging, Dry Deposition and Resuspension" (H. R. Pruppacher, R. G. Semonin, and W. G. N. Slinn, eds.), Vol. 1. Elsevier, New York, 1983.

Lee, Y. N., Senum, G. I., and Gaffney, J. S., Peroxyacatyl nitrate (PAN) stability, solubility, and reactivity-implications for tropospheric nitrogen cycles and precipitation chemistry. *Int. Conf. Comm. Atmos. Chem. Global Pollut., Symp. Trop. Chem.* Oxford, England, *5th,* 1983.

Le Henaf, P., Methodes d'étude et propriétés des hydrates, hemiacetals et hemiacetals dérivés des aldehydes et des cetones. *Bull. Soc. Chim. Fr.*, p. 4687 (1968).

Lelieveld, J., and Crutzen, P. J., Influences of cloud photochemical processes on tropospheric ozone. *Nature (London)* **343**, 227 (1990).

Lelieveld, J., and Crutzen, P. J., The role of clouds in tropospheric photochemistry. *J. Atmos. Chem.* **12**, 229 (1991).

Lightfoot, P. D., Cox, R. A., Crowley, J. N., Destriau, M., Hayman, G. D., Jenkin, M. E., Moortgat, G. K., and Zabel, F., Organic peroxy radicals: Kinetics, spectroscopy and tropospheric chemistry. *Atmos. Environ.* **26A**, 1805 (1992).

Lind, J. A., and Kok, G. L., Henry's law determinations for aqueous solutions of hydrogen peroxide, methylhydroperoxide, and peroxyacetic acid. *J. Geophys. Res.* **91**, 7889 (1986).

Lind, J. A., and Lazrus, A. L., Aqueous-phase oxidation of Sulfur(IV) by some organic peroxides. *EOS, Trans.* **64**, 670 (1983).

Liu, S. C., Cicerone, R. J., Donahue, T. M., and Chameides, W. L., Sources and sinks of atmospheric N_2O and the possible ozone reduction due to industrial fixed nitrogen fertilizers. *Tellus* **29**, 251 (1977).

Logan, J. A., Nitrogen oxides in the troposphere: Global and regional budgets. *J. Geophys. Res.* **88**, 10785 (1983).

Logan, J. A., Tropospheric ozone: Seasonal behavior, trends and anthropogenic influence. *J. Geophys. Res.* **90**, 10463 (1985).

Logan, J. A., Ozone in rural areas of the United States. *J. Geophys. Res.* **94**, 8511 (1989).

Logan, J. A., Prather, M. J., Wofsy, S. C., and McElroy, M. B., Tropospheric chemistry: A global perspective. *J. Geophys. Res.* **86**, 7210 (1981).

Loomis, A. G., Solubilities of gases in water. *In* "International Critical Tables," Vol. III, p. 255. McGraw-Hill, New York, 1928.

Lurmann, F. W., and Main, H. H., "Analysis of the Ambient VOC Data Collected in the Southern California Air Quality Study," Final report, Contract No. A832-130. State of California Air Resources Board, Sacramento, 1992.

Maahs, H. G., Kinetics and mechanism of the oxidation of S(IV) by ozone in aqueous solution with particular reference to SO_2 conversion in nonurban tropospheric clouds. *J. Geophys. Res.* **88**, 10721 (1983).

Mackay, D., "Multimedia Environmental Models: The Fugacity Approach." Lewis Publishers, Chelsea, MI, 1991.

Magnotta, F., and Johnston, H. S., Photodissociation yields for the NO_3 free radical. *Geophys. Res. Lett.* **7**, 769 (1980).

Marsh, A. R. W., and McElroy, W. J., The dissociation constant and Henry's law constant of HCl in aqueous solution. *Atmos. Environ.* **19**, 1075 (1985).

Martin, L. R., Kinetic studies of sulfite oxidation in aqueous solution. *In* "SO_2, NO, and NO_2 Oxidation Mechanisms: Atmospheric Considerations" (J. G. Calvert, ed.), p. 63. Butterworth, Stoneham, MA, 1984.

Martin, L. R., and Damschen, D. E., Aqueous oxidation of sulfur dioxide by hydrogen peroxide at low pH. *Atmos. Environ.* **15**, 1615 (1981).

Martin, L. R., and Good, T. W., Catalyzed oxidation of sulfur dioxide in solution: The iron-manganese synergism. *Atmos. Environ.* **25A**, 2395 (1991).

Martin, L. R., and Hill, M. W., The iron catalyzed oxidation of sulfur: Reconciliation of the literature rates. *Atmos. Environ.* **6**, 1487 (1987a).

Martin, L. R., and Hill, M. W., The effect of ionic strength on the manganese catalyzed oxidation of sulfur(IV). *Atmos. Environ.* **21**, 2267 (1987b).

Martin, L. R., Hill, M. W., Tai, A. F., and Good, T. W., The iron catalyzed oxidation of sulfur(IV) in aqueous solution: Differing effects of organics at high and low pH. *J. Geophys. Res.* **96**, 3085 (1991).

McArdle, J. V., and Hoffmann, M. R., Kinetics and mechanism of the oxidation of aquated sulfur dioxide by hydrogen peroxide at low pH. *J. Phys. Chem.* **87**, 5425 (1983).

Menichini, E., Urban air pollution by polycyclic aromatic hydrocarbons: Levels and sources of variability. *Sci. Total Environ.* **116**, 109 (1992).

Mount, G. H., and Eisele, F. L., An intercomparison of tropospheric OH measurements at Fritz Peak Observatory, Colorado. *Science* **256**, 1187 (1992).

Munger, J. W., Jacob, D. J., and Hoffmann, M. R., The occurrence of bisulfite-aldehyde addition products in fog- and cloudwater. *J. Atmos. Chem.* **1**, 335 (1984).

NASA, Chemical kinetics and photochemical data for use in stratospheric modeling. Evaluation No. 6, Demore W. B., Margitan, J. J., Molina, M. J., Watson, R. J., Golden, D. M., Hampson, R. F., Kurylo, M. J., Howard, C. J., Ravishankara, A. R., *JPL Publ.* **85-37**, (1985).

NASA, Chemical kinetics and photochemical data for use in stratospheric modeling. *JPL Publ.* **87-41**, Evaluation No. 8, (1987).

National Research Council, "Rethinking the Ozone Problem in Urban and Regional Air Pollution." National Academy Press, Washington, DC, 1991.

Neftel, A., Beer, J., Oeschger, H., Zürcher, F., and Rinkel, R. C., Sulfate and nitrate concentrations in snow from South Greenland 1895–1978. *Nature (London)* **314**, 611 (1985).

Pandis, S. N., and Seinfeld, J. H., Sensitivity analysis of a chemical mechanism for aqueous-phase atmospheric chemistry. *J. Geophys. Res.* **94**, 1105 (1989a).

Pandis, S. N., and Seinfeld, J. H., Mathematical modeling of acid deposition due to radiation fog. *J. Geophys. Res.* **94**, 12911 (1989b).

Pandis, S. N., Paulson, S. E., Seinfeld, J. H., and Flagan, R. C., Aerosol formation in the photooxidation of isoprene and β-pinene. *Atmos. Environ.* **25A**, 997 (1991).

Pandis, S. N., Seinfeld, J. H., and Pilinis, C., Heterogeneous sulphate production in an urban fog. *Atmos. Environ.* **26**, 2509 (1992).

Pankow, J. F., Review and comparative analysis of the theories on partitioning between the gas and aerosol particulate phases in the atmosphere. *Atmos. Environ.* **21**, 2275 (1987).

Pankow, J. F., A simple box model for the annual cycle of partitioning of semi-volatile organic compounds between the atmosphere and the earth's surface. *Atmos. Environ.* **27A**, 1139 (1993).

Paulson, S. E., Flagan, R. C., and Seinfeld, J. H., Atmospheric photooxidation of isoprene. Part 1. The hydroxyl radical and ground state atomic oxygen reactions. *Int. J. Chem. Kinet.* **24**, 79 (1991a).

Paulson, S. E., Flagan, R. C., and Seinfeld, J. H., Atmospheric photooxidation of isoprene. Part 2. The ozone-isoprene reaction. *Int. J. Chem. Kinet.* **24**, 103 (1991b).

Penkett, S. A., Oxidation of SO_2 and the other atmospheric gases by ozone in aqueous solution. *Nature (London)* **240**, 105 (1972).

Penkett, S. A., Jones, B. M. R., Brice, K. A., and Eggleton, A. E. J., The importance of atmospheric ozone and hydrogen peroxide in oxidizing sulfur dioxide in cloud and rainwater. *Atmos. Environ.* **13**, 123 (1979).

Penner, J. E., Atherton, C. S., Dignon, J., Ghan, S. J., Walton, J. J., and Hameed, S., Tropospheric nitrogen: A three-dimensional study of sources, distribution, and deposition. *J. Geophys. Res.* **96**, 959 (1991).

Perrin, D. D., "Ionization Constants of Inorganic Acids and Bases in Aqueous Solution," 2nd ed. Pergamon, New York, 1982.

Pilinis, C., Seinfeld, J. H., and Grosjean, D., Water content of atmospheric aerosols. *Atmos. Environ.* **23**, 1601 (1989).

Ridley, B. A., Recent measurements of oxidized nitrogen compounds in the troposphere. *Atmos. Environ.* **25A**, 1905 (1991).

Ross, A. B., and Neta, P., "Rate Constants for Reactions of Inorganic Radicals in Aqueous Solution," NSRDS-NBS 65. U.S. Department of Commerce, Washington, DC, 1979.

Sakugawa, H., and Kaplan, I. R., H_2O_2 and O_3 in the atmosphere of Los Angeles and its vicinity. *J. Geophys. Res.* **94**, 12957 (1989).

Sakugawa, H., Kaplan, I. R., Tsai, W., and Cohen, Y., Atmospheric hydrogen peroxide. *Environ. Sci. Technol.* **24**, 1452 (1990).

Savoie, D. L., Prospero, J. M., Merrill, J. T., and Nematsu, M., Nitrate in the atmospheric boundary layer of the tropical South Pacific: Implications regarding sources and transport. *J. Atmos. Chem.* **8**, 391 (1988).

Schmidt, K. H., Electrical conductivity techniques for studying the kinetics of radiation induced chemical reactions in aqueous solutions. *Int. J. Radiat. Phys. Chem.* **4**, 439 (1972).

Schwartz, S. E., Gas- and aqueous-phase chemistry of HO_2 in liquid water clouds. *J. Geophys. Res.* **89**, 11589 (1984).

Schwartz, S. E., and Freiberg, J. E., Mass transport limitation to the rate of reaction of gases in liquid droplets: Application in oxidation of SO_2 in aqueous solution. *Atmos. Environ.* **15**, 1129 (1981).

Schwartz, S. E., and White, W. H., Solubility equilibrium of the nitrogen oxides and oxyacids in dilute aqueous solution. *Adv. Environ. Sci. Eng.* **4**, 1 (1981).

Scoles, G., and Willson, R. L., γ-radiolysis of aqueous thymine solutions. Determination of relative reaction rates of OH radicals. *Trans. Faraday Soc.* **63**, 2982 (1967).

Sehested, K., Rasmussen, O. L., and Fricke, H., Rate constants of OH with HO_2, O_2^-, and $H_2O_2^+$ from hydrogen peroxide formation in pulse-irradiated oxygenated water. *J. Phys. Chem.* **72**, 626 (1968).

Sehested, K., Holcman, J., and Hart, E. J., Rate constants and products of the reactions of e_{aq}^-, O_2^-, and H with ozone in aqueous solutions. *J. Phys. Chem.* **87**, 1951 (1983).

Seila, R. L., Lonneman, W. A., and Meeks, S. A., "Determination of C_2 to C_{12} Ambient Air Hydrocarbons in 39 U.S. Cities from 1984 Through 1986," EPA/600/3-89/058. Atmospheric Research and Assessment Laboratory, U.S. Environ. Prot. Agency, Research Triangle Park, NC, 1989.

Seinfeld, J. H., "Atmospheric Chemistry and Physics of Air Pollution." Wiley, New York, 1986.

Seinfeld, J. H., Ozone air quality models. A critical review. *J. Air Pollut. Control Assoc.* **38**, 616 (1988).

Shepson, P. B., Kleindienst, T. E., Edney, E. O., Namie, G. R., Pittman, J. H., Cupitt, L. T., and Claxton, L. D., The mutagenic activity of irradiated toluene/NO_x/H_2O/air mixtures. *Environ. Sci. Technol.* **19**, 249 (1985).

Shepson, P. B., Bottenheim, J. W., Hastie, D. R., and Venkatram, A., Determination of the relative ozone and PAN deposition velocities at night. *Geophys. Res. Lett.* **19**, 1121 (1992).

Smith, R. M., and Martell, A. E., "Critical Stability Constants," Vol. 4. Plenum, New York, 1976.

Snider, J. R., and Dawson, G. A., Tropospheric light alcohols, carbonyls, and acetonitrile: Concentrations in the southwestern United States and Henry's law data. *J. Geophys. Res.* **90**, 3797 (1985).

Solomon, P. A., Fall, T., Salmon, L., Cass, G. R., Gray, H. A., and Davidson, A., Chemical characteristics of PM_{10} aerosols collected in the Los Angeles area. *J. Air Pollut. Control Assoc.* **39**, 154 (1989).

Sorensen, P. E., and Andersen, V. S., The formaldehyde-hydrogen sulphite system in alkaline aqueous solution: Kinetics, mechanism, and equilibria. *Acta Chem. Scand.* **24**, 1301 (1970).

Stelson, A. W., Friedlander, S. K., and Seinfeld, J. H., A note on the equilibrium relationship between ammonia and nitric acid and particulate ammonium nitrate. *Atmos. Environ.* **13**, 369 (1979).

Stockwell, W. R., and Calvert, J. G., The mechanism of NO_3 and HONO formation in the nighttime chemistry of the urban troposphere. *J. Geophys. Res.* **88**, 6673 (1983).

Stumm, W., and Morgan, J. J., "Aquatic Chemistry." Wiley, New York, 1981.

Taylor, W. D., Allston, T. D., Moscato, M. J., Fazekas, G. B., Kozlowski, R., and Takacs, G. A., Atmospheric photodissociation lifetimes for nitromethane, methyl nitrite and methyl nitrate. *Int. J. Chem. Kinet.* **12**, 231 (1980).

Thompson, A. M., and Cicerone, R. J., Possible perturbations to atmospheric CO, CH_4 and OH. *J. Geophys. Res.* **91**, 10853 (1986).

Tie, X. X., Kao, C.-Y. J., and Mroz, E. J., Net yield of OH, CO, and O_3 from the oxidation of atmospheric methane. *Atmos. Environ.* **26A**, 125 (1992).

Treinin, A., and Hayon, E., Absorption spectra and reaction kinetics of NO_2, N_2O_3, and N_2O_4 in aqueous solutions. *J. Am. Chem. Soc.* **92**, 5821 (1970).

Tuazon, E. C., and Atkinson, R., A product study of the gas-phase reaction of isoprene with the OH radical in the presence of NO_x. *Int. J. Chem. Kinet.* **22**, 1221 (1990).

Tuazon, E. C., Atkinson, R., Plum, C. N., Winer, A. M., and Pitts, J. N., Jr., The reaction of gas phase N_2O_5 with water vapor. *Geophys. Res. Lett.* **10**, 953 (1983).

Tuazon, E. C., Sanhueza, E., Atkinson, R., Carter, W. P. L., Winer, A. M., and Pitts, J. N., Jr., Direct determination of the equilibrium constant at 298 K for the $N_2 + NO_3 \rightleftarrows N_2O_5$ reactions. *J. Phys. Chem.* **88**, 3095 (1984).

Tuazon, E. C., MacLeod, H., Atkinson, R., and Carter, W. P. L., α-Dicarbonyl yields from the NO_x-air photooxidation of a series of aromatic hydrocarbons in air. *Environ. Sci. Technol.* **20**, 383 (1986).

Tyndal, G. S., and Ravishankara, A. R., Atmospheric oxidation of reduced sulfur species. *J. Phys. Chem.* **23**, 483 (1991).

Van Valin, C. C., Ray, J. D., Boatman, J. F., and Gunter, R. L., Hydrogen peroxide in air during winter over the south-central United States. *Geophys. Res. Lett.* **14** 1146 (1987).

Wagman, D. D., Evans, W. H., Parker, V. B., Schumm, R. H., Halow, I., Bailey, S. M., Churney, K. L., and Nuttall, R. L., The NBS tables of chemical thermodynamic properties. *J. Phys. Chem. Ref. Data* **11**, 2.1 (1982).

Wallington, T. J., and Japar, S. M., Atmospheric chemistry of diethyl ether and ethyl tert-butyl ether. *Environ. Sci. Technol.* **25**, 410 (1991).

Wallington, T. J., and Kurylo, M. J., The gas-phase reactions of hydroxyl radicals with a series of aliphatic alcohols over the temperature range 240–440K. *Int. J. Chem. Kinet.* **19**, 1015 (1987).

Wallington, T. J., Liu, R., Dagaut, P., and Kurylo, M. J., The gas-phase reactions of hydroxyl radicals with a series of aliphatic ethers over the temperature range 240–440K. *Int. J. Chem. Kinet.* **20**, 41 (1988a).

Wallington, T. J., Dagaut, P., Liu, R., and Kurylo, M. J., The gas phase reaction of hydroxyl radicals with a series of esters over the temperature range 240–44K. *Int. J. Chem. Kinet.* **20**, 177 (1988b).

Wallington, T. J., Dagaut, P., Liu, R., and Kurylo, M. J., Gas-phase reactions of hydroxyl radicals with the fuel additives methyl tert-butyl ether and tert-butyl alcohol over the temperature range 240K–440. *Environ. Sci. Technol.* **22**, 842 (1988c).

Wallington, T. J., Andino, J. M., Skewes, L. M., Siegl, W. O., and Japar, S. M., Kinetics of the reaction of OH radicals with a series of ethers under simulated atmospheric conditions at 295K. *Int. J. Chem. Kinet.* **21**, 993 (1989).

Wallington, T. J,. Dagaut, P., and Kurylo, M. J., Ultraviolet absorption of cross sections and reaction kinetics and mechanisms for peroxy radicals in the gas phase. *Chem. Rev.* **92**, 667 (1992).

Wang, S. C., Paulson, S. E., Grosjean, D., Flagan, R. C., and Seinfeld, J. H., Aerosol formation and growth in atmospheric organic/NO_x systems: I. Outdoor smog chamber studies of C_7 and C_8 hydrocarbons. *Atmos. Environ.* **26A**, 403 (1992a).

Wang, S. C., Flagan, R. C., and Seinfeld, J. H., Aerosol formation and growth in atmospheric organic/NO_x systems: II. Aerosol dynamics. *Atmos. Environ.* **26A**, 421 (1992b).

Warneck, P., "Chemistry of the Natural Atmosphere." Academic Press, San Diego, 1988.

Warneck, P., Chemical reactions in clouds. *Fresenius J. Anal. Chem.* **340**, 585 (1991).

Warneck, P., Chemistry and photochemistry in atmospheric water drops. *Ber. Bunsen ges. Phys. Chem.* **96**, 454 (1992).

Wayne, R. P., "Chemistry of Atmospheres." Oxford Univ. Press, Oxford, 1991.

Wayne, R. P. *et al.*, The nitrate radical: Physics, chemistry and the atmosphere. *Atmos. Environ.* **25A**, 1 (1991).

Weeks, J. L., and Rabani, J., The pulse radiolysis of deaerated aqueous carbonate solutions. I. Transient optical spectrum and mechanism. II. pK for OH radicals. *J. Phys. Chem.* **70**, 2100 (1966).

Wu, Y. I., Davidson, C. I., Dolske, D. A., and Sherwood, S. I., Dry deposition of atmospheric contaminants: The relative importance of aerodynamics, boundary layer, and surface resistances. *Aerosol. Sci. Technol.* **16**, 65 (1992).

Yin, F., Grosjean, D., and Seinfeld, J. H., Photooxidation of dimethyl sulfide and dimethyl disulfide. I: Mechanism development. *J. Atmos. Chem.* **11**, 309 (1990a).

Yin, F., Grosjean, D., Flagan, R. C., and Seinfeld, J. H., Photooxidation of dimethyl sulfide and dimethyl disulfide. II: Mechanism evaluation. *J. Atmos. Chem.* **11**, 365 (1990b).

Zetzsch, C., Koch, R., Siese, M., Witte, F., and Devolder, P., *in* "Proceedings of the Fifth European Symposium on the Physico-Chemical Behavior of Atmospheric Pollutants," p. 320. Reidel Publ., Dordrecht, The Netherlands, 1990.

INDEX

B

C

I

J

K

L

Q

R

Contents of Volumes in This Serial

ISBN 0-12-008519-4

90051

9 780120 085194